HOST DEFENSES AND IMMUNOMODULATION TO INTRACELLULAR PATHOGENS

ADVANCES IN EXPERIMENTAL MEDICINE AND BIOLOGY

Recent Volumes in this Series

A Continuation Order Plan is available for this series. A continuation order will bring delivery of each new volume immediately upon publication. Volumes are billed only upon actual shipment. For further information please contact the publisher.

HOST DEFENSES AND IMMUNOMODULATION TO INTRACELLULAR PATHOGENS

Edited by

Toby K. Eisenstein
Temple University School of Medicine
Philadelphia, Pennsylvania

Ward E. Bullock
University of Cincinnati College of Medicine
Cincinnati, Ohio

and

Nabil Hanna
Smith Kline and French Laboratories
Philadelphia, Pennsylvania

With the Editorial Assistance of

Linda Miller
Publications Committee Chairperson
Eastern Pennsylvania Branch of the
American Society for Microbiology
Philadelphia, Pennsylvania

SPRINGER SCIENCE+BUSINESS MEDIA, LLC

Library of Congress Cataloging in Publication Data

Host defenses and immunomodulation to intracellular pathogens / edited by Toby K. Eisenstein, Ward E. Bullock, and Nabil Hanna.
p. cm.—(Advances in experimental medicine and biology: v. 239)
"Based on the proceedings of the Eastern Pennsylvania Branch of the ASM Symposium on Host Defenses and Immunomodulation to Intracellular Pathogens, held November 19-20, 1986, in Philadelphia, Pennsylvania"—T.p. verso.
Includes bibliographical references and index.
ISBN 978-1-4757-5423-0 ISBN 978-1-4757-5421-6 (eBook)
DOI 10.1007/978-1-4757-5421-6
1. Immunity—Congresses. 2. Host-parasite relationships—Immunological aspects—Congresses. 3. Immune response—Regulation—Congresses. 4. Intracellular pathogens—Congresses. I. Eisenstein, Toby K. II. Bullock, Ward E. III. Hanna, Nabil. IV. Eastern Pennsylvania Branch of the ASM Symposium on Host Defenses and Immunomodulation to Intracellular Pathogens (1986: Philadelphia, Pa.) V. American Society for Microbiology. Eastern Pennsylvania Branch. VI. Series.
QR185.3.H67 1988 88-25164
599′.029—dc19 CIP

Based on the Proceedings of the Eastern Pennsylvania Branch of the ASM Symposium on Host Defenses and Immunomodulation to Intracellular Pathogens, held November 19-20, 1986, in Philadelphia, Pennsylvania

ORGANIZING COMMITTEE

Convenors

Toby K. Eisenstein, Ph.D.
Temple University School of Medicine
Philadelphia, Pa.

Ward E. Bullock, M.D.
University of Cincinnati Medical Center
Cincinnati, Oh.

Nabil Hanna, Ph.D.
Smith Kline & French Laboratories
Philadelphia, Pa.

Conference Committee

Carl Abramson, Ph.D.
Pennsylvania College of Podiatric Medicine
Philadelphia, Pa.

Paul Actor, Ph.D.
Smith Kline & French Laboratories
Philadelphia, Pa.

Alison Badger, Ph.D.
Smith Kline & French Laboratories
Philadelphia, Pa.

Josephine Bartola, J.D.
Bureau of Laboratories
Pennsylvania Department of Health
Lionville, Pa.

Walter S. Ceglowski, Ph.D.
Temple University School of Medicine
Philadelphia, Pa.

Kenneth R. Cundy, Ph.D.
Temple University School of Medicine
Philadelphia, Pa.

Bruce Kleger, Ph.D.
Bureau of Laboratories
Pennsylvania Department of Health
Lionville, Pa.

Linda Ann Miller, Ph.D.
Holy Redeemer Hospital and Medical Center
Meadowbrook, Pa.

ACKNOWLEDGMENTS

This conference was held under the sponsorship of the Eastern Pennsylvania Branch of the American Society for Microbiology, as one in a continuing series of Basic Science Symposia. The untiring volunteer efforts of the members of the Symposium Committee are deeply appreciated. The Bureau of Laboratories of the Pennsylvania Department of Health was a cosponsor and generously provided staff and secretarial services to handle the difficult task of registration. The Departments of Microbiology and of Microbiology and Immunology at the five medical schools in Philadelphia—Temple University School of Medicine, Medical College of Pennsylvania, Thomas Jefferson University, Hahnemann University, and the University of Pennsylvania—were academic cosponsors, and the support of the Chairpersons and the faculties are gratefully acknowledged. The Department of Microbiology and Immunology at Temple University deserves special thanks for providing secretarial and office support that made the program and this volume possible.

Smith Kline & French Laboratories was a cosponsor and also provided a generous financial contribution that was a major ingredient in bringing the Symposium to fruition. The Branch, the speakers, and the attendees extend their sincere gratitude to SK&F for supporting this endeavor.

The editors wish to acknolwedge Linda Miller, who as Chairperson of the Branch Publications Committee helped immeasurably in assembling this Proceedings. We also want to thank Mr. Greg Harvey for his expert typing and editorial advice, and Dr. Joyce M. Greene for supervising the final preparation of the volume.

PREFACE

This Symposium is a sequel to one on "Host Defenses to Intracellular Pathogens" held in Philadelphia in 1981. At that time, the impetus for holding a meeting on this topic was the lack of a forum for scientists addressing similar questions about immunity to intracellular pathogens, but using diverse organisms. Historically, investigators have tended to present their findings at Society meetings, which traditionally are structured around the microbe (virology, mycology, parasitology) or the discipline (microbial pathogenesis, immunology, infectious diseases). It was apparent that advances in immunology, mammalian genetics, and cell biology could be applied to understanding how the host copes with a wide array of intracellular pathogens, but more intense cross-fertilization between fields was needed. In 1981, major issues addressed were 1) the relationship between delayed-type hypersensitivity (DTH) and cellular immunity; 2) the capacity of spleen cell fractions to transfer immunity or DTH; 3) the role of T-cells in activating macrophages and in killing virally infected targets; 4) the description of differences among inbred strains of mice in their capacity to control growth of intracellular pathogens, with definition and mapping of the relevant genes; 5) the biochemistry governing microbicidal levels in phagocytes; and 6) elucidation of mechanisms of phago-lysosome fusion.

In the six intervening years, developments in our understanding of how the host copes with intracellular organisms have progressed rapidly, with major advances stemming from application of an array of new techniques. Among the most powerful tools now at our disposal is the capacity to generate T-cell clones of various subsets _in vitro_. These can be transferred _in vivo_, to allow the phenotypes which mediate cellular immunity and/or DTH to be definitively established in some cases. The ability to clone viral antigens and express them individually on the surface of target cells has provided a new means of probing precisely the antigenic specificity recognized by cytotoxic T-cells. Our understanding of the nature of microbial epitopes recognized by lymphocytes has also been greatly advanced by the wide-spread use of monoclonal antibodies, directed either against the organism or the T-cell receptors. The possibility of producing synthetic peptides and glycolipids which mimic microbial antigens, as probes of the specificity of the immune system, is still another new approach finding wide application in defining the specificity of cellular immune reactions.

Enormous advances in delineating the basic intricacies in cell-cell interactions within the immune system have been rapidly applied to our understanding of host defenses. For example, elucidation of T-suppressor cell circuits has opened a new aspect of immunoregulation that may be applicable in unraveling anergic manifestations of diseases such as leprosy and tuberculosis. Definition and cloning of monokines and lymphokines, including interleukin-1, interleukin-2, γ-interferon, and BSF-1, have provided an array of defined immunomodulators that are being used to probe the circuitry by which microbes induce or suppress immune responses.

Indeed the rate of progress in acquisition of biological knowledge seems to be increasing exponentially. As we move rapidly forward, there is a real need to exchange information, so investigators can keep abreast of advances in the basic areas, as well as applications using microbes other than the ones which they are studying. The uniqueness of the Symposium held in Philadelphia is its interdisciplinary nature, bringing together immunologists, infectious disease researchers, mammalian geneticists, and investigators trained in microbial pathogenesis. The manuscripts assembled in this volume present approaches at the cellular, biochemical, and genetic levels.

As we explore further the delicate balance between the invaders and the dispatchers of the host's defenses, there is an almost palpable excitement at the mosaic of interactions which are revealed, and the possibility of capturing and taming elements in the various immune pathways for the prevention and cure of infectious diseases.

Toby K. Eisenstein, Ph.D.
Professor of Microbiology and Immunology
Temple University School of Medicine

Ward E. Bullock, M.D.
Head, Division of Infectious Diseases
University of Cincinnati Medical Center

Nabil Hanna, Ph.D.
Director, Department of Immunology and
Anti-infectives Therapy
Smith Kline & French Laboratories

CONTENTS

I. Phagocytes as Effector Cells

II. T-Cells, NK Cells and Host Defenses

III. Mediators, Macrophages and Host Defenses

LYMPHOKINE REGULATION OF MACROPHAGE EFFECTOR ACTIVITIES

Carol A. Nacy, Miodrag Belosevic, Robert M. Crawford, Alison T. Healy, Robert D. Schreiber, and Monte S. Meltzer

Department of Immunology, Walter Reed Army Institute of Research, Washington, D.C., 20307-5100, and Washington University, St. Louis, MO, 63110

INTRODUCTION

Host reaction to the changes in homeostatic balance induced by infection or neoplasia is characterized by a complex, but carefully orchestrated series of events called inflammation. Cells involved in this process communicate with their environment, and themselves, through multi-directional networks of inflammatory signals (cytokines) that induce, amplify, or suppress particular responses. Analysis of the cells that are involved in inflammation repeatedly points to a single cell in control: the macrophage. These cells serve not only as the initiators of antigen-specific immunity through antigen processing and presentation, but also as effector cells for elimination of the offending pathogen once immunity has been established. Of particular interest in recent years has been the signals and sequence of events that regulate the onset of nonspecific cytotoxic effector reactions of macrophages. This interest initiated from the original studies of Mackaness, who observed that mice infected with one bacterium were able to survive normally lethal infections with completely unrelated bacteria. After years of experimental analysis, it became clear that the cellular basis for this nonspecific resistance had two obligate components: T lymphocytes and macrophages. Immune T cells respond to antigen in context of histocompatability antigens on the macrophage, and release hormone-like cytokines (lymphokines, LK), that regulate macrophage function. A subset of these LK, in turn, activates macrophages to become nonspecific killer cells. These activated cells can now eliminate not only the inciting infectious agent that induced the immune response, but also a wide variety of completely unrelated viral, bacterial, fungal, parasitic, and neoplastic targets. The activation of macrophages for nonspecific cytotoxic effector functions occurs early in the evolution of an immune response, and constitutes the host's first opportunity for containment of the invading microorganism.

Like inflammation, regulation of macrophage activation for nonspecific cytotoxic effector functions is remarkably complex, and is accomplished through the interaction of cells, signals, and targets in a defined sequence of events. We use two very different targets, a fibrosarcoma, TU-5, and an obligate intracellular protozoan, the amastigote of Leishmania major, to illustrate events that lead to nonspecific killing reactions. The recent availability of recombinant LK has simplified the task of sorting out events that induce activated macrophages capable of killing these two targets: a single LK can be assessed without the obvious complications of interactive LK in culture supernatants of antigen- or mitogen-stimulated spleen cells, the conventional source of LK. At the same time, the use of single LK has highlighted both the complexity and the uniqueness of regulatory events in the induction of each effector reaction, as well as pointed out the requirement for cooperation between LK for the induction of certain of these reactions. With the two targets, the fibrosarcoma TU-5 and the amastigote of L. major, and a variety of recombinant or spleen cell-derived LK, we can now classify macrophage activating LK into three broad, overlapping categtories:

(1) LK that induce **qualitatively different** changes in macrophage function; ie, they act by themselves to induce phenotypically similar killing reactions, but by distinct pathways,

(2) LK that induce **quantitative** changes in macrophages; these changes can be amplified or suppressed by second signals, and

(3) LK that **cooperate** to induce certain effector reactions; individual LK have no effect.

We present data for LK (Table 1) that induce maximal activity in each assay.

Table 1. LK assessed for macrophage activating capacities

LK	Culture supernatants of PPD-stimulated spleen cells from BCG-infected mice, 1/10 final concentration. IFN-gamma concentration was 100 IRU/ml.
MAF	LK depleted of gamma interferon by immunoaffinity chromatography, 1/10 final concentration.
IFN	Recombinant gamma interferon, 50 IRU/ml; gift of Genentech, South San Francisco, CA.
IL-2	Recombinant interleukin 2, 50 U/ml, Genzyme, Boston, MA.
IL-3	Purified interleukin 3, 100 U/ml, Genzyme, Boston, MA.
CSF	Recombinant granulocyte-macrophage colony stimulating factor, 100 U/ml, Genzyme, Boston, MA.
BSF-1	Purified B cell stimulating factor 1, 30 U/ml, gift of Dr. W. Paul, NIH, Bethesda, MD.

The effector reactions of macrophages for extracellular destruction of tumor cells and for intracellular killing of L. major share many characteristics. Each effector activity is (a) rapid in onset; observed as early as 4 hr after LK addition, (b) short-lived; capacity to interpret LK signals, or express effector reaction, decays after 24 hr in culture, (c) a multi-stage reaction; two discrete steps can be distinguished in the activation process, and (d) induced by factors in LK (7). Although there are other features (maturational state of the macrophage, genetic control of macrophage function) that can be used to dissociate these two killing activities, none illustrates the individuality of the two effector reactions better than the analysis of LK that regulate intracellular and extracellular killing (Figure 1).

The capacity of macrophages to kill extracellular targets, such as the TU-5 fibrosarcoma, can be demonstrated in cells exposed to whole LK, as well as several recombinant LK: IFN, GM-CSF, and BSF-1 (Figure 2, hatched bars). The macrophage activating capacity of IFN has been documented in a variety of systems, and IFN is thought to be the primary activation factor in LK for extracellular killing. In fact, MAF, LK depleted of IFN, failed to induce tumor cytotoxicity in these studies. Recent reports show, however, that recombinant GM-CSF also induces human monocyte tumoricidal activity, and GM-CSF was effective in induction of macrophage extracellular killing of TU-5 cells in our murine assay, as well. The ability of macrophages exposed to BSF-1 to kill tumor targets was quite a surprise. The details of the interaction of BSF-1 with macrophages are given in another Chapter (see Crawford, et al), but a brief survey of these interactions suggests that BSF-1 may be as potent a regulator of macrophage function as it is B cell function.

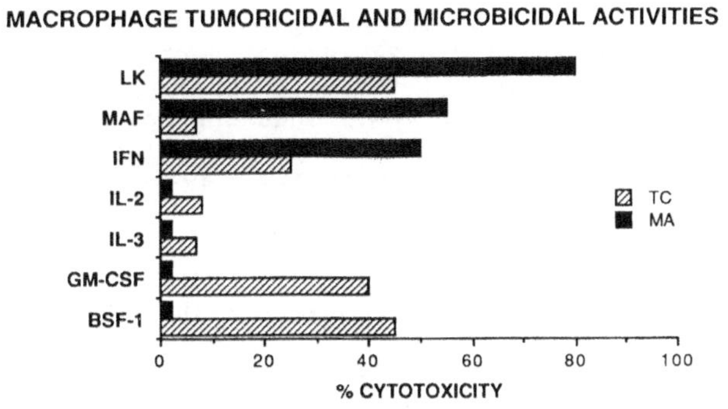

Figure 1. Tumoricidal activity (TC) was assessed 48 hr after culture of macrophages, targets, and LK, and is expressed as % total label released from TdR prelabeled TU-5 cells. Microbicidal activity (MA) was assessed 72 hr after culture of infected macrophages with LK, and is expressed as % reduction infected cells in treated cultures compared to medium controls.

If we compare the effect of the same set of LK for induction of microbicidal effector functions, we find a very different pattern of activity (Figure 2, solid bars). Whole LK, of course, induce potent intracellular killing, with microbicidal activity consistently in the range of 80%. Removal of IFN by immunoaffinity chromatography affects the plateau of intracellular killing (now at 45-55%), but the dose response remains the same (9). IFN by itself induces intracellular killing, again at the 45-55% level. Despite the ability of several recombinant LK to induce tumoricidal activity, we could not demonstrate any microbicidal activity in macrophages treated with factors other than MAF and IFN (Figure 2). Thus, there are several factors that by themselves induce tumoricidal activity in the absence of any effect on microbicidal activity (CSF, BSF-1), and at least 1 that induces microbicidal activity in the absence of tumoricidal activity (MAF).

LK THAT INDUCE QUALITATIVELY DIFFERENT EFFECTOR ACTIVITIES OF MACROPHAGES

Macrophage activation for intracellular killing and tumoricidal activity occurs as a series of reactions, much like the complement or clotting systems (2,3,12). We can demonstrate at least two steps in the activation process *in vitro* by treating macrophages sequentially with low concentrations of LK (inactive for induction of the effector reaction) followed by a high dose LK pulse. This series of reactions we call "priming" and "triggering", although these are strictly operational definitions. Neither priming nor triggering have been defined on a molecular level. Priming *in vitro* occurs in the low dose LK incubation step, and is characterized by an absolute requirement for a minimum 4 hr exposure to LK at 37°C. Although primed macrophages are not yet cytotoxic, priming does lower the threshold of the cell for a second signal, the trigger, that actually induces expression of the effector activity. Triggering requires only a short interaction of primed macrophages with the second signal, from 15 min to 1 hr. The trigger signal can be factors in LK or can be certain bacterial products, such as LPS. Once priming and triggering has occurred, the inducing agents can be removed completely from the culture system and the reaction, be it microbicidal or tumoricidal activity, proceeds at maximal levels. With the availability of pure recombinant reagents, we can address the issue of the interaction of different LK in induction of macrophage effector activities. One possibility for the change in dose response plateau of macrophage microbicidal activity with MAF and IFN compared to whole LK (Figure 2) is that certain cells exposed to whole LK may be primed with IFN, but these IFN-primed macrophages will accept a trigger signal from either MAF or IFN. Thus the optimal priming signal in LK may be IFN. To test this hypothesis we primed cells with either IFN or MAF, and triggered these primed cells with the homologous activation agent, or the heterologous agent (Table 2).

Table 2. Activation of macrophages with IFN or MAF

PRIME 4 HR WITH:	TRIGGER 1 HR WITH:	% INTRACELLULAR KILLING	
MAF, 1/10	MAF, 1/10	50	*
1/100	1/100	15	
1/100	MAF, 1/10	55	*
1/100	IFN, 12 U	20	
IFN, 12 U	IFN, 12 U	60	*
1 U	1 U	15	
1 U	IFN, 12 U	80	*
1 U	MAF, 1/10	15	

* microbicidal activity exceeds 95% confidence limits of control cultures.

Both MAF and IFN activate macrophages in sequential steps, but more importantly, priming is specific for the activation agent. Neither MAF nor IFN were capable of priming cells for trigger with the heterologous factor. Through systematic analysis of this model of macrophage activation for microbicidal activity, we have developed the following schema for events that occur in the presence of MAF and IFN (Figure 2):

We know that certain suppressor factors that are released from phorbol myristate acetate-treated EL-4 thymoma cells (8) will block the induction of macrophage activation by both MAF and IFN. Kinetics of this EL-4 suppressor activity suggest that activation is blocked in the priming phase, and occurs within 1-2 hr after addition of the activation agent. After this time, however, the suppressor factor is no longer able to affect the expression of intracellular killing. We conclude from these studies that MAF and IFN must have at least one step in common in the pathways for induction of intracellular killing, and that this common step occurs very early during priming. After an hour or two, however, the cells become irreversibly committed to the activation cascade initiated by the specific activation agent, and can no longer interpret the trigger signals generated by exposure to a heterologous activation agent. Thus MAF and IFN are two examples of macrophage activation agents that induce phenotypically similar, but **qualitatively different** effector activities. Whether the distinct metabolic events induced by the two activation agents result in two different intracellular killing mechanisms, or are complementary pathways for the same effector mechanism, is simply not known.

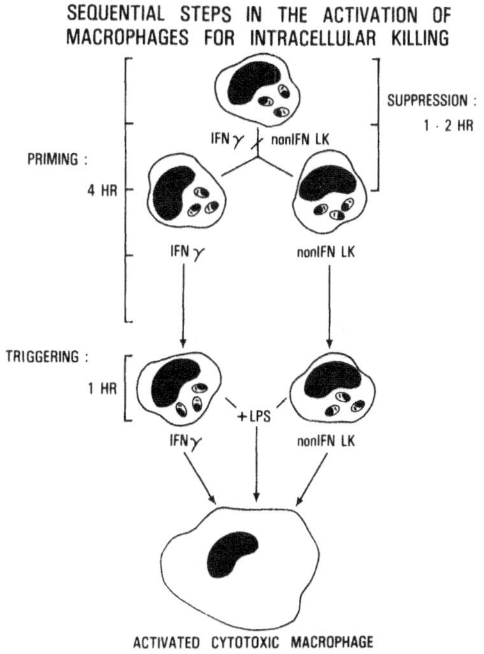

Figure 2. Macrophage activation for intracellular destruction of *L. major* amastigotes by IFN and nonIFN MAF.

It is interesting that both activation agents can induce intracellular killing, but neither does so as well as unfractionated LK (9, Figure 1): the dose response plateau for each single reagent is substantially less (approximately 50% microbicidal activity) than the level reached with whole LK (80% microbicidal activity). The different activation agents may interact with discrete, but overlapping subpopulations of macrophages. That most, if not all macrophages exposed to a single activation agent can develop cytotoxic activity under the appropriate circumstances is demonstrated in Figure 3, where LPS is used to amplify the effects of single activation agents: here virtually 100% of infected cells are able to eliminate intracellular amastigotes.

LYMPHOKINES THAT INDUCE QUANTITATIVE CHANGES IN MACROPHAGE FUNCTION

One exogenous factor that can act as a trigger agent for microbicidal activity induced by both IFN and MAF is LPS (Figure 2). The interaction of LPS and LK has been studied in detail for tumoricidal activities of activated macrophages, and LPS is thought to be an obligatory second signal for macrophage killing of certain tumor targets. In Figure 3, we examine the interaction of the various recombinant and purified LK with LPS for induction of both microbicidal and tumoricidal activities. In each case, the addition of nanogram amounts of LPS dramatically amplifies the effects of active LK for induction of the effector activity: maximal levels of tumoricidal activity increase from an average of 35% to 65% with LK, IFN, and BSF-2; maximal levels of microbicidal activity increase from 55% to nearly 100% for IFN and MAF. LPS by itself is not active in induction of these effector reactions. Moreover, LPS is not effective in making a nonactive LK active. Thus, we can demonstrate with both intracellular and extracellular killing the powerful synergistic interaction of LPS with a variety of LK. Each of the activation agents we have examined induces **quantitative** changes in the macrophage that can be amplified by second signals, such as LPS. Yet there remain LK that induce one effector reaction without affecting expression of a second effector reaction: BSF-1 fails to induce microbicidal activity and MAF fails to induce tumoricidal activity.

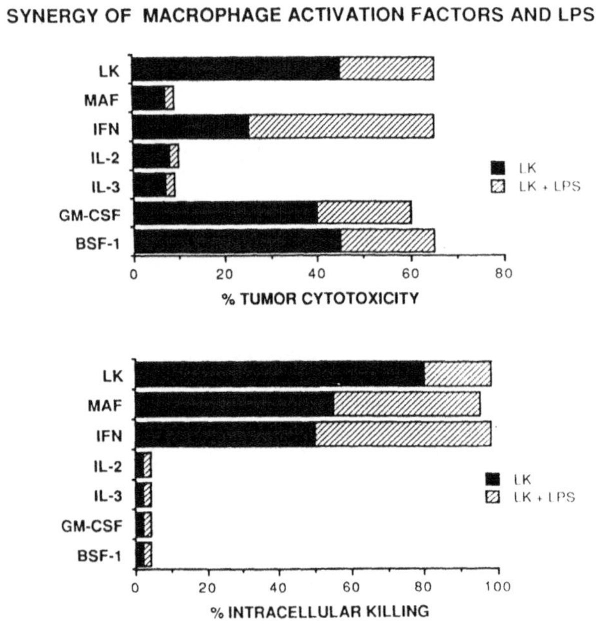

Figure 3. Synergistic interaction of LPS and LK. Macrophages were exposed to targets and LK (see Table 4 for concentrations), with or without 10 ng/ml LPS. Tumoricidal activity was assessed at 48 hr; microbicidal activity was assessed at 72 hr.

LYMPHOKINES THAT COOPERATE TO INDUCE CHANGES IN MACROPHAGE FUNCTION

To examine the cooperation of LK for induction of effector functions, we need to introduce a third effector activity of activated macrophages: resistance to infection. We demonstrate this effector activity by treating cells with LK before we introduce amastigotes of L. major. Cells pretreated with LK ingest fewer parasites than medium-treated controls, and it is this decrease in uptake of parasites that we call "resistance to infection" (11). The actual mechanism involved in this macrophage resistance is unknown, but is thought to be extracellular killing of the parasite at diffusion-limited junctions during attachment of the parasite to the macrophage membrane. Resistance to infection is (a) rapid in onset; observed as early as 4 hr after treatment of cells with LK (11), (b) long-lived; activity persists for 72 to 96 hr in culture (11), (c) not parasite specific; has been observed with a variety of obligate and facultative intracellular microorganisms (4,5), and (d) induced by factors in LK (4,6). The major characteristic of resistance to infection that distinguishes it from intracellular killing of amastigotes and extracellular killing of tumor targets is the persistence of this effector activity with time: cells treated with LK for 4 hr undergo a stable change in phenotype, and have enhanced resistance to infection for as long as we observe them in vitro. Since IFN is a macrophage activation factor that induces a variety of effector reactions, and macrophage resistance to infection is reminiscent of viral interference, we assumed that IFN played a role in induction of this effector reaction as well. As it turned out, we were right, but the induction of resistance to infection is markedly more complex, and consequently more interesting, than we had originally envisioned.

The details of macrophage activation for resistance to infection are presented in another Chapter (Belosevic, et al). Induction of resistance to infection requires the interaction of macrophages and at least 2 factors in LK: IFN and another nonIFN macrophage activation agent; each factor by itself is inactive. Unlike priming and triggering for the effector reactions

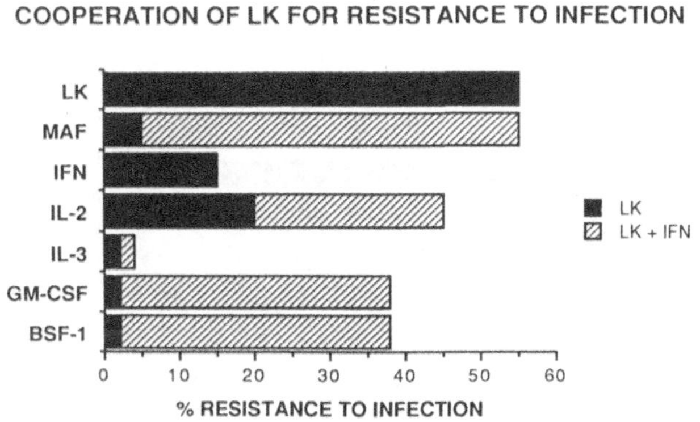

Figure 4. Induction of resistance to infection. Cells were treated with LK alone, or in combination with IFN, for 6 hr, washed, and exposed to amastigotes for 2 hr. Results are expressed as percent decrease in infected cells 2 hr after infection in treated cultures compared to medium-treated controls.

described above, the order to addition of the factors for induction of resistance to infection is not critical. And, finally, very little IFN is required as a cofactor for induction of this effector activity: 25 U/ml IFN is sufficient to initiate the reaction in the presence of MAF. What are the nonIFN macrophage activation factors in LK that cooperate with IFN for the induction of resistance to infection? Figure 4 shows the results of a combination of IFN and purified or recombinant LK. While none of the LK, including IFN, are capable of stimulating resistance to infection by themselves (Figure 4, solid bars), adding IFN to several of the purified and recombinant LK restores the capacity of these activation agents to induce expression of the effector activity (Figure 4, hatched bars). MAF, IL-2, GM-CSF, and BSF-1 are all capable of inducing this activity. This is the first effector reaction of macrophages that has an absolute requirement for two endogenous mediators. It is also the first macrophage effector reaction in which IL-2 is an active participant. Recent reports document IL-2 receptors on human monocytes, and an upregulation of IL-2 receptors by IFN. The role IFN plays in the induction of this effector reaction may be to increase the number of receptors of the second obligate mediator so that there is a more efficient intracellular signal generated. With purified recombinant reagents we may now begin to understand the molecular mechanisms that underlie the regulation of macrophage resistance to infection.

That resistance to infection is the result of **cooperation** between LK and not simply amplification (LK that induce **quantitative** changes) is shown by the lack of participation of LPS in these reactions (Figure 5):

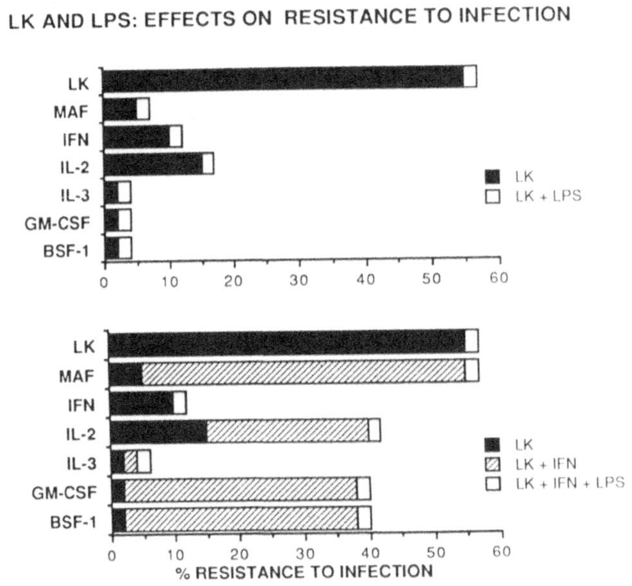

Figure 5. Addition of 50 ng/ml LPS to macrophage cultures treated with LK alone (A), or in combination with 50 U/ml IFN (B) for induction of macrophage resistance to infection.

In contrast to macrophage extracellular destruction of tumor targets or intracellular killing of amastigotes (Figure 3), LPS failed to synergize with LK, or even the combination of LK and IFN, for induction of macrophage resistance to infection (Figure 5).

That cooperation by multiple LK for induction of an effector reaction is the exception, not the rule, is shown in Figure 6. Both BSF-1 and IFN by themselves induce macrophage tumoricidal activity. The extracellular killing activity of macrophages exposed to the combination of BSF-1 + IFN, however, was actually less than that of cells exposed to either activation agent alone. In contrast, neither IFN nor BSF-1 by themselves had activity for induction of macrophage resistance to infection, but the combination of LK was effective.

The **cooperation** of LK, then, can best be illustrated by macrophage resistance to infection with obligate or facultative intracellular parasites. The LK that cooperate to induce this effector reaction are IFN and either MAF, IL-2, GM-CSF, or BSF-1.

SUMMARY

Our concept of the regulation of macrophage activation is ever expanding and contracting. In regard to the number of LK that regulate macrophages killing activities, we have entered a new phase. In the beginning there was one macrophage activation factor, MIF; then there were many macrophage activation factors, most uncharacterized and bearing a variety of names. Then came IFN, a genetically cloned single reagent that induced destruction of virtually every target assessed; all activities of macrophages were assumed

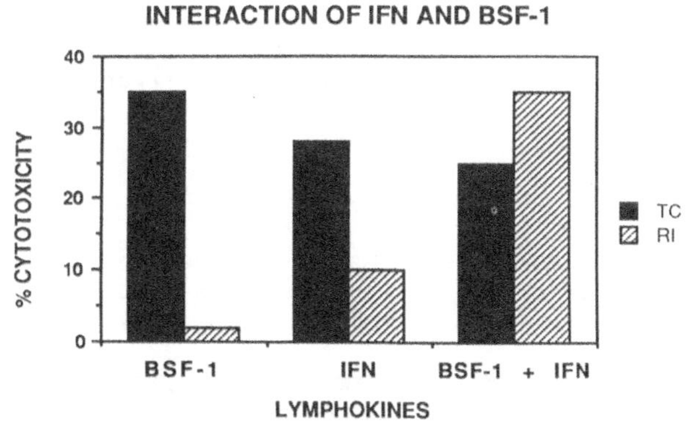

Figure 6. Addition of multiple LK for induction of macrophage effector activities. Cells were treated with BSF-1, IFN, or BSF-1 + IFN for 6 hr, washed, and then exposed to TU-5 or amastigotes of <u>L. major</u>. Tumoricidal activity was assessed at 48 hr, and was expressed as % total label released from prelabeled TU-5 cells. Resistance to infection was assessed 2 hr after addition of parasites, and was expressed as percent decrease in number of cells with intracellular amastigotes compared to medium-treated controls.

to be regulated by IFN. Once again, however, the LK universe is expanding: the number of single, cloned reagents that induce macrophage killing activities is amazing. With just two targets, a fibrosarcoma cell and an intracellular amastigote of L. major, we can identify 5 different macrophage activation factors, four of which are cloned and sequenced. As more recombinant reagents become available, the story of macrophage activation is likely to become even more complex. It is fascinating not only that certain of the LK are capable of inducing single effector reactions in the absence of effects on other effector activities, but also that at least one effector reaction requires the cooperation of several molecularly distinct LK.

The complexity of LK activation factors that regulate a single effector reaction in vitro is compounded by the complexity in effector cell populations. For example, inflammatory macrophages exposed to LK kill the fibrosarcoma tumor target 5 to 10-fold better than an equal number of resident peritoneal macrophages (3). In contrast, LK treated resident macrophages eliminate intracellular amastigotes of leishmania far more efficiently than inflammatory cells (1). Thus, changes in cell populations dramatically affect the capacity to demonstrate a single effector reaction. Further, simple changes in assay conditions also determine whether an effector reaction can be observed in vitro (3). And superimposed upon all these layers of complexity is the target itself. The mechanisms a macrophages uses to block the replication of a virus may be totally ineffective in the destruction of a multicellular helminth, such as Schistosoma mansoni (7). And there is no reason to suspect that the extracellular destruction of a tumor target occurs by the same means that the macrophage uses to kill an intracytoplasmic bacterium, such as a rickettsia. Is there a "unifying hypothesis" in macrophage activation? Probably not. The number of infectious and neoplastic agents confronted by the macrophage are simply too numerous to rely on a single activation agent or a single effector reaction: these critical activities would be far too easy to subvert. As it is, many of the successful parasites have found ways to subvert the potent effects of activated macrophages, and thus pose the greatest challenge for the infected host. Somehow we have to identify overriding signals that restore the ability of the macrophage to contain infection. Identification of different LK that induce selective but potent killing mechanisms effective against these parasites is but the first step in this process. The next major hurdle in the understanding of macrophage activation will be to determine where and when these activation factors operate in vivo, and design transport systems to deliver the activation agent to the appropriate site.

REFERENCES

1. Hoover, D.L. and C.A. Nacy. 1984. Macrophage activation to kill Leishmania tropica: defective intracellular destruction of amastigotes by macrophages elicited by sterile inflammatory agents. J. Immunol. 132:1487-1493.
2. Meltzer, M.S. and C.A. Nacy. 1985. Macrophage cytotoxicity against tumor cell and microbial targets: genetic control of the activation network. Prog. Leuk. Biol. 3:595-604.
3. Meltzer, M.S., D.L. Hoover, M.J. Gilbreath, R.D. Schreiber, and C.A. Nacy. 1986. Experimental variables for induction of activated cytotoxic macrophages. Ann. Inst. Pasteur/Immunol. 137C:206-211.
4. Nacy, C.A., M.S. Meltzer, E.J. Leonard, and D.J. Wyler. 1981. Intracellular replication and lymphokine-induced destruction of Leishmania tropica in C3H/HeN mouse macrophages. J. Immunol. 127:2381-2386.
5. Nacy, C.A. and M.S. Meltzer. 1979. Macrophages in resistance to rickettsial infection: macrophage activation in vitro for killing of Rickettsia tsutsugamushi. J. Immunol. 123:2544-2549.

6. Nacy, C.A., E.J. Leonard and M.S. Meltzer. 1981. Macrophages in resistance to rickettsial infections: characterization of lymphokines that induce rickettsiacidal activity in macrophages. J. Immunol. 126:204-207.
7. Nacy, C.A., C.N. Oster, S.L. James, and M.S. Meltzer. 1984. Activation of macrophages for destruction of intracellular and extracellular parasites. Cont. Topics Immunobiol. 14:147-170.
8. Nacy, C.A. 1984. Macrophage activation to kill _Leishmania tropica_: identification of a soluble T cell factor that suppresses lymphokine-induced intracellular killing of amastigotes. J. Immunol. 133:448-453.
9. Nacy, C.A., A.H. Fortier, M.S. Meltzer, N.A. Buchmeier, and R.D. Schreiber. 1985. Macrophage activation to kill _Leishmania tropica_: macrophages can be activated to kill amastigotes by both interferon gamma and non-interferon lymphokines. J. Immunol. 135:3505-3511.
10. Nacy, C.A., C.E. Davis, B.A. Mock, M.J. Gilbreath, and M.S. Meltzer. 1986. Regulation of macrophage antimicrobial activities by lymphocyte products. Clin. Immunol. Newsletter 7:65-69.
11. Oster, C.N. and C.A. Nacy. 1984. Macrophage activation to kill _Leishmania tropica_: kinetics of macrophage response to lymphokines that induce microbicidal activities against _Leishmania tropica_ amastigotes. J. Immunol. 132:1494-1500.
12. Pappas, M.G., C.N. Oster, and C.A. Nacy. 1982. Intracellular destruction of _Leishmania tropica_ by macrophages activated _in vivo_ with _Mycobacterium bovis_ strain BCG. Adv. Exp. Med. Biol. 162:425-431.

WHAT T CELLS TELL MACROPHAGES TO DO DURING RESISTANCE TO LISTERIOSIS

Priscilla A. Campbell

Department of Medicine
National Jewish Center for Immunology and Respiratory Medicine
Denver, Colorado

INTRODUCTION

Current understanding of cell-mediated immunity originated with the elegant experiments of Mackaness and colleagues (1,2). These investigators recognized that antigen-specific thymus-derived lymphocytes, T cells, stimulated non-specific macrophages to express high levels of anti-microbial activity. These experiments, completed in the 1960's, laid the foundations for a model still widely accepted today. However, as with most biologic processes, we have come to understand that events are more complicated than they originally seemed. Recent evidence suggests that while this model may describe T cell-mediated activation of macrophages to kill tumor cells and obligate intracellular microbes, it may not describe the events which occur during induction of resistance to infection by facultative intracellular organisms, particularly facultative intracellular bacteria. The discussion below describes experiments conducted by us and by others which suggest that the primary role of T cells in resistance to infection by *Listeria monocytogenes*, a facultative intracellular bacterium, is not to activate the macrophage. Rather, the major role of the T cell seems to be to cause recruitment of inflammatory cells, both macrophages and neutrophils, which express high levels of bactericidal activity. Many of these ideas have been expressed in a recent article (3).

CLASSICAL (ACTIVATION) MODEL FOR CELL-MEDIATED IMMUNITY AGAINST MICROORGANISMS

The classical model proposes that an antigen, for instance listeria, is taken up by antigen-presenting cells. These cells process the antigen and present it on the surface of the antigen-presenting cell in intimate contact with class II major histocompatibility complex (MHC) molecules. Understanding of this process of antigen-presentation derives largely from studies by Unanue and colleagues using listeria antigens (4-6). Antigen presented on the cell surface in the context of class II MHC molecules can then be seen by antigen specific T cells, which have a receptor capable of recognizing this combination of antigen and Ia molecules (6,7). The expression of Class II MHC molecules (Ia

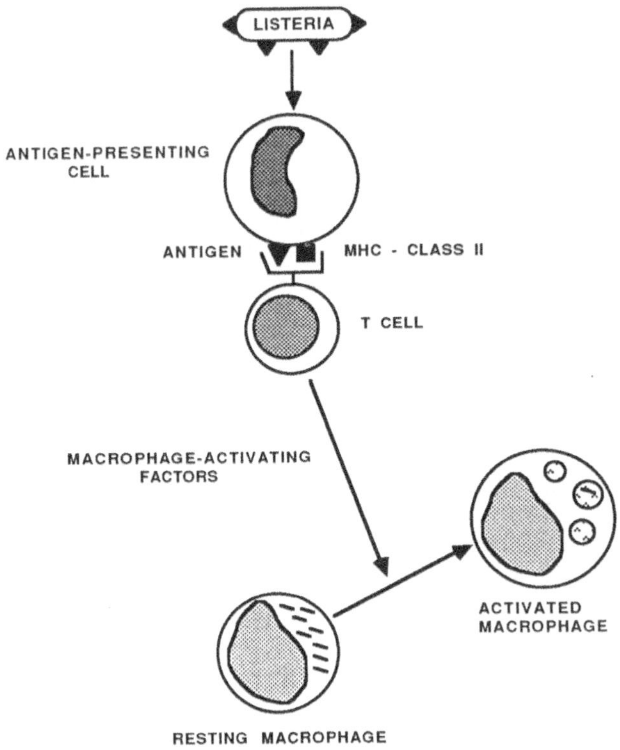

Fig. 1. Classical (activation) model for cell-mediated immunity against facultative intracellular bacteria.

antigens) on the surface of macrophages is itself controlled by T cell-derived lymphokines, particularly by gamma-interferon (IFN_γ) (6,8). IFN_γ is probably secreted by both natural killer cells and antigen-specific T cells. The helper T cell, of the CD4 phenotype (T4 in man, L3T4 in the mouse), binds by its receptor to the antigen-MHC complex, and becomes activated. It then expresses increased amounts of receptor for the T cell growth factor interleukin-2 (IL-2) (9). Then this T cell divides in response to IL-2 secreted either by itself or by other CD4-positive cells, producing an increased number of effector cells. These effector cells secrete many lymphokines, including a family of lymphokines called macrophage-activating factors (10). Macrophage-activating factors, alone or in conjunction with other molecules, stimulate quiescent macrophages to express high levels of biologic activity, including the ability to kill internalized microbial pathogens (10-13). A simplified version of this model is depicted in Figure 1.

ALTERNATE (RECRUITMENT) MODEL FOR CELL-MEDIATED IMMUNITY AGAINST FACULTATIVE INTRACELLULAR BACTERIA

If the above model were true, one would predict that T cell-secreted factors could easily activate macrophages *in vitro* to express heightened

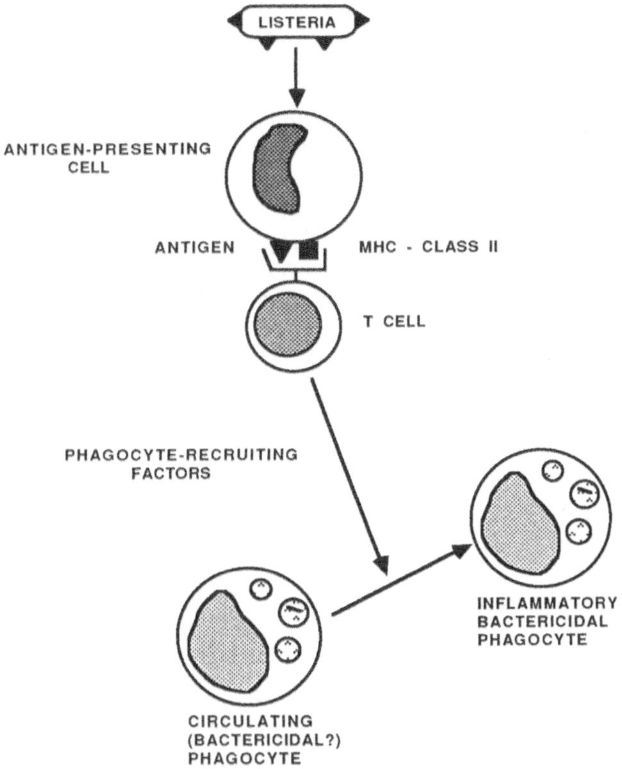

Fig. 2. Alternate (recruitment) model for cell-mediated immunity against facultative intra-cellular bacteria.

levels of activity. This has been shown to be true for tumor cell cytotoxicity and for microbicidal activity against obligate intra-cellular microorganisms (12,13). In fact, some of the activating molecules have been sequenced, and the genes cloned and expressed. But it has been surprisingly difficult to identify molecules which can activate macrophages to express high levels of bactericidal activity against facultative intracellular bacteria. For this reason and because of the findings described below, we propose that the major role of the T cell in mediating resistance to infection by these bacteria is not to activate the macrophage to enhanced levels of bactericidal activity, but rather to cause recruitment of cells which express high levels of bactericidal activity. Figure 2 depicts a simplified version of this model for induction of resistance to listeria. In this model triggering of antigen-specific T cells occurs as described above for the classical model - that is, listeria antigen is taken up by macrophages and re-expressed on the surface in association with class II MHC molecules. The expression of class II MHC molecules on the surface on macrophages is itself controlled by T cell-derived lymphokines, particularly by IFN_{γ}. In the absence of IFN_{γ}, Ia antigen expression on antigen-presenting macrophages is not increased, and T cells recognize and respond to antigen poorly. The IFN_γ which induces Ia expression may be secreted by natural killer cells or by listeria-reactive T cells. Once stimulated, T cells, probably CD4-positive helper T cells, are triggered to express IL-2 receptors, and to expand under the influence of IL-2. They then secret lymphokines, including factors which directly or indirectly cause recruitment of bactericidal phagocytes, both neutrophils and macrophages. These inflammatory cells, once recruited to the site of antigenic challenge, already express high levels of bactericidal activity and cannot readily be induced to express higher levels of activity. Thus, according to this model, the major role of listeria-reactive T cells is to mediate recruitment of bactericidal neutrophils and macrophages, not to activate quiescent macrophages to express bactericidal activity. These T cells also secrete IFN_γ (14), which helps maintain the high levels of Ia on antigen-presenting cells required for continuation of the immune response.

EVIDENCE IN SUPPORT OF THE RECRUITMENT MODEL

Immunologically-elicited and inflammatory macrophages are equally bactericidal

A prediction of the classical model is that secretory products of listeria-specific T cells will activate macrophages to heightened bactericidal activity. Over the years this has been surprisingly difficult to demonstrate, suggesting that the model may not be entirely correct. As an alternate approach, we conducted experiments to test whether macrophages stimulated *in vivo* by T cell-dependent mechanisms express better bactericidal activity *in vitro* than do non-immunologically-elicited inflammatory macrophages (15). The data showed that when inflammatory macrophages and macrophages harvested from the peritoneal cavities of listeria-immune mice following antigen injection were titrated for their ability to kill listeria, both cell populations killed listeria equally well. That is, immunologically-elicited macrophages, presumably stimulated by T cells and T cell factors, were no better than non-immunologically elicited macrophages at killing listeria.

However, since the immunized mice were extremely resistant to challenge with live listeria organisms, what enhanced functions did they express? The immune animals were able to recruit more neutrophils and more macrophages to their peritoneal cavities in response to challenge with antigen than were non-immune animals. Others have also reported enhanced accumulation of peritoneal macrophages in immune mice challenged with listeria antigen (16). These data suggest that an important component of resistance is acquisition of the ability to recruit more bactericidal cells to a site of infection.

Neutrophils may be involved

The experiments described above predict that a population of T cells which transfers resistance to infection should also be able to transfer the ability to recruit macrophages and neutrophils to a site of infection. We conducted experiments to test this hypothesis (17). Earlier experiments from several laboratories had shown that spleen T cells could transfer resistance to listeria infection (17-19). We asked whether spleen T cells from mice resistant to listeria infection, when injected into the peritoneal cavity and challenged with antigen, could cause recruitment of neutrophils and macrophages. The data showed that intraperitoneal injection of immune T cells plus antigen caused a T cell dose-dependent accumulation in the peritoneal cavity of neutrophils at 18 hrs and of macrophages at 48 hrs. This provides further evidence that the major role of the listeria-immune T cell is not to stimulate the macrophages to express increased bactericidal activity, but rather to recruit more inflammatory cells.

The experiments described above raise an interesting point: T cells seem to solicit the help of neutrophils as well as macrophages as effector cells in resistance to listeriosis. Yet historically, the suggestion has been that the neutrophil is not an important mediator of acquired resistance to infection by *Listeria monocytogenes*. Data presented here suggest that this may not be true. In the first place, neutrophils from both mice and men (15,20) express excellent bactericidal activity against listeria *in vitro*. This is true whether the neutrophils are assayed in a suspension assay as we have used throughout most of the experiments described here, or whether they are assayed adherent to plastic or glass (unpublished observations). In the second place, neutrophils as well as macrophages appear in the peritoneal cavity in greater numbers in immune mice than normal mice (14). And third, in an antigen-dependent, dose-dependent manner, T cells from immune mice transfer the ability to accumulate neutrophils to a site of antigenic challenge.

Perhaps the neutrophil participates in resistance to infection by listeria and other facultative intracellular organisms such as *Salmonella typhimurium* and *Escherichia. coli* at two levels. First, neutrophils rapidly accumulate at a site of bacterial infection, drawn perhaps by bacterial chemotactic factors, perhaps because bacteria activate the alternative pathway, or perhaps because of the inflammatory process (2,21-23). This early, non-specific influx of neutrophils results in perhaps 80-90% of the organisms being destroyed. Since simultaneously macrophages and other antigen-presenting cells are probably phagocytosing and processing bacterial antigens, immune responses are being initiated as well. Second, two or three days later, there are high numbers of antigen-specific immune T cells which could induce the second neutrophil-mediated event in resistance: recruitment of low numbers of neutrophils and high numbers of macrophages to the site of infection. Although these neutrophils may constitute no more than 10% of the cells responding to T cell stimuli, they express high levels of bactericidal activity and could contribute significantly to immunologically-mediated acquisition of resistance.

Genetically-susceptible mice recruit effector cells poorly

Additional evidence suggesting that recruitment of effector phagocytes plays an important role in resistance to infection comes from experiments using mice genetically-susceptible and genetically-resistant to listeria. Experiments by Skamene and colleagues and by us indicate that the major defect in listeria-susceptible mice is in their ability to recruit cells to the peritoneal cavity (24-26). Once recruited, macrophages and neutrophils from both strains of mice kill listeria well (26,27).

Macrophage bactericidal and tumoricidal activities can be dissociated

Macrophage activation has often been thought of as a continuum in which the most highly-activated cells express both tumoricidal and microbicidal activity. Yet very few studies have tested directly whether a cell stimulated to express tumoricidal activity necessarily also expresses bactericidal activity and vice versa. Wing and colleagues (28,29) demonstrated that macrophages from trichinella- and toxoplasma-infected mice showed different abilities to kill tumor cells and intracellular parasites depending on the length of *in vitro* macrophage cultivation. Nacy and colleagues (30) used different lymphokine fractions *in vitro* to demonstrate that tumoricidal activity could be dissociated from the ability of macrophages to limit intracellular growth of rickettsia. Sedimentation velocity separation was used by Hopper and Cahill (30) to demonstrate that macrophages with bactericidal activity could be separated from those with tumoricidal activity following secondary infection with *Salmonella enteritidis*. We showed (32) that macrophages harvested from the peritoneal cavities of mice or hamsters injected 2-9 weeks earlier with BCG expressed high levels of tumoricidal activity against three different targets, but showed little anti-bacterial activity against listeria or *E. coli*. Proteose peptone-elicited macrophages, on the other hand, were bactericidal for listeria and *E. coli*, but were not tumoricidal. Thus, macrophages stimulated to express tumoricidal activity do not necessarily express bactericidal activity, and macrophages stimulated to express bactericidal activity do not necessarily express tumoricidal activity.

WHAT IS THE ROLE OF IFN_{γ} IN RESISTANCE TO LISTERIA INFECTION?

The stimuli which induce macrophages to express tumoricidal activity recently have been more carefully characterized. It has been shown that IFN_{γ} provides a priming stimulus while other agents, such as lipopolysaccharide (LPS), provide triggering stimuli to induce cells to express tumoricidal activity (10,12,33,34). Moreover, there is compelling evidence in the literature to indicate that IFN_{γ} can activate macrophages to express microbicidal activity against obligate intracellular organisms such as leishmania, toxoplasma, and rickettsiae (30,34,35). Yet other experiments indicate that IFN_{γ} is not able to stimulate human macrophages to express bactericidal activity against *Mycobacterium tuberculosis*, even though these same cells become tumoricidal and leishmanicidal (36).

We have recently conducted experiments which demonstrate that peritoneal macrophages elicited 24 hr earlier with 10% fetal calf serum and then incubated overnight with 200-2000 U/ml IFN_{γ} express tumoricidal but not bactericidal activity (P.A.Campbell and J.L. Cook, submitted for publication). That is, macrophages stimulated in a IFN_{γ}-dependent manner to express tumoricidal activity do not express bactericidal activity. Macrophages harvested from mice injected with proteose peptone 48 hrs earlier express bactericidal activity before and after overnight incubation, ruling out the trivial possibility that the overnight incubation per se eliminates bactericidal activity.

Yet these *in vitro* findings must be reconciled with experiments which demonstrate that injection of monoclonal anti-IFN_{γ} antibodies into mice results in decreased resistance to infection by listeria (38,39). Schreiber and colleagues have shown that monoclonal antibodies to IFN_{γ} inhibit two important IFN_{γ}-mediated functions. They inhibit priming of macrophages for non-specific tumoricidal activity, and they inhibit expression of cell-mediated immune responses by inhibiting IFN_{γ}-dependent induction of class II MHC antigen expression on macrophages required for efficient antigen presentation (40,41). It is quite clear that the ability of macrophages to present listeria antigens is dependent on their ability to express Ia antigens. Thus it is conceivable that injection of anti-IFN_{γ} antibodies inhibits resistance to listeriosis because these antibodies prevent induction of an effective immune response to listeria, and not because they prevent the activation of macrophages to express enhanced bactericidal activity. Whether the IFN_{γ} required for antigen presentation is secreted by natural killer cells or by immune T cells is not yet known.

Taken together, the data obtained thus far seem to indicate that IFN_{γ} secretion is necessary for resistance to infection by listeria and perhaps by other facultative intracellular bacteria. Its role may be to promote effective antigen presentation in order to trigger T cells to secrete factors required for recruitment of effector cells, rather than to activate effector macrophages to express high levels of bactericidal activity. On the other hand, it is possible that IFN_{γ} influences effector cell function during resistance to infection, but its role may be indirect. It is conceivable, for instance, that IFN_{γ} could stimulate on macrophages to secret IL-1 or other mediators which would cause enhanced accumulation of bactericidal inflammatory effector cells. It is also possible that IFN_{γ} does activate macrophages to express listericidal activity, but in a manner different from the way in which it stimulates cells to express tumoricidal activity. If this were true, this heightened bactericidal activity must not be able to be detected in a suspension assay such as we have used - this seems an unlikely possibility, but can not formally be ruled out at this time.

SUMMARY

We have presented 5 experimental observations which support a model for resistance to infection by the facultative intracellular bacterium, L. monocytogenes, in which the primary role for listeria-specific effector T cells is to cause recruitment of heightened numbers of macrophages and neutrophils which express potent anti-bacterial activity.

These observations are:

1. Both macrophages and neutrophils, from mice and men, are bactericidal for listeria, salmonella, and E. coli.

2. When titrated, inflammatory macrophages and neutrophils have as much bactericidal activity as do immunologically-elicited macrophages and neutrophils. Thus "activated" macrophages are no better than inflammatory macrophages at killing bacteria.

3. Spleen T cells which transfer resistance to listeria also transfer, in a dose-dependent manner, the ability to accumulate enhanced numbers of neutrophils and macrophages following antigenic challenge. Phagocytes which accumulate following injection of immune vs. normal T cells kill bacteria equally well.

4. The major defect in mice which are genetically-susceptible to listeria is that they accumulate fewer macrophages and neutrophils in response to challenge with antigen or with an inflammatory agent than do mice which are genetically-resistant to listeria.

5. Macrophages induced to express bactericidal activity are not necessarily tumoricidal, and macrophages induced to express tumoricidal activity are not necessarily bactericidal. Thus bactericidal and tumoricidal properties of macarophages can be dissociated. Moreover, macrophages stimulated by recombinant

IFN$_\gamma$ to express tumoricidal activity do not express bactericidal activity.

ACKNOWLEDGEMENTS

The authors thank Kelly Crumrine for typing the manuscript.

REFERENCES

1. Mackaness, G.B. 1964. The immunological basis of acquired cellular resistance. J. Exp. Med. 120:105.

2. Mackaness, G.B. and R.V. Blanden. 1967. Cellular Immunity Progr. Allergy 11:89.

3. Campbell, P.A. 1986. Are inflammatory phagocytes responsible for resistance to facultative intracellular bacteria? Immunol. Today 7:70.

4. Farr, A.G., J.-M. Kiely and E.R. Unanue. 1979. Macrophage-T cell interactions involving Listeria monocytogenes - role of the H-2 gene complex. J. Immunol. 122:2395.

5. Ziegler, K. and E.R. Unanue. 1981. Identification of a macrophage antigen-processing event required for I region-restricted antigen presentation to T lymphocytes. J. Immunol. 127:1869.

6. Unanue, E.R. 1984. Antigen-presenting function of the macrophage. Ann. Rev. Immunol. 2:395.

7. Haskins, K., J. Kappler and P. Marrack. 1984. The major histocompatibility complex-restricted antigen receptor on T cells. Ann. Rev. Immunol. 2:51.

8. Steeg, P.S., R.N. Moore, H.M. Johnson and J.J. Oppenheim. 1982. Regulation of murine Ia antigen expression by a lymphokine with gamma interferon activity. J. Exp. Med. 156:1780.

9. Habu, S. 1986. IL2 receptor expression on differentiating lymphocytes in the murine thymocyte. Immunol. Rev. 92:67.

10. Schreiber, R.D. 1984. Identification of gamma-interferon as a murine macrophage-activating factor for tumor cytotoxicity. Contemp. Topics Immunobiol.: Macrophage Activation 13:171.

11. Murray, H.W. 1984. Macrophage Activation: Enhanced oxidative and antiprotozoal activity. Contemp. Topics Immunobiol: Macrophage Activation 13:97.

12. Adams, D.O. and T.A. Hamilton. 1984. The cell biology of macrophage activation. Ann. Rev. Immunol. 2:283.

13. Nacy, C.A., S.L. James, C.N. Osler and M.S. Meltzer. 1984. Activation of macrophages to kill Rickettsiae and Leishmania: Dissociation of intracellular microbicidal activities and extracellular destruction of neoplastic and Helminth targets. Contemp. Topics Immunobiol.: Macrophage Activation 13:147.

14. Kaufmann, S.H.E., H. Hahn, R. Berger and H. Kirchner. 1983.

Interferon-γ production by Listeria monocytogenes specific T cells active in cellular antibacterial immunity. Eur. J. Immunol. 13:265.

15. Czuprynski, C.J., P.M. Henson and P.A. Campbell. 1984. Killing of Listeria monocytogenes by inflammatory neutrophils and mononuclear phagocytes from immune and nonimmune mice. J. Leukocyte Biol. 35:193.

16. Czuprynski, C.J., P.M. Henson and P.A. Campbell. 1985. Enhanced accumulation of inflammatory neutrophils and macrophages mediated by transfer of T cells from mice immunized with Listeria monocytogenes. J. Immunol. 134:3449.

17. Lane, F.C. and E.R. Unanue. 1972. Requirement of thymus (T) lymphocytes for resistance to listeriosis. J. Exp. Med. 135:1104.

18. Blanden, R.V. and R.E. Langman. 1972. Cell-mediated immunity to bacterial infection in the mouse. Thymus-derived cells as effectors of acquired resistance to Listeria monocytogenes. Scand. J. Immunol. 4:379.

19. North, R.J. 1973. Importance of thymus-derived lymphocytes in cell-mediated immunity to infection. Cell. Immunol. 7:166.

20. Czuprynski, C.J., P.A. Campbell and P.M. Henson. 1983. Killing of Listeria monocytogenes by human neutrophils and monocytes, but not by monocyte-derived macrophages. J. Reticuloendothel. Soc. 34:29.

21. North, R.J. 1970. The relative importance of blood monocytes and fixed macrophages to the expression of cell-mediated immunity to infection. J. Exp. Med. 132:521.

22. Mandel, B.F. and C. Cheers. 1980. Resistance and susceptibility of mice to bacterial infection: Histopathology of listeriosis in resistant and susceptible strains. Infect. Immun. 30:851.

23. Baker, L.A., P.A. Campbell and J.R. Hollister. 1977. Chemotaxigenesis and complement fixation by Listeria monocytogenes cell wall fractions. J. Immunol. 119:1723.

24. Stevenson, M.M., P.A.L. Kongshavn and E. Skamene. 1981. Genetic linkage of resistance to Listeria monocytogenes with macrophage inflammatory responses. J. Immunol. 127:402.

25. Gervais, F., M. Stevenson and E. Skamene. 1984. Genetic control of resistance of Listeria monocytogenes: Regulation of leukocyte inflammatory responses by the Hc locus. J. Immunol. 132:2078.

26. Czuprynski, C.J., B.P. Canono, P.M. Henson and P.A. Campbell. 1985. Genetically determined resistance to listeriosis is associated with increased accumulation of inflammatory neutrophils and macrophages which have enhanced listericidal activity. Immunol. 55:511.

27. Gervais, F., A. Morris-Hooke, T.A. Tran and E. Skamene. 1986. Analysis of macrophage bactericidal function in genetically resistant and susceptible mice by using the temperature-sensitive mutant of Listeria monocytogenes. Inf. and Immun. 54:315.

28. Wing, E.J., I.D. Gardner, F.W. Ryning and J.S. Remington. 1977. Dissociation of effector functions in populations of activated macrophages. Nature 268:642.

29. Wing, E.J., J.L. Krahenbuhl and J.S Remington. 1979. Studies of macrophages function during Trichonella spiralis infection in mice. Immunol. 36:479.

30. Nacy, C.A., E.J. Leonard and M.S. Meltzer. 1981. Macrophages in resistance to rickettsial infections: Characterization of lymphokines that induce rickettsiacidal activity in macrophages. J. Immunol. 126:204.

31. Hopper, K.E. and J.M. Cahill. 1983. Immunoregulation by macrophages. II. Separation of mouse peritoneal macrophages having tumoricidal and bactericidal activities and those secreting PGE and interleukin 1. J. Reticuloendothel. Soc. 33:443.

32. Campbell, P.A., C.J. Czuprynski, and J.L. Cook. 1984. Differential expression of macrophage effector functions: Bactericidal versus tumoricidal activities. J. Leukocyte Biol. 36:293.

33. Hibbs, J.B., Jr., R.R. Taintor, H.A. Chapman, Jr. and J.B. Weinberg. 1977. Macrophage tumor killing: Influence of the local environment. Science 197:279.

34. Ruco, L.P. and M.S. Meltzer. 1978. Macrophage activation for tumor cytotoxicity: development of macrophage cytotoxic activity requires completion of a sequence of short lived intermediary reactions. J. Immunol. 121:2035.

35. Nathan, C.F., H.W. Murray, M.E. Wiebe and B.Y. Rubin. 1983. Identification of interferon-γ as the lymphokine that activates human macrophage oxidative metabolism and antimicrobial activity. J. Exp. Med. 158:670.

36. Murray, H.W., G.L. Spitalny, and C.F. Nathan. 1985. Activation of mouse peritoneal macrophages in vitro by interferon-γ. J. Immunol. 134:1619.

37. Douvas, G.S., D.L. Looker, A.E. Vatter and A.J. Crowle. 1985. Gamma interferon activates human macrophages to become tumoricidal and leishmanicidal but enhances replication of macrophage-associated mycobacteria. Inf. and Immun. 50:1.

38. Kaufmann, S.H.E., H. Hahn, R. Berger and H. Kirchner. 1983. Interferon-γ production by Listeria monocytogenes-specific T cells active in cellular antibacterial immunity. Eur. J. Immunol. 13:265.

39. Buchmeier, N.A. and R.D. Schreiber. 1985. Requirement of endogenous interferon-γ production for resolution of Listeria monocytogenes infection. Proc. Natl. Acad. Sci. 82:7404.

40. Schreiber, R.D., L.J. Hicks, A. Celada, N.A. Buchmeier and P.W. Gray. 1985. Monoclonal antibodies to murine γ-interferon which differentially modulate macrophage activation and antiviral activity. J. Immunol. 134:1609.

41. Schreiber, R.D. 1987. This book.

GENETIC BASIS OF HOST RESISTANCE AND SUSCEPTIBILITY TO INTRACELLULAR PATHOGENS

Emil Skamene and Adrien Forget*

Division of Clinical Immunology and Allergy, Montreal General Hospital, Montreal, Quebec H3G 1A4, and *Department of Microbiology and Immunology, University of Montreal, Montreal, Quebec H3C 3J7

INTRODUCTION

History provides numerous examples of variable susceptibility of human populations to viral, bacterial and parasitic infections, both during epidemics and in the endemic areas of the world. Although the influence of environmental factors must be considered in any explanation of such variability, it has recently become clear, mainly on the basis of studying experimental infections in inbred animals, that genetic factors play decisive role in individual susceptibility.

In principle, the entire basis of susceptibility or resistance to infection is genetically determined but, because of the immense variety of offenders and the complexities of host defenses, few common patterns of resistance are discernible. Thus, we are compelled to study step-wise processes affecting individual microorganisms with the hope of extending the studies to other infections and other hosts. It furthermore follows that no natural infection could be expected to be solely regulated by a single gene. It is true that a possession of a particular allele at one genetic locus may dramatically influence the course of disease in certain individuals but at the level of whole population many genes would be expected to be responsible for the, often spectral, disease profile which is frequently observed in infections with intracellular pathogens.

Genetic basis of susceptibility and resistance to these infections must, therefore, be viewed as a composite interplay of inherited mechanisms which manifest themselves as a programmed sequence of events. Only by separating the particular pattern of host response to a given pathogen into discrete steps may we reconstruct its genetic regulation. This paper will deal with the strategy of such analysis, using as an example the model of genetic variation of mice to infection with *Mycobacterium bovis*, strain BCG.

GENETIC VARIATION OF RESISTANCE/SUSCEPTIBILITY TO INFECTION

The prerequisite of the genetic analysis is a variation, quantitative or qualitative, in the host response to pathogen. When found among inbred mouse strains which are kept under controlled environmental conditions, such variation is usually the result of either mutation or a polymorphism at one or more chromosomal loci. It is important at that point of the study to define well the character to be studied. While death of the infected animal is often used as a typing criterion for susceptibility, it is preferable to use simpler (in biologic terms) end points, such as the number of microorganisms in the tissue at various times post-infection or the size and appearance of tissue lesions (necrosis, granuloma etc.). It is often seen that such variables as the dose of infectious agent, virulence of the pathogen or route of inoculation alter dramatically the observed genetic variation in the response of the host (Fig. 1). This fact was alluded to by Gowen (1) but it is often ignored when seemingly discrepant results from different laboratories are being compared. In order to be able to probe one variable (i.e. host genes) one has to fix the other side of the equation (i.e. make the conditions of infection standardized) and thus transform the three-dimensional problem into a two-dimensional one.

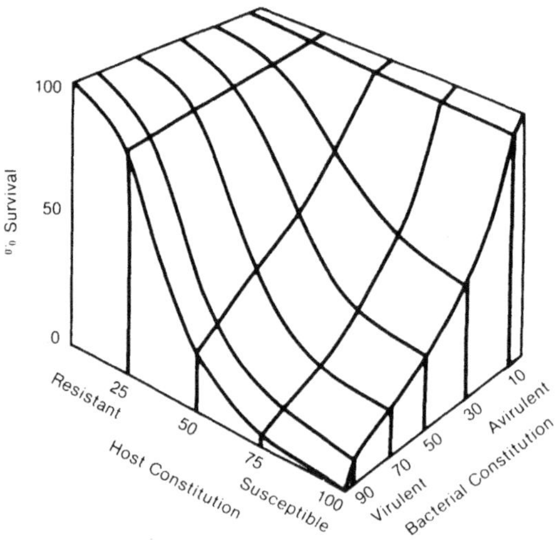

Fig. 1. Interaction of the host genotype and the microbial genotype in the outcome of infection (Adapted from ref. 1).

When mice of various inbred mouse strains are infected intravenously with a small dose (10^4 colony forming units, CFU) of Mycobacterium bovis BCG, strain Montreal and the number of bacillary colonies in their spleens is studied at time after infection two patterns of response can be seen (Fig. 2). Approximately half of the strains are resistant, not having allowed any bacterial proliferation to occur. There is a logarithmic growth of mycobacteria in the spleens of the other half of inbred strains, the difference between the two groups often being significant as early as 24 hours after the infection. The most impressive variation in this genetic character is seen at 2-3 weeks post infection. Such a clear, discontinuous, inter-strain pattern of response immediately suggests that the character may be under single gene control (2). It is of interest to note that this pattern is seen only with some substrains of BCG and with some other mycobacteria which seem to be of intermediate virulence (e.g. BCG Montreal, BCG Pasteur, BCG Tice, Mycobacterium kansasii, Mycobacterium intracellulare, and Mycobacterium lepraemurium). Infection with those BCG substrains which are relatively avirulent (e.g. BCG Japan) result in almost undetectable bacterial growth in all strains tested, with some genetic advantage seen in the resistant group of mice as a pattern of more rapid bacterial elimination (3). The more virulent mycobacterial strains (e.g. M. tuberculosis H37Rv) fail to exhibit two distinct patterns of infection and the inbred mouse strains infected with such pathogens form a discontinuous spectrum of responses where, clearly, additional genetic influences are operating (4).

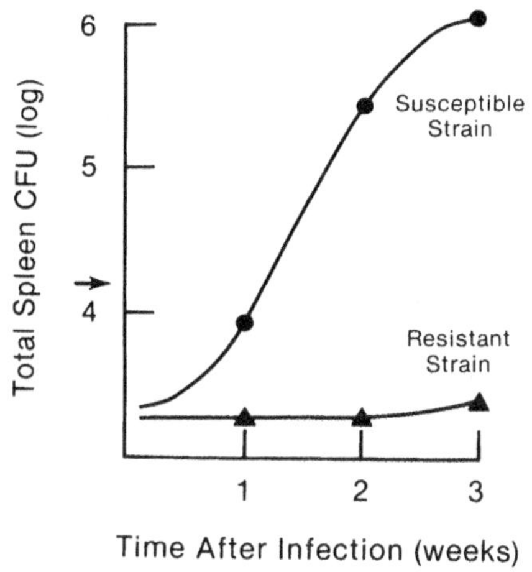

Fig. 2. Genetic variation in the control of BCG proliferation in vivo (arrow = dose of BCG injected)

SEGREGATION MENDELIAN ANALYSIS OF RESISTANCE/SUSCEPTIBILITY

Having defined a discontinuous variation in the phenotype of resistance and susceptibility among inbred strains one may embark on further analysis which aims at the estimation of the number of genetic loci involved in the control of such trait. This means setting up numerous crosses of the typical resistant and susceptible progenitors and to type the individual animals of the segregating populations (F2 and backcrosses) for the trait of resistance/susceptibility. These studies must have redundancy built into their design since, often, quantitative traits with certain threshold characteristics are being studied. Where the distribution of a given trait in mice of prog-nitor strains can clearly be differentiated from that of Fl hybrids (without the occurrence of an overlap), single locus control of resistance leads to a bimodal distribution of resistant and susceptible animals among the backcross progeny. Such is the case of genetic resistance to M. bovis BCG where individuals of numerous segregating populations always express one of the parental types with the proportion of susceptible and resistant phenotypes approaching the predicted mendelian ratio for monogenic control (5).

More often than not, however, such clear distinction of variant phenotypes is not seen and a considerable degree of overlap in the expression of the traits of resistance and susceptibility exists in the genetically homogenous populations of parental and Fl strains. Understandably, the distributions of phenotypic classes in the segregating generations also overlap extensively in those situations. Goodness-of-fit tests are often applied inappropriately to a subset of data selected by arbitrary rules (e.g. the use of 2 standard deviations [SD] from the parental mean to type backcross individuals as being like the parental strain "with 95% confidence"). These types of data are being obtained in the genetic studies of resistance and susceptibility to infection much more frequently than the clear segregations into distinct phenotypic categories. Their analysis requires thorough familiarity with the principles of quantitative genetics that have statistical foundations. Excellent examples of treatment of such data in the field of genetic resistance have recently been provided by Curtis et al. (6) and by McCall (7).

MAPPING OF THE GENES OF HOST RESISTANCE/SUSCEPTIBILITY TO INFECTION

An identification, by segregation analysis, of a single gene which controls the phenotype of resistance or susceptibility, leads to an immediate temptation to search for its chromosomal location. One may ask at this particular point of investigation whether the gene mapping is likely to advance our knowledge of the genetic basis of resistance and susceptibility? There is no doubt that the gene mapping has its intrinsic value as it adds a definitive and an elegant quality to any studies of host resistance. It also helps the mouse geneticists (and, by extension the human geneticists) to fill blanks on the chromosomal maps of murine or human genome. However, there are several much more important reasons why it is useful to embark on a long and often difficult path to look for a chromosomal location of the host resistance gene. These reasons are summarized in Table 1 and will be expanded using the Bcg gene as an example.

Table 1. Why map genes of host resistance to infection?

(1) To uncover a pleoiotropic effect of the gene (this may contribute to our understanding of the mechanism of genetic control).

(2) To map the host resistance gene to a previously identified locus carrying an already known gene which codes for a product that may be involved in the phenotype of resistance/susceptibility.

(3) To identify closely-linked chromosomal markers which are useful in (a) typing for resistance/susceptibility; (b) creation of congenic lines; (c) search for the gene using the tools of molecular biology.

(4) To search for conservation of homologous domains containing the same host resistance gene in different species.

There are two feasible ways of mapping genes of host resistance to infection. The classical one employs the strategy of linkage analysis using the known linkage groups and it is based on the search for a co-segregation of the phenotype of host resistance with one of the previously identified allotypic markers in the backcross and F2 generation. This approach has successfully been used by Plant and Glynn in the location of Ity gene which controls innate resistance to Salmonella typhimurium (8). The practical problem with that methodology is the necessity to make precise measurements of the variable phenotype (resistant vs susceptible) on single, individual animals of the segregating progeny and it is, therefore, applicable only in those circumstances where there is a well-defined, "tight", typing method available. Once typed by exposure to destructive infection, that same animal is never available for repeated measurements. The other limitation is the availability of only a small number of testing stocks with appropriately-identified linkage groups. For this reason, a newer genetic tool, namely recombinant inbred (RI) strains have widely been used in the analysis of genetic control of resistance to a variety of infectious agents.

RI mouse strains are derived by inbreeding the F_2 progeny of a cross between two inbred parental strains. Once inbred, such set of RI strains can be thought of as stable segregant population. Unlinked genes are randomized in the RI strains while linked genes will tend to become fixed in the same (parental) combination as they entered the cross. The recombination of segments of parental chromosomes is thus random but it can be detected by typing the different RI strains for the parental phenotypes of known genes which are allelic in the progenitor strains. If the parental strains carry different alleles at a locus one wants to map, its chromosomal location may be determined by typing, in each RI strain, for the presence of one or the other parental allele.

A basic feature of analyzing data sets derived from typing RI strains for given character is the assignment of one of the progenitor phenotypes to each of the RI strains in order to determine a strain distribution pattern (SDP) for the RI set. For a trait controlled by a single gene one may expect a bimodal distribution of parental phenotypes among the RI mice. By comparing the SDP of the new locus to a table of SDPs for other already known loci, one determines whether alleles at any other loci are inherited in a similar fashion. The more closely two loci are linked, the more likely it is that their SDP's will be identical or nearly identical.

In the case of resistance to M. bovis BCG this bimodal pattern clearly emerged when animals of BXD, BXH and BXA sets (B = susceptible C57BL/6J progenitor, D, H, A = resistant DBA/2, C3H/HeJ and A/J progenitors) were examined. The SDP of this trait was concordant (but not identical) with the SDP of two Chromosome 1 genes, namely Idh-1 and Pep-3. The recombination frequency of the gene of resistance to

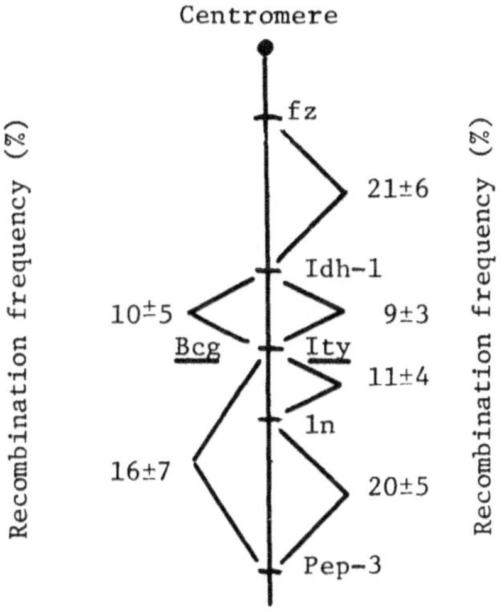

Fig. 3. Mapping of Bcg and Ity loci on Chromosome 1.

M. bovis BCG (named the Bcg gene at that point) with the Idh-1 and Pep-3 loci signaled a putative location of Bcg gene on the Chromosome 1, in the vicinity of those 2 marker genes (Fig. 3).

The RI strain analysis of the resistant (Bcg^r) and susceptible (Bcg^s) phenotype had, furthermore, resulted in the most valuable appreciation of an absolute concordance between the Bcg^r/Bcg^s pattern and the SDP of resistant and susceptible alleles of two more host resistance genes identified previously, namely the Ity (Salmonella typhimurium resistance gene) and the Lsh (a gene controlling innate resistance to Leishmania donovani, 10). This was one of the most tangible pieces of evidence attesting to the value of gene mapping for our understanding of the genetic mechanisms of resistance and susceptibility: a single gene was found which controlled innate resistance to a group of immunologically-distinct and taxonomically-unrelated pathogens. Already at this early stage of the genetic studies it was suggested that perhaps the inherited mechanism operates via macrophages since all 3 pathogens identified as being genetically restricted by this gene are intracellular parasites of the macrophage (11).

The RI approach to gene mapping is not always as straightforward as described in the example of Ity-Lsh-Bcg locus. The assignment of an SDP to the RI strains becomes problematic when a continuous gradation of responses is observed between the RI and parental strains and when the distribution of phenotypes into resistant and susceptible group is blurred. Several statistical approaches have recently been devised to alleviate this problem and to make a linkage analysis possible. Among them is the discriminant function analysis which allows for the identification of the least variable characters or attributes for the discrimimation of progenitor phenotypes (12) and the adaptation of two sample rank test which makes a non-parametric analysis of data and can thus deal with measurements that do not follow a normal distribution pattern (13).

CONGENIC LINES FOR HOST RESISTANCE GENES

The mapping of the gene of host resistance makes the task of creating lines congenic for that locus much easier. The common way of propagating such lines is to select, by typing for the parental phenotype of resistance or susceptibility, the resistant heterozygotes of the segregating backcross progeny which are then allowed to mate with the susceptible progenitor. In the case of monogenic control, the single gene should breed true and the result of such mating is a population segregating approximately 50:50 into susceptible homozygotes and resistant heterozygotes in each subsequent generation of backcrossing. The problem with that approach is that the selection method involves an infection and there is always a danger of vertical transfer of either microorganisms themselves or components of immune response (e.g. antibodies) along with the appropriate genes. The cumbersome way around that dilemma is the selection of resistant heterozygotes by progeny testing but this manouever delays by 100% the progress of creating the congenic line.

The knowledge of the chromosomal location of the host resistance gene in question allows us to construct the congenic line, at least in the initial stages of backcrossing, by selection for closely-linked flanking chromosomal markers present in their allelic forms in the parental animals. Furthermore, already existing congenic lines, developed for other reasons can be screened for the presence of allelic forms of the host resistance gene. The example of the latter approach is the emergence of Bcg (Ity,Lsh) congenic mouse strain in the collection of BALB/c (Bcg^s) congenics carrying different parts of the DBA/2 (Bcg^r) genome. These strains were developed by Dr. M. Potter in his search for the genes of resistance to plasmacytomas (14). One of those strains, C.D2 - $Idh\text{-}1^b\text{-}Pep\text{-}3^b$ carried a piece of DBA/2 chromosome 1 which, theoretically, should have included the Bcg^r allele of DBA/2 origin on, otherwise susceptible, BALB/c background. The experimental evidence was obtained to prove that hypothesis (15) and, without any effort on their own part, the students of the Bcg-Ity-Lsh gene had at their disposal lines congenic for this locus (with flanking segments of Chromosome 1). These strains have then been used extensively in the search for the phenotypic expression of this gene.

Conceptually similar approach has often been used where mouse strains carrying known mapped mutations were employed in studies of genetic resistance to infection. The best known example are the C3H/HeJ mice carrying the Lps^d allele on Chromosome 4 which alters dramatically the response of these mutants to variety of biological effects of lipid A component of LPS (16). This mutation is responsible for innate susceptibility to a number of pathogens including *Salmonella typhimurium* (17). Another interesting example is the congenic A2G strain, a result of an illegitimate mating of an unwanted visitor into otherwise purebred A colony in England. The result of this experiment of nature (in the true sense of the word) was a line which proved to be extremely resistant to myxovirus infection and which served, together with its congenic susceptible A partner, to unravel yet the best analyzed case of host resistance gene, the Mx gene (18).

The use of congenic and mutant strains is also extremely useful in dissecting the action of different genes which result in a phenotypically similar alteration of host resistance. For example, the C3HeB/FeJ substrain is phenotypically identical to the Lps-defective C3H/HeJ substrain in its extreme susceptibility to *Salmonella*. Yet, breeding studies set up to assess the possible complementation effects resulted in the clear distinction of the gene controlling *Salmonella*-susceptibility of C3HeB/FeJ strain from the Lps gene and from all other genes known until that point to regulate the *Salmonella* response (19).

PHENOTYPIC EXPRESSION OF HOST RESISTANCE GENES

The availability of mutant and congenic lines which were developed or discovered in the course of genetic analysis of the host resistance, allows us to embark on functional studies dealing with the control mechanisms. These can be performed without the interfering effect of the rest of the genome which is always a problem when functional correlates of resistance and susceptibility are looked for in regular inbred strains exhibiting the alternate resistant or susceptible phenotypes. The search for the phenotypic expression of Bcg(Ity,Lsh) gene in congenic mice revealed that the genetic mechanism was operating very early after infection, with its clear effects being seen already at 24 hours (20, 21). The functional depletion of T cell, B cell and NK cell subsets has not influenced the phenotype of genetic resistance. Bcg^r mice remained resistant even after having been irradiated with 550R and 900R of total body radiation. Experiments with reciprocal $Bcg^s \rightarrow Bcg^r$ radiation lymphopoietic chimeras clearly documented that the cell population expressing the resistant phenotype originated from bone marrow. Finally, the only manoeuver which was able to transform the genetically resistant mouse strain into the phenotypically susceptible one was a chronic treatment with silica (21). All these indirect lines of evidence pointed out to the mature macrophage as the cell expressing the resistant or susceptible forms of the *Bcg* gene (Table 2).

Table 2. Phenotypic expression of *Bcg* gene

T cell independent.
B cell independent.
NK cell independent.
Radiation-resistant.
Bone marrow - derived.
Sensitive to chronic treatment with silica.

Conclusion: Mature macrophage

Subsequent series of investigation confirmed this hypothesis. It was demonstrated that in all the models where the host resistance patterns *in vivo* followed the distribution of Bcg^r and Bcg^s alleles, the macrophage-pathogen interaction *in vitro* was controlled by this locus. The Bcg^r macrophages explanted from the peritoneal cavity of normal, noninfected donors were shown to be superior to Bcg^s macrophages in their ability to interfere with the intracellular growth of BCG as detected by the assay of uracil incorporation into BCG (22) or by the plating efficiency of the BCG microorganisms released from those two macrophage types (23). Similar experiments using temperature-sensitive mutant of Salmonella (24) or its wild type (25) showed the identical pattern of genetic restriction as an intrinsic function of the resident (peritoneal) macrophage. Interaction of *Leishmania donovani* with macrophages *in vitro* (*Lsh* gene) also follows the same pattern except for the superior activity of liver macrophages compared to peritoneal macrophages (26). A most interesting observation, not made in the *Bcg* or *Ity* models, was reported by the group of Blackwell in the system of natural resistance to *L. donovani*: There was a definite 2-3 day time lag between the infection and the expression of the resistance in the macrophages either *in vivo* or in Kupfer cells *in vitro*. Furthermore, the resistance of the Lsh^r congenic mice was selectively enhanced following pre-treatment with *S. typhimurium* LPS or with purified *L. donovani* membranes *in vivo*. These effects could not be demonstrated in Lsh^s congenic mice. A hypothesis has been advanced that the chromosome 1 *Lsh* (*Bcg*,*Ity*) gene regulated some form of T cell independent macrophage activation process (26).

PLEIOTROPIC EFFECT OF BCG GENE: MACROPHAGE PRIMING FOR ACTIVATION

Studies of macrophage physiology became one of recent interests of several groups of investigators dealing with genetic resistance to infections with intracellular pathogens. Since it is now clear that a macrophage - from the peritoneal cavity, spleen or the liver - is intrinsically able to express the Bcg^r or Bcg^s form of the gene without any influence of other cell populations, the question arose what particular process of macrophage function is regulated by this gene. The data of Blackwell et al. (26) suggested indirectly the possibility that this gene might be involved in the process of macrophage activation.

Another line of evidence supporting this concept experimentally (albeit with a different interpretation) came from the laboratory of

Zwilling (27). Their work showed that BCG infection induces continuous I-A expression in the macrophages from *Bcg*^{r} mice while the I-A expression in the *Bcg*^{s} macrophages is a transient event. The continuous I-A expression was not due to contamination of cultures with lymphocytes nor did it require a continued presence of bacteria.

We have seen, in our laboratory, a conceptually similar phenomenon, in a different experimental system. Our observation was made in the course of routine genetic monitoring of *Bcg* congenic lines where a reciprocal negative mixed leukocyte culture in the *Bcg*^{r} → *Bcg*^{s} congenic system was used as a marker of genetic purity of these lines. An interesting result triggered our interest in the possibility that the macrophage accessory role in the alloantigen presentation may be different in the *Bcg*^{s} and *Bcg*^{r} congenic mice. The *Bcg*^{r} macrophages supported a one-way MLR against histoincompatible targets quantitatively much better than *Bcg*^{s} macrophages (Fig. 4).

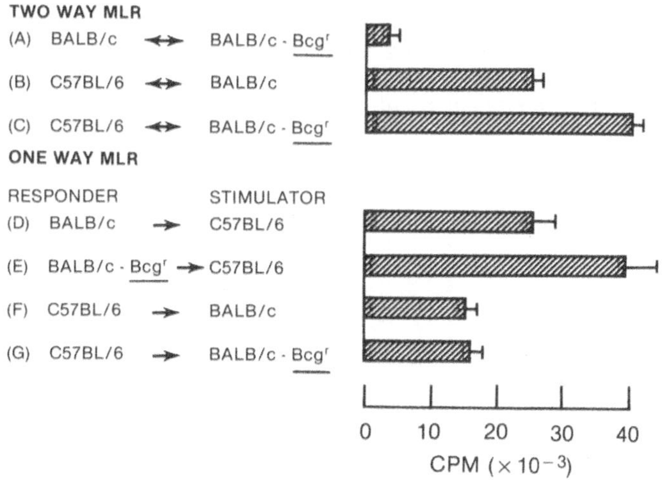

Fig. 4. *Bcg* gene effect in the macrophage support of MLR

This observation led to series of experiments which clearly established that the accessory role of *Bcg*^{r} macrophages (compared with that of *Bcg*^{s} congenic counterparts) was superior not only in response to alloantigens but also to mitogens, and to bacterial antigens such as BCG, *Salmonella typhimurium*, *Brucella abortus* and *Listeria monocytogenes* (28). These accessory functions vary quantitatively with the density of Ia antigens on the macrophage surface. The upregulation of Ia antigens being one of the markers of macrophage activation we have investigated the presence of other markers associated with that event, in the *Bcg*^{r} and *Bcg*^{s} macrophages. Among those examined was the downregulation of membrane ectoenzyme 5'nucleotidase and an enhanced respiratory burst in the macrophages. A functional corollary of macrophage activation, namely the listericidal activity was also examined. Results of those studies are summarized in Table 3. Briefly, in all instances which were tested so far, the *Bcg*^{r} macrophages, when compared with their *Bcg*^{s} controls, showed quantitatively enhanced ability to become activated by a variety of specific and nonspecific stimuli (29, 30, 31, 32).

Table 3. Pleiotropic effects of Bcg gene

MACROPHAGE FUNCTION	**Bcg^r**	**Bcg^s**
Support of MLC	+++	+
Antigen presentation	+++	+
Support of mitogenesis	+++	+
Upregulation of Ia	+++	+
Downregulation of 5' nucleotidase	+++	+
H_2O_2 and O_2^- production	+++	+
Listericidal activity	+++	+
Antimycobacterial activity	+++	+

Macrophage activation is a stepwise chain of events in which cells in different stages of maturation and/or differentiation become receptive to priming and activating signals to acquire cytotoxic effector responses against intracellular and extracellular microbial and neoplastic targets (33). In its simplified form the cascade involves the stimulation of responsive macrophages into the primed state by molecules such as interferon γ. Primed macrophages are then able to respond to a variety of membrane stimuli, among them lipopolysaccharide and other components of bacterial cell wall, to become activated for microbicidal function. According to this concept and based on our results and those of others, the difference between the Bcg^r and Bcg^s macrophages may be thought of as follows (Fig. 5).

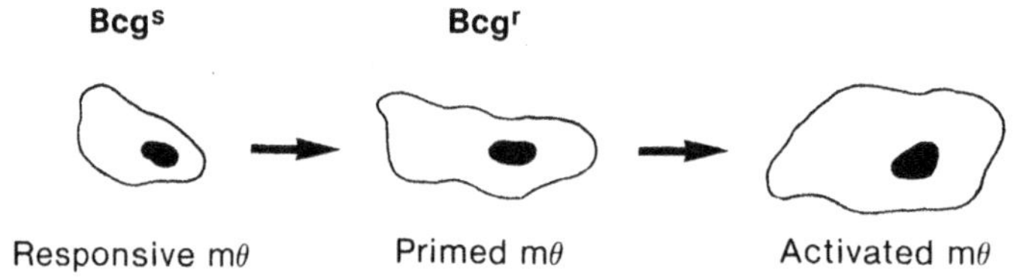

Fig. 5. Proposed mechanism of Bcg gene control at the cellular level.

The Bcg^r macrophage is at a more advanced level in the activation sequence; descriptively it seems to have many characteristics of a **primed** cell. The phagocytosis of BCG or an interaction with other activating stimuli leads to membrane perturbation and to a cascade of events which are characteristic of activated macrophages: upregulation of Ia, downregulation of 5'nucleotidase, increased oxidative burst, enhanced nonspecific bacteriostatic and bactericidal activity. It should be pointed out that these processes should only be considered- **markers** of the activated state of the macrophage - it is not implied that any one of these particular markers is actually **the** expression of the resistant phenotype at a molecular level.

The Bcg^s macrophage, on the other hand, is quantitatively lower in the cascade of macrophage activation; descriptively it appears to be in the responsive, but not yet primed, state. The phagocytosis of BCG or of any other intracellular pathogen does not lead to the full activation of the Bcg^s macrophage - the stage of priming in that cell has not yet been achieved under natural conditions. The Bcg^s

macrophage does, however, have the capacity to develop into a fully activated cell when exposed to such priming stimuli as, for example, T cell derived lymphokines in the course of acquired immunity. The Bcg^s mice are able to control BCG load later on in the course of natural infection, in its immune phase, through the process of T cell-dependent macrophage activation. It just seems that the Bcg^r macrophage can respond, by activation, to the phagocytic BCG stimulus already very early on in the course of infection, without the need for priming by the specifically sensitized T cell. To unravel the molecular basis of the immunologically non-specific priming of Bcg^r macrophages (effective membrane processing of priming signal such as γ-interferon?, resistance to inhibition of priming by AA metabolites?, etc.) is the experimental challenge for the near future.

DOES A HUMAN EQUIVALENT OF THE Bcg GENE EXIST?

The genetic locus discussed in this chapter seems to have a considerable biological significance considering the fact that it regulates natural resistance to infections with a great variety of intracellular pathogens. The resistant allele of the Bcg(Ity,Lsh) gene confers a survival advantage to the mouse as attested by the fact that, so far, wild mice from a variety of locations all over the world were typed as resistant to infection (34). One would intuitively expect that mouse gene with such a survival advantage for *Mus musculus* might have its homology in other species including man. Genetic polymorphism in the resistance and susceptibility to tuberculosis in rabbits has been well characterized by pioneering studies of Lurie (35) and found to have its basis in the differential macrophage handling of virulent mycobacteria. Resistance of human populations to tuberculosis has often been postulated to have a genetic basis and the twin studies as well as familial segregation of the disease support that hypothesis (36). Similarly, there are multiple lines of evidence suggesting that the spectral character of several other diseases with intracellular pathogens such as leprosy and leishmaniasis may have a genetic basis.

There are three possible approaches to the search for the Bcg gene homologue in other species. The first one would take an advantage of our current knowledge of the phenotypic expression of Bcg gene and would apply to other species the techniques of macrophage-pathogen interaction, which were developed to recognize the resistant and susceptible macrophage phenotypes in the mouse. Such studies are now in progress in several laboratories. Another possibility would be to isolate the murine Bcg gene as a biochemical entity and then to probe the genome of other species for homologous sequences. That, obviously, is a major task and one that will not be easily accomplished given the fact that the Bcg gene product is still, in 1987, an elusive molecule. In fact, the direct identification of primary gene products responsible for the traits of host resistance to infection has successfully been achieved in only two instances, namely, the xid gene (37) and the Mx gene (38). The strategy proposed for the isolation and characterization of the Bcg gene is based on the use of genetic linkage techniques to identify the DNA sequences which encode these genes (39). This approach involves the saturation of the region of the chromosome surrounding the Bcg locus with genetic markers which are defined by specific cloned DNA segments. The location of the Bcg gene within a cloned segment of DNA can then be determined by examining its segregation pattern in genetic linkage studies with respect to other markers defined by DNA probes within that chromosomal segment.

This line of investigation has led to the recent discoveries of new polymorphisms in the vicinity of the Bcg gene. The Len-1 gene (coding for the polymorphic variants of the γ-crystallin protein of the lens) was found to be located a few centimorgans proximal to the Bcg gene (40) and the Fib gene coding for the fibronectin variants seems to map almost precisely (by the RI strain analysis) to the Bcg locus (Skow, personal communication). The examination of this sequence of linked genes on the Chromosome 1 in the approximate order Idh-1 - Len-1 - Fib - Bcg reveals a striking homology with a similar linkage group which is preserved on the long arm of the human chromosome 2 (Fig. 6). An attractive hypothesis raised by this finding of syntheny between the mouse and the man is that the presence of the gene of host resistance in this region is the reason for the conservation of this chromosomal segment. This hypothesis, further supported by the fact that a similar sequence homology is also found in the bovine (Womack, personal communication), is now being tested by examination of co-segregation of these chromosomal markers with the pattern of resistance and susceptibility to tuberculosis in families living in endemic areas of the world.

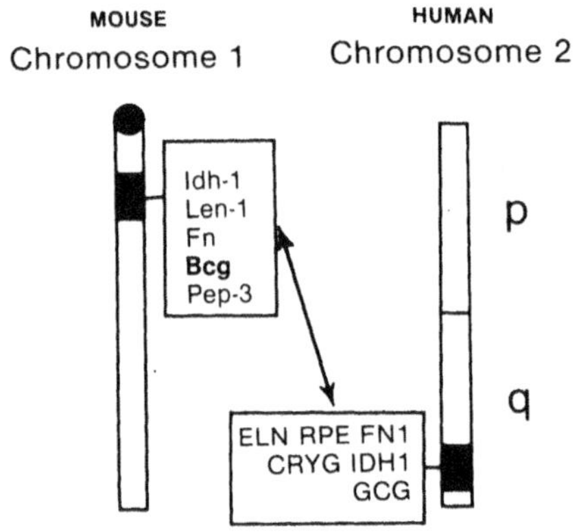

Fig. 6. Conservation of murine and human linkage groups (Len-1 is a γ-crystallin gene, homologous to GRYG).

CONCLUSION

The purpose of this contribution was to discuss the strategies of genetic analysis of host resistance and susceptibility to intracellular pathogens and to justify the use of genetics by amateurs in this field, namely by immunologists. It is becoming clear that our ability to identify genetic variations in the phenotypes of effective or defective host defenses in the inbred mouse models, with the subsequent definition of the mode of inheritance and with gene mapping greatly advances our knowledge of the innate basis of resistance and susceptibility. Beyond that, this approach allows us to find markers for the genetically susceptible individuals in population which can eventually be used in the programs of genetic epidemiology with the aim of identifying those persons which are particularly prone to the development of severe infections. Measures of prevention and early detection of those diseases should eventually be developed based on this information. Of even greater value will be the elucidation of the physiological and biochemical determinants of genetic susceptibility as a basis for specifically-targeted vaccination and other therapeutic measures.

REFERENCES

1. Gowen, J.W. 1960. Genetic effects in nonspecific resistance to infectious disease. Bact. Rev. 24:192-200.
2. Forget, A., E. Skamene, P. Gros, A.C. Miailhe, and R. Turcotte. 1981. Strain differences in the response to infection with small dispersed doses of Mycobacterium bovis BCG among inbred mice. Infect. Immun. 32:42-48.
3. Denis, M., A. Forget, M. Pelletier, R. Turcotte, and E. Skamene. 1986. Control of the Bcg gene of early resistance in mice to infections with BCG substrains and atypical mycobacteria. Clin. exp. Immunol. 63:517-525.
4. Nickonenko, B.V., A.S. Apt, A.M. Moroz and M.M. Averbakh. 1985. Genetic analysis of susceptibility of mce to H37RV tuberculosis infection: Sensitivity versus relative resistance. Prog. Leukocyte Biol. 3:291-298.
5. Gros, P., E. Skamene, and A. Forget. 1981. Genetic control of natural resistance to Mycobacterium bovis (BCG) in mice. J. Immun. 127:2417-2423.
6. Curtis, J., C.F. Curtis, and N.H. Barton. 1985. Methodology for testing the hypothesis of single locus control of host resistance. Prog. Leukocyte Biol. 3:65-70.
7. McCall, R.D. 1985. A maximum likelihood alternative to genetic analysis of quantitative immunologic data from inbred strains. Prog. Leukocyte Biol. 3:71-81.
8. Plant, J., and A.A. Glynn. 1979. Locating Salmonella resistance gene on mouse chromosome 1. Clin. exp. Immunol. 37:1-6.
9. Skamene, E., A. Forget, P. Gros, and P.A.L. Kongshavn. 1982. Chromosome 1 locus: a major regulator of natural resistance to intracellular pathogens. p. 313-318. In R.B. Herberman (ed). NK cells and other natural effector cells. Academic Press, New York.
10. Bradley, D.J., B.A. Taylor, J.M. Blackwell, E.P. Evans, and J. Freeman. 1979. Regulation of Leishmania populations within the host. III. Mapping of the locus controlling susceptibility to visceral leishmaniasis in the mouse. Clin Exp. Immunol. 37:7-14.
11. Skamene, E., P. Gros, A. Forget, P.A.L. Kongshavn, C. St. Charles, and B.A. Taylor. 1982. Genetic regulation of resistance to intracellular pathgens. Nature 297:506-510.
12. Mock, B.A., E. Russek-Cohen, J. Hilgers, and C.A. Nacy. 1985. Discriminant function analysis of genetic traits associated with Leishmania major infection in the CXS recombinant inbred strains. Prog. Leukocyte Biol. 3:83-95.
13. Briles, D.E., W.H. Benjamin, W.J. Huster, and B. Posey. 1986. Genetic approaches to the study of disease resistance, with special emphasis on the use of recombinant inbred mice. Curr. Top. Microbiol. Immunol. 124:21-36.
14. Potter, M., and J.S. Wax. 1981. Litton Bionetics Report. Mouse News Letter 64:62.
15. Potter, M., A. O'Brien, E. Skamene, P. Gros, A. Forget, P.A.L. Kongshavn, and J.S. Wax. 1983. A BALB/c congenic strain of mice that carries a genetic locus (Ity^r) controlling resistance to intracellular parasites. Infect. Immun. 40:1234-1235.
16. Watson, J., K. Kelly, M. Largen, and B.A. Taylor. 1978. The genetic mapping of a defective LPS response gene in C3H/HeJ mice. J. Immunol. 120:422-424.
17. O'Brien, A.D., D.L. Rosenstreich, I. Scher, G.H. Campbell, R.P. MacDermott, and S.B. Formal. 1980. Genetic control of susceptibility to Salmonella typhimurium in mice: Role of the LPS gene. J. Immunol. 124:20-24.

18. Haller, O. 1981. Inborn resistance of mice to orthomyxoviruses. Curr. Top. Microbiol. Immunol. 92:25-52.
19. O'Brien, A.D., and D.L. Rosenstreich. 1983. Genetic control of the susceptibility of C3HeB/FeJ mice to Salmonella typhimurium is regulated by a locus distinct from known Salmonella response genes. J. Immunol. 131:2613-2615.
20. Swanson, R.N., and A.D. O'Brien. 1983. Genetic control of the innate resistance of mice to Salmonella typhimurium: Ity gene is expressed in vivo by 24 hours after infection. J. Immunol. 131:3014-3020.
21. Gros, P., E. Skamene, and A. Forget. 1983. Cellular mechanisms of genetically controlled host resistance to Mycobacterium bovis (BCG). J. Immunol. 131:1966-1972.
22. Stach, J-L., P. Gros, A., Forget, and E. Skamene. 1984. Phenotypic expression of genetically-controlled natural resistance to Mycobacterium bovis (BCG). J. Immunol. 132:888-892.
23. Stokes, R.W., I.M. Orme, I.M., and F. Collins. 1986. Role of mononuclear phagocytes in expression of resistance and susceptibility to Mycobacterium avium infection in mice. Infect. Immun. 54:811-819.
24. Lissner, C.R., R.N. Swanson, and A.D. O'Brien. 1983. Genetic control of the innate resistance of mice to Salmonella typhimurium: expression of the Ity gene in peritoneal and splenic macrophages in vitro. J. Immunol. 131:3006-3013.
25. van Dissel, J.T., J.J.M. Stikkelbroeck, W. Sluiter, P.C.J. Leijh, and R. van Furth. 1985. Course of an intraperitoneal inflammation during a Salmonella typhimurium infection in Salmonella-resistant CBA and Salmonella-susceptible C57BL/10 mice. Prog. Leukocyte Biol. 3:245-255.
26. Crocker, P.R., J.M. Blackwell, and D.J. Bradley. 1984. Expression of the natural resistance gene Lsh in resident liver macrophages. Infect. Immun. 43:1033-1040.
27. Zwilling, B.S., S. Johnson, L. Vespa, and M. Kwasniewski. 1985. BCG infection induces continuous I-A expression in BCG resistant mice. Prog. Leukocyte Biol. 3:299-304.
28. Denis, M., E. Buschman, A. Forget, M. Pelletier, and E. Skamene, 1986. Pleiotropic effects of the Bcg gene: Regulation of Ia dependent macrophage functions (Abstract). 6th International Congress of Immunology, Toronto.
29. Denis, M., A. Forget, M. Pelletier, A. Jodoin, and E. Skamene. 1987. Pleiotropic effects of the Bcg gene. I. Antigen-presentation in genetically - susceptible and resistant congenic mouse strains. J. Immunol. submitted.
30. Denis, M., A. Forget, A. Jodin, M. Pelletier, and E. Skamene. 1987. Pleiotropic effects of the Bcg gene. II. Genetic restriction of non-specific mitogenesis. J. Immunol. submitted.
31. Denis, M., A. Forget, M. Pelletier, and E. Skamene. 1987. Pleiotropic effects of the BCG gene. III. Hydrogen peroxide production in BCG - congenic mice. Clin. Exp. Immunol. submitted.
32. Denis, M., A. Forget, A. Jodoin, E. Skamene, and M. Pelletier. 1987. Pleiotropic effects of the Bcg gene. IV. Listericidal activity of Bcg^r and Bcg^s macrophages. Infect. & Immunol. submitted.
33. Meltzer, M.S., and C.A. Nacy. 1985. Macrophage cytotoxicity against tumor cell and microbial targets: Genetic control of the activation network. Prog. Leukocyte Biol. 3:595-604.
34. Blackwell, J.M. 1983. Regulation of Leishmania populations within the host. V. Resistance to L. donovani in wild mice. J. Trop. Med. Hyg. 86:17-22.

35. Lurie, M.B. 1964. Resistance to tuberculosis: experimental studies in native and acquired defensive mechanisms. Harvard University Press, Cambridge.
36. Skamene, E. 1986. Genetic control of resistance to mycobacterial infection. Curr. Topics Microbiol. Immunol. 124:49-66.
37. Cohen, D.I., S.M. Hedrick, E.A. Nielsen, P. D'Eustachio, F. Ruddle, A.D. Steinberg, W.E. Paul, and M.M. Davis.1985. Isolation of cDNA clone corresponding to an X-linked gene family (XLR) closely linked to the murine immunodeficiency disorder. Nature 314:369-372.
38. Staeheli, P., O. Haller, W. Boll, J. Lindenmann, and C. Weissmann. 1986. Mx protein: constitutive expression in 3T3 cells transformed with cloned Mx cDNA confers selective resistance to influenza virus. Cell 44:147-158.
39. Housman, D.E., P. Gros. 1985. Isolation of host resistance genes: A general strategy based on recombinant DNA and genetic linkage techniques. Prog. Leukocyte Biol. 3:101-107.
40. Skow, L.C. 1982. Location of a gene controlling electrophoretic variation in mouse γ-1 crystallins. Exp. Eye Res. 34:509-516.

EFFECTS OF BONE MARROW ABLATION ON COMPARTMENTAL PROSTAGLANDIN SYNTHESIS BY MONONUCLEAR PHAGOCYTES

A. Volkman*, Y. Shibata*, W. Dempsey†, and P.S. Morahan†

*Department of Pathology, East Carolina University School of Medicine, Greenville, NC 27858, and †Department of Microbiology and Immunology, Medical College of Pennsylvania, Philadelphia, PA 19129

INTRODUCTION

It is well known that comparisons of populations or compartments of mononuclear phagocytes show considerable diversity of cellular function. In the case of resident-type macrophages (Mϕ), such differences are widely believed to result from influences characteristic of individual compartments exerted on less specialized immigrant monocytes following their ongoing influx from the blood into tissues and tissue spaces. In this connection, data supporting the compartmental regulation of Mϕ arachidonic acid metabolism, at least in the pleural and the peritoneal cavities, were recently reported (1). The data we present show that in the spleen, Mϕ arachidonic acid metabolism is in part an expression of regulatory mechanisms at a distant site, the bone marrow. This demonstration required a model of bone marrow ablation and monocyte depletion, the principles of which are described below.

BACKGROUND

Ongoing monocyte emigration is popularly regarded as the principal mechanism for the renewal of resident macrophages (Mϕ) under steady state conditions (2). Although some proponents of this idea have more recently presented data for a small degree of local proliferation (3). It is remarkable, however, that virtually all the information concerning monocyte emigration relates to agents generated in the inflammatory process or by molecules which simulate them. Mechanisms for the putative "physiological" or steady state emigration of blood monocytes, remain to be elucidated. There seems to be a curious acceptance by default of the notion that "physiological" emigration is mechanistically the same as in inflammation and conversely, that monocyte emigration in inflammation is a localized numerical enhancement of the "physiological" process. It is clear that more information is needed concerning the blood monocyte and its relationship to resident Mϕ populations and their functions. We approached this problem by studying the impact of monocyte depletion for selected functions of mononuclear phagocyte compartments. One would predict, from the prevailing concepts, that if the output of blood monocytes from the bone marrow were severely impaired for a sufficiently long period Mϕ populations should themselves become depleted at rates reflecting the lifespans characteristic of an individual compartment.

One would also expect demonstrable alterations of Mϕ function if only on the basis of changes in age distributions. If, however, a Mϕ population were to persist in the face of a profoundly reduced blood monocyte pool certain explanations would have to be considered: 1. Local proliferation and formation of Mϕ, 2. Selective emigration of residual blood monocytes, 3. Increased monocyte formation due to enhanced extramedullary hemopoiesis (along with a decreased transit time in the blood), or 4. An exceedingly long compartmental turnover time. Combinations of these conditions might also occur. It is important, however, that the agents employed for the purpose of monocyte depletion should not have wide-ranging direct effects associated with whole body irradiation (4) and the administration of high doses of adrenal glucocorticoids (6).

The ^{89}Sr Model of Bone Marrow Ablation and Monocyte Depletion

The model employed in the studies described takes advantage of the radiosensitivity of monocyte precursors (4), the fact that nearly all monocyte precursors are located in the bone marrow (5) and the bone-seeking property of the radioactive isotope, ^{89}Sr ($E_{\beta\ max}$ 1.3 MeV; T 1/2, 50.4 days). Since over 90% of the energy emitted by ^{89}Sr is dissipated within 2 mm of soft tissue (7) cells beyond the immediate proximity of bone marrow are spared. In the intestinal epithelium and the spleen, for example, mitotic activity is undiminished (8). The regimen of ^{89}Sr administration we employ in the mouse consists of a single iv dose of 2-4 μCi per gram of body weight. In some experiments a second dose of ^{89}Sr is administered 21-28 days after the first one (9). Some of the major consequences of the regimen of ^{89}Sr administration employed by us are summarized in Table 1. Effects of bone marrow destruction with other regimens of ^{89}Sr administration have been studied extensively by Bennett and Kumar and their co-workers and are summarized in ref 10.

It is worth noting (Table 1) that following the administration of ^{89}Sr blood monocyte output in the mouse is profoundly impaired for 30 days and longer and that elicitation of inflammatory monocyte Mϕ into the peritoneal cavity is trivial or absent. This observation is additionally important because it suggests that there are not enough monocytes available for maintenance of the demonstrably unaffected resident Mϕ. Abundant but unrecognizable (by inference, "masked monocytes"), an explanation for a source of renewal of the persisting resident Mϕ in the ^{89}Sr mouse, suggested by Bennett and Kumar (10), is implausible because failure of elicitation clearly showed effective monocyte depletion (19) unless one wants to plead the case for masked Mϕ. Neither can the persistence of resident alveolar and peritoneal Mϕ for over 30 days in monocyte-depleted mice be attributed to long turnover times of these populations; mean turnover times of alveolar and resident peritoneal Mϕ of 6 and 15 hours, respectively, have recently been reported by van Furth and Sluiter (11). A splenic origin for resident Mϕ cannot be invoked since earlier splenectomy has little effect on monocytes or Mϕ in ^{89}Sr treated mice (12). Taken together, our observations suggest that there may be some serious flaws in the concept that the influx of blood monocytes is an important mechanism of resident Mϕ population renewal.

Assessments of proliferative activity among alveolar and peritoneal Mϕ based on 30-60 minute incorporation of ^{3}H-TdR have yielded observed labeling indices (LI) ranging from 1.5 - 4% among control and ^{89}Sr treated mice (8). This range is consistent with a capacity for self-renewal. In addition, one should take into account the important and neglected observation that hemopoietic stem cells are present among unstimulated peritoneal cell populations in the mouse (13). Although the reported frequency of these stem cells in peritoneal lavage samples was low it is possible that their pool is extramesothelial and thus underestimated. In this connection, other investigators have presented evidence for a proliferative pool of Mϕ precursors in the

Table 1. Some Consequences of ^{89}Sr Administration to Mice

Massive destruction of the bone marrow.
Rapid fall in total white blood cell count.
Reduction of blood monocyte counts by 80->99% within 72 hours.
Increase in M-CFC in spleen (10-20 fold).
Increase in total phagocytic Mϕ in spleen (~2 fold).
Monocyte-Mϕ elicitation with i.p. thioglycollate, *C. parvum* or *L. monocytogenes* ineffective.
Induction of PGE-forming Mϕ in spleen by *C. parvum* ineffective.
Resident peritoneal and alveolar Mϕ maintain normal numbers and ^{3}HTdR incorporation.

milky spots of the omentum (14). The foregoing possibilities, could represent mechanisms for self-renewal in the peritoneal cavity; it is possible that analogous situations obtain in other populations of tissue Mϕ.

Another interesting feature of the ^{89}Sr mouse indicated in Table 1 is the rapid increase in splenic hemopoiesis along with an increase in macrophage colony-forming cells (M-CFC) and in phagocytic Mϕ (12, 15). These findings suggest that unlike Mϕ in the peritoneal and pleural cavities (1), those in the spleen may be dependent on extracompartmental factors.

Arachidonic Acid Metabolism in the ^{89}Sr-Treated Mouse

To pursue the foregoing idea we focussed our attention on the response of splenic Mϕ to the activating agent *C. parvum*. Following the intraperitoneal administration of formalized *C. parvum* vaccine (Parvovax, Burroughs-Wellcome), 56 mg/kg, suppressor Mϕ are detectable within the spleen as early as 72 hrs later and reach a peak in activity at about 7 days (22). Activity is taken as the capacity to suppress, in a dose dependent manner, the response of T-lymphocytes to mitogens. This suppressor activity is indomethacin sensitive and correlates with the release of PGE_2 into the medium (as measured by radioimmunoassay) by splenic Mϕ cultured *in vitro*. Neither unstimulated nor elicited peritoneal Mϕ nor bone marrow Mϕ behave in this manner (15, 16). Bone marrow Mϕ do respond to the administration of *C. parvum* but with distinctly different kinetics of PGE_2 release (unpublished data). Resident peritoneal Mϕ release relatively large quantities of PGE_2 and other eicosanoids after stimulation by agents such as zymosan, calcium ionophore A23187, phorbol esters or bacterial lipopolysaccharide (16). Immigrant Mϕ elicited into the peritoneal cavity of the mouse by thioglycollate, *C. parvum* or BCG, release substantially less PGE_2 and other eicosanoids than do the resident cells (16). In the ^{89}Sr treated mouse, spenic Mϕ despite their increase in total number, failed to respond to *C. parvum*, and PGE_2 release did not exceed background levels.

^{3}H-PGE_2 release following the uptake of ^{3}H-arachidonic acid by membrane phospholipids was determined by thin-layer chromatography. PGE_2 production by splenic prostaglandin-releasing suppressor macrophages (PGSM) in intact mice increased ten-fold by 7 days after ip *C. parvum* to levels as high as 45-62 ng/3 x 10^6 cells. A distinct difference was found, however, in the ^{89}Sr treated mice. Neither the suppressor nor the PGE_2 responses could be induced in splenic Mϕ isolated from these mice despite an increase in the total number of splenic Mϕ following *C. parvum* administration. Treatment of splenic Mϕ *in vitro* with either Con A, zymosan, calcium ionophore A23187 or phorbol ester likewise failed to stimulate the release of PGE_2. An additional finding was that no release of LTC_4 was detectable in splenic Mϕ from either intact or bone marrow-depleted mice (17). This observation contrasts sharply with the LTC_4-releasing capacity of peritoneal Mϕ (18) and underscores the heterogeneous nature of Mϕ function. Uptake of ^3H-arachidonic acid was comparable, however, in the control and ^{89}Sr treated mice. The distribution of ^3H-arachidonic acid in membrane phospholipids, as measured by thin-layer chromatography, was virtually identical in control and test mice (24).

In contrast to their effect on splenic Mϕ, bone marrow deprivation and monocyte depletion had no observable influence on PGE_2 and LTC_4 release by resident peritoneal Mϕ. Thus, an increased release of PGE_2 was induced, as usual, upon in vitro stimulation of resident peritoneal Mϕ with zymosan and A23187.

Another finding of interest was that cell suspensions prepared from the spleens of ^{89}Sr treated mice can restore hemopoiesis in lethally irradiated syngenic recipients (17, and unpublished data). In these mice, supranormal levels of blood monocytes are found by 2 weeks and the splenic PGSM response can be detected by 3 weeks following bone marrow infusion. Thus, the failure of splenic hemopoiesis to generate normal hemopoietic elements and PGE_2-forming Mϕ in ^{89}Sr mice cannot be attributed to the absence of appropriate stem cells. It is therefore reasonable to suggest that the formation of blood monocytes and the expression of PGE_2-releasing splenic Mϕ (PGSM) have an obligatory dependence on bone marrow. It is an obvious speculation that PGSM in the spleen are derived from the bone marrow and migrate to the spleen. Preliminary studies show that the kinetics of PGE_2 release by bone marrow Mϕ differ from those of splenic Mϕ. It may be that both the environments of the spleen and the bone marrow are necessary for phenotypic expression characteristic of splenic Mϕ. An alternative possibility is that a regulatory agent or cytokine is formed by a bone marrow cell and acts on splenic Mϕ to facilitate the synthesis of PGE_2. We are currently unable to choose between these alternatives.

COMMENTS

These studies described have delineated at least 3 distinct populations of mononuclear phagocytes. One, represented by circulating blood monocytes, apparently has an obligatory dependence on the bone marrow but seems to be a dispensable population as far as the maintenance of resident Mϕ is concerned. A second, resident peritoneal Mϕ, and probably alveolar Mϕ, appears to represent autonomous populations which can maintain themselves in the face of long standing bone marrow deprivation and profound monocytopenia. For reasons given earlier the apparent self-maintenance of these populations cannot be attributed to longevity. A third population of mononuclear phagocytes represented by splenic Mϕ, appears to be divided into subsets with one population independent of bone marrow and blood monocytes, but incapable of differentiation to PGE_2-releasing Mϕ. A second splenic subset functionally expressed as PGSM depends upon a function of bone marrow and may possibly be formed in the bone marrow. A relationship between these splenic Mϕ and blood monocytes is uncertain but experiments in the monocyte depleted $S1/S1^d$ mouse with demonstrable PGSM suggest that these Mϕ are not directly derived from the blood monocyte (19). In any case, the regulation of prostaglandin synthesis by splenic Mϕ appears to be determined by extra, as well as intracompartmental factors.

SUMMARY

Mononuclear phagocyte functions were studied in mice selectively deprived of bone marrow and rendered profoundly monocytopenic by the administration of the bone seeking isotope, ^{89}Sr. Characteristics of such mice include severe impairment of monocyte-Mϕ elicitation, ablation of *C. parvum* induction of PGSM but the persistence of resident peritoneal and pulmonary alveolar Mϕ populations; splenic Mϕ increase in number concommitantly with splenic hemopoiesis. Studies on compartmental regulation in this model suggest that the capacity of splenic Mϕ to synthesize and release PGE_2 is dependent upon a function of the bone marrow and is not wholly determined by the local environment. The relationship of blood monocytes to PGSM is uncertain. In contrast to splenic Mϕ, the capacity of resident peritoneal Mϕ for eicosanoid synthesis appears to be independent of bone marrow function. Monocyte influx, moreover, does not appear necessary for the maintenance of the resident peritoneal and alveolar Mϕ populations. We do not yet know whether bone marrow ablation destroys a migratory precursor of PGSM or the source of a crucial regulatory agent. In conclusion, the observations discussed show that prostaglandin metabolism within the spleen is subject to extracompartmental influence. It is clearly important to determine the regulatory characteristics of individual Mϕ compartments and generalizations about functional properties of mononuclear phagocytes should be made with circumspection.

REFERENCES

1. Fels, A., N. Pawlowski, E. Abraham and Z. Cohn. 1986. Compartmentalized regulation of macrophage arachidonic acid metabolism. J. Exp. Med. 163:752-757.
2. van Furth, R., Z.A. Cohn, J.G. Hirsch, J.H. Humphrey, W.G. Spector and H.L. Langevoort. 1972. The mononuclear phagocyte system: a new classification of macrophages, monocytes and their precursor cells. Bull. WHO 46:845.
3. van Furth, R., L. Diesselhoff and M. Dulk. 1984. Dual origin of mouse spleen macrophages. J. Exp. Med. 160:1273.
4. Volkman, A., and J.L. Gowans. 1965. The production of macrophages in the rat. Br. J. Exp. Path. 50.
5. Volkman, A., and J.L. Gowans. 1965. The origin of macrophages from bone marrow in the rat. Br. J. Exp. Path. 46:62.
6. Thompson, J., and R. van Furth. 1970. The effect of glucocorticosteroids on the kinetics of mononuclear phagocytes. J. Exp. Med. 131:429.
7. Raper, J.R. 1964. Beta rays: biologic effects, *in*: "Medical Physics II," O. Glasser, ed., p. 66, Chicago, The Year Book Publishers, Inc.
8. Sawyer, R.T., P.H. Strausbauch and A. Volkman. 1982. Resident macrophage proliferation in mice depleted of blood monocytes by strontium-89. Lab. Invest. 46:165.
9. Morahan, P.S., W.L. Dempsey, A. Volkman and J. Connor. 1986. Antimicrobicidal activity of various immunomodulators: independence from normal levels of circulating monocytes and natural killer cells. Infect. Immun. 51:87.
10. Bennett, M., and V. Kumar. 1983. ^{89}Sr-induced bone marrow aplasia: effects on seed (stem cells) and soil (inductive microenvironment). Lab. Invest. 49:235.
11. van Furth, R., and W. Sluiter. 1985. Macrophages as autoregulators of mononuclear phagocyte proliferation, *in*: "Macrophage Biology," R. Sand and M. Kojuma, ed., p. 111-123, Alan R. Liss, New York.
12. Volkman, A., N.C. Chang, P.H. Strausbauch and P.S. Morahan. 1983. Differential effects of chronic monocyte depletion on macrophage populations. Lab. Invest. 49:291.
13. Goodman, J.W. 1963. Transplantation of peritoneal fluid cells. Transplantation 3:334-346.
14. DeBakker, J.M., A.W. deWit, J.J.M. Onderwater, L.A. Ginsel and W.T. Daems. 1985. On the origin of peritoneal resident macrophages. II. Recovery of the resident macrophage population in the peritoneal

cavity and in the milky spots after peritoneal cell depletion. J. Submicroscop. Cytol. 17:141.
15. Shibata, Y., and A. Volkman. 1985. The effect of bone marrow depletion on prostaglandin E-producing suppressor macrophages in mouse spleen. J. Immunol. 135:3897-3904.
16. Humes, J.L., S. Burger, M. Galavage, F.A. Kuehl, Jr., P.D. Wightman, M.E. Dahlgren, P. Davies and R.J. Bonney. 1980. The diminished production of arachidonic acid oxygenation products by elicited mouse peritoneal macrophages: possible mechanisms. J. Immunol. 124:2110-2116.
17. Shibata, Y., A.P. Bautista, S.N. Pennington, J.L. Humes and A. Volkman. 1986. Eicosanoid production by peritoneal and splenic macrophages in mice depleted of bone marrow by ^{89}Sr. Am J. Path., accepted for publication.
18. Rouzer, C.A., W.A. Scott, A.L. Hamill and Z.A. Cohn. 1982. Synthesis of leukotriene C and other arachidonic acid metabolites by mouse pulmonary macrophages. J. Exp. Med. 155:720-733.
19. Shibata, Y., and A. Volkman. 1985. The effect of hemopoietic microenvironment on splenic suppressor macrophages in congenitally anemic mice of genotype Sl/Sld. J. Immunol. 135:3905-3910.

RECOGNITION AND BINDING OF PATHOGENIC YEASTS BY ADHESION MOLECULES OF HUMAN MACROPHAGES

Ward E. Bullock and Samuel D. Wright

From the Department of Internal Medicine
University of Cincinnati College of Medicine
Cincinnati, OH and The Laboratory of Cellular
Physiology and Immunology, The Rockefeller University
New York, NY

INTRODUCTION

The dimorphic zoopathogenic fungus, Histoplasma capsulatum (Hc) is distributed worldwide and causes a broad spectrum of disease in man and other mammals. The vast majority of infections are acquired by inhalation of spores or fragments of the mycelial phase that is present in contaminated soil. After lodging within the pulmonary alveoli, spores or mycelial fragments convert to the yeast form of Hc that causes all subseqent disease manifestations. During the initial phase of infection, patches of pneumonitis are observed that contain a predominance of macrophages (MO) within which the Histoplasma yeasts appear to multiply with a generation time estimated to be 9-11 hours.[1-4] Thus, during primary infection of the lung, pulmonary MO presumably bind and phagocytose Hc yeasts in the absence of significant opsonizing activity thereby providing a favorable intracellular environment for multiplication of the organisms.

As the multiplication cycle continues within MO, Hc yeasts are disseminated from the lung to other sites by the lympho-hematogenous route. After antigen-specific mechanisms of cell mediated immunity become detectable approximately 10-20 days after inoculation, both the primary lesions in lung and those at peripheral locations begin to heal slowly. It is apparent therefore, that the process of initial recognition and attachment of Hc yeasts by phagocytic cells is a crucial event for both the pathogen and the host. It is by means of this binding mechanism that yeasts secure access to an environment favorable to the replicative events necessary for establishment of infection. Later however, after activation of cell mediated defense mechanisms, Hc yeasts that have been bound and ingested by MO are now exposed to a hostile intracellular milieu in which they appear to be inhibited or killed.

In an attempt to better delinate the initial interaction between this fungal pathogen and host cells, we have studied the receptor-ligand interactions between unopsonized Hc yeasts and human MO derived from peripheral blood monocytes (PBM) obtained from donors who were non-immune to Hc. The results from some of these studies are summarized here and their relevance to the interactions between host phagocytic cells and other pathogenic yeasts is discussed. Additional information has been presented elsewhere.[5]

GENERAL METHODOLOGY

The yeast phase of Hc, strain 217B, and a clinical isolate of the yeast, *Torulopsis glabrata*, were employed. The yeasts were grown in brain/heart infusion broth (Difco Laboratories Inc., Detroit, MI) at 37°C with a gyrorotatory speed of 180 rpm. Cultures of Hc and *T. glabrata* were harvested after 36 h and 18 h, respectively, and washed twice with phosphate buffered saline (PBS) by centrifugation at 327 g for 5 min. A final centrifugation at 30 g for 1 min allowed for removal of larger cell aggregates. The yeasts were counted in a hemocytometer and resuspended in PBS to 2.2 x 10^8 organisms/ml for addition to MO monolayers.

Human monocytes were purified from buffy coats on Percoll gradients and cultured in 12.5% human serum in Teflon beakers as described previously.[6] Sheep erythrocytes (E) coated with C3b (EC3b), C3bi (EC3bi), or IgG (EIgG) were prepared as described.[6]

To study attachment of unopsonized yeasts and ligand-coated erythrocytes, MO were harvested from teflon beakers after 4-7 d, then were washed, and suspended at 0.5-1.0 x 10^6/ml in PBS containing 3 mM glucose, 0.5 mg/ml human serum albumin (HSA) and 0.3 U/ml aprotinin. Terasaki tissue culture plates (Miles Laboratories Inc., Naperville, IL) were coated with HSA (1 mg/ml) by a 60-min incubation at 20°C or monoclonal antibodies (mAbs) (20-50 ug/ml) directed against various surface receptors of MO. The culture surfaces were washed, 5 μl of MO suspension were added per well, and cells were allowed to spread at 37°C for 45 min. Attachment of test particles to monolayers of MO was determined by adding 10^6 yeasts or 5 x 10^5 ligand-coated E per well and incubating for 45 min at 37°C. The attachment of particles to MO was then scored by phase microscopy. Results are expressed as the attachment index (AI) i.e., the percent of phagocytes that attached particles multiplied by the average number of particles per phagocyte. This figure includes both the attached and ingested yeasts. All assays were performed in triplicate and at least 100 cells were counted.

RESULTS AND DISCUSSION

As a first step, the kinetics of MO attachment to unopsonized Hc yeasts were studied at 4°C and 37°C respectively. At 4°C there was almost no binding of yeasts by MO even after coincubation for 90 min. On the other hand, binding of yeasts by MO was extensive at 37°C with the maximum AI of 698 achieved at 60 min. Binding activity progressed very rapidly such that 43% of the maximum AI was achieved after only 5 min of incubation. Subsequently, studies were performed to determine if divalent cations played a role in binding of Hc yeasts. Five-day cultured MO were incubated with yeasts (washed and suspended in cation-free medium) in the presence or absence of Ca and Mg ions. The results demonstrated that both divalent cations are essential for optimal binding of Hc yeasts by MO.[5]

The requirement for divalent cations and a warm temperature for attachment of yeasts were of great interest since precisely the same requirements are necessary for optimal binding of C3bi-coated particles to MO.[7] Conversely, the binding of IgG or C3b-coated particles by MO requires neither warm temperatures nor the presence of divalent cations. These findings suggest that the C3bi receptor or related molecules on the MO surface might bind to a ligand(s) on Hc. More specifically, MO express a family of heterodimeric cell surface glycoproteins that function in cell adhesion. CR3 (the C3bi receptor) mediates attachment of C3bi-coated particles and LFA-1 mediates binding to tumor and endothelial cells.[8-10] The precise function of a third glycoprotein, p150,95, has not yet been defined. All three molecules of the CR3/LFA-1/p150,95 family are expressed in approximately equal numbers on MO surfaces. Each consists of a unique α subunit that is associated non-covalently with a common β subunit (M_r, 95,000) in an $\alpha_1 \beta_1$ configuration. Both the α chains and, β chain are surface exposed.

To assess directly the putative role of CR3, LFA-1, and p150,95 in the binding of unopsonized Hc, a series of mAbs directed against α chains or the common β chain of these adherence molecules were added individually to separate sets of test wells containing adherent MO immediately before addition of yeasts. Antibodies directed specifically against the α chains of the CR1, LFA-1, and p150,95 glycoprotein molecules respectively, each caused a small but consistent reduction of the AI. However, mAbs 1B4 and 60.3, both directed against the β chain of this family, invariably reduced the binding of Hc to MO by 80% or more of control values. Importantly, mAb directed against low avidity Fc receptors (3G8) did not reduce the AI.

The role played by each member of the family of leukocyte adhesion molecules (LAM), was analyzed further by taking advantage of the fact that mononuclear cell surface receptors diffuse freely in the plain of the plasma membrane and function independently of one another in particle binding. When MO are plated on surfaces coated with a monoclonal-antireceptor antibody, there is specific down modulation of the target antigen from the apical portion to the substrate-adherent domain of the cell; thus, the apical surface of the cell is depleted of a single receptor.

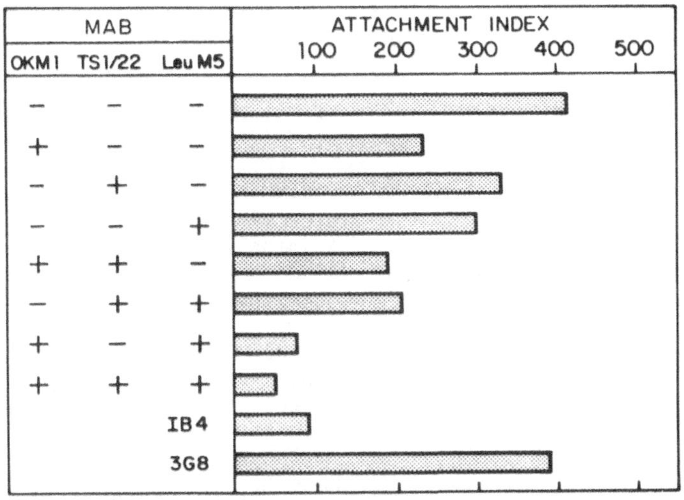

Fig. 1. Effect on Hc yeast binding of down regulating MO surface target antigens by mAb coated surfaces. mAbs against α chains of the CR3/LFA-1, p150,95 family were used singly or in combination in a concentration of 50 μg/ml; IB4 and 3G8 were used singly at 50 μg/ml. The data shown are representative of four experiments. Reproduced by permission from reference 5.

As shown in Figure 1, plating of MO on surfaces coated with mAb directed against the α chain of any one of the three adherence glycoproteins reduced the attachment of Hc yeasts by a small amount. When MO were plated on surfaces coated with any two of the anti-α chain directed mAbs, a greater reduction of the AI was achieved. However, the most severe and consistent reduction of AI was observed when MO were plated on surfaces coated with all three mAbs directed against the specific α chains. In other studies, removal of all three members of the CR3/LFA-1/p150,95 family by the same technique using a mAb against the common β chain (1B4) also caused profound reduction of the AI. In a control experiment, removal of Fc receptors from the apical portions of MO by surface bound mAb3G8 also failed to reduce the binding of yeasts. Taken together, these results indicate that each of the members of the CR3/LFA-1/p150,95 family is capable of binding the organism independently.

All components of the classical complement cascade and of the alternative pathway are synthesized and secreted by MO (11). Thus, it is possible that MO may opsonize particles in close proximity by means of an endogenous store of complement components. To examine the possibility that MO-derived C3 played a role in recognition of Hc yeasts, binding assays were conducted in the presence of Fab anti-C3 antibody. At a concentration of 50 μg/ml, the antibody nearly abolished binding of E coated with approximately 80,000 molecules of C3b.[5] Conversely, 100 μg/ml of Fab anti-C3 did not diminish the binding of yeasts. Therefore, it is quite unlikely that MO binding of Hc yeasts can be explained by opsonization of these organisms with C3 of MO origin and subsequent binding to CR3 receptors via C3bi.

It has been observed that various particulate activators of the alternative complement pathway are recognized by a MO receptor that can be blocked with soluble β-glucan.[12] Since Hc yeasts can activate the alternative complement pathway[13] we attempted to block MO binding of Hc by β-glucan. However, a concentration of 100 μg/ml of this polysaccharide exerted no effect on the AI. Thus, the β-glucan receptor does not mediate binding of MO to these yeasts[5].

In view of the fact that the cell wall of Hc yeasts is composed of polymeric carbohydrates, we sought to determine if a sugar or an aminosugar in the cell wall might serve as a recognition site for MO receptors. Repeated attempts to induce significant blockade of MO binding to Hc yeasts with high concentrations (100 mM) of galactose, N-acetyl-galactosamine, fucose, mannose, α-methyl mannoside, N-acetyl glucosamine, and glucuronic acid were without significant effect[5]. These findings suggest that the MO receptors that recognize Hc do not act as lectins for these sugar specificities.

The observation that D-mannose did not block binding of Hc yeasts was of importance since MO also expressed a receptor that recognizes mannose and fucose. This mannosyl/fucosyl (M/F) receptor is known to play a major role in MO attachment to zymosan particles[14], to *Candida krusei*[15] and promastigotes of *Leishmania donovani*.[16] In view of these facts, we performed comparative studies of the effects of M/F receptor blockade on MO binding to Hc and to the opportunistic pathogen, *T. glabrata*. The latter is a yeast that does not form germ tubes and is similar in size to a Hc yeast forms. Addition of either mannan (1,000 μg/ml) or mannosylated BSA (50 μg/ml) to the serum-free medium employed for co-incubation of *T. glabrata* and MO substantially reduced the AI. Conversely, neither agent decreased the binding of Hc yeasts by MO. Moreover, addition of mAb 1B4 to wells containing MO and yeasts had no effect upon the binding of *T. glabrata* whereas binding of Hc yeasts was greatly reduced as expected.[5]

Freshly isolated human monocytes do not express the M/F receptor. However, it is highly expressed on the surfaces of monocyte-derived MO.[17]

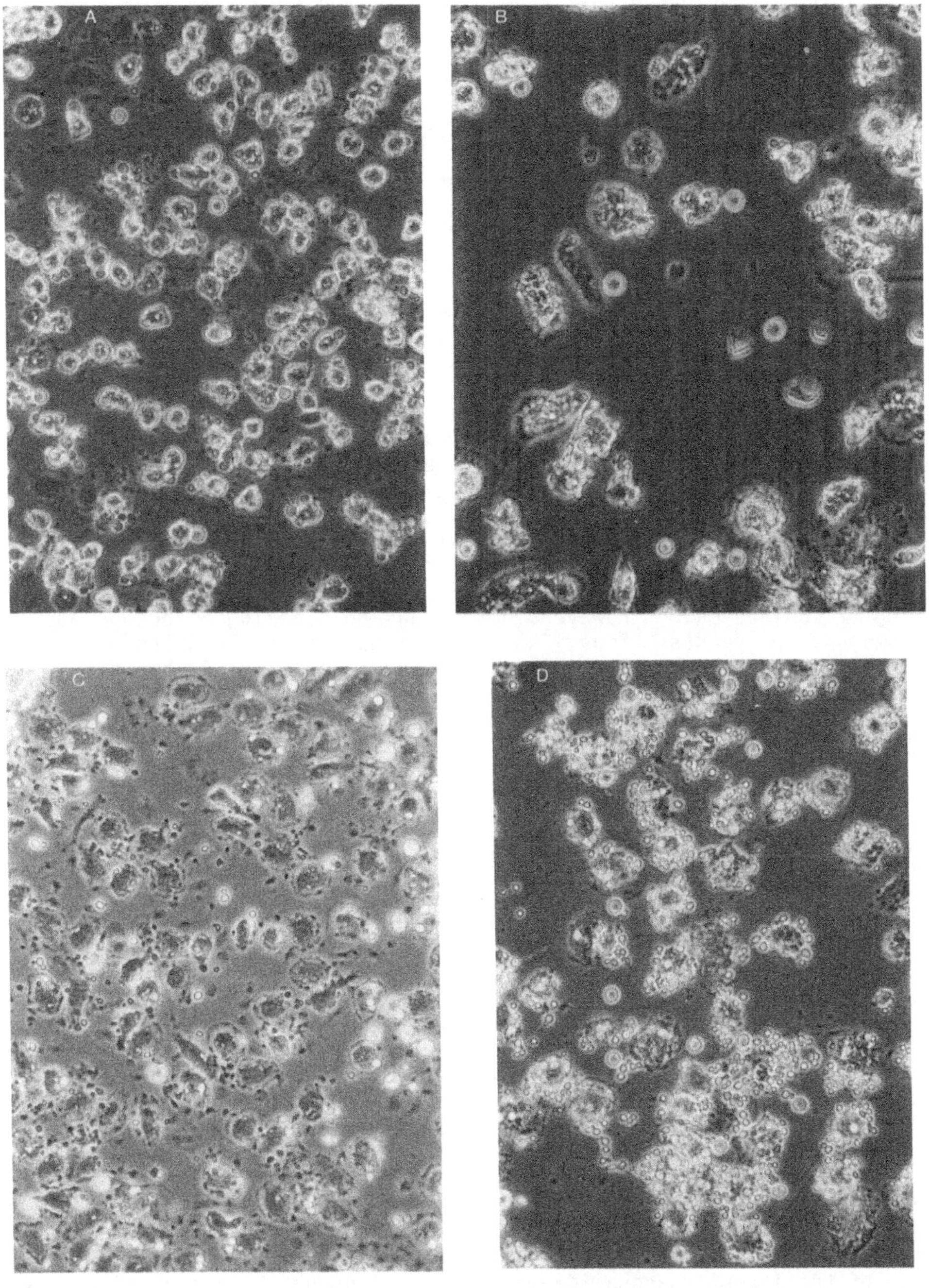

Fig. 2. Binding of Hc yeasts by freshly isolated monocytes (A) and 7 day monocyte-derived MO (B) and binding of T. glabrata by monocytes (C) and MO (B) respectively. The small, dark granular forms in monocyte preparations (A and C) are platelets. Phase photomicrographs at 275 X magnification.

CR3 receptors, on the other hand, are present on blood monocytes and they increase in number during maturation in vitro.[6] Therefore, to provide additional confirming evidence that unopsonized Hc and T. glabrata are bound by entirely different MO surface receptors, we measured the binding of Hc and T. glabrata by fresh monocytes and by 7-day-cultured MO. As seen in Figure 2A, there was extensive binding of Hc yeasts to monocytes (AI=380) whereas there was very little attachment of T. glabrata (AI=31) as shown in Figure 2C. By contrast, after 7 days in culture, monocyte-derived MO displayed high levels of binding activity to T. glabrata; in fact, the AI of 467 was quite similar to that obtained when 7 day MO were coincubated with Hc yeasts (Figures 2B, 2D). These data provide strong evidence that T. glabrata is bound by the M/F receptor but is not recognized by the CR3/LFA-1/p150,95 protein family. Conversely, Hc yeasts are bound by these adherence molecules but not by the M/F receptor.

The studies summarized above have established that unopsonized Hc yeasts are bound to MO by the CR3/LFA-1/p150,95 adherence glycoproteins. At present, the structural basis for the finding that all three members of the family share the ability to recognize Hc is not clear. One possibility is that the Hc ligand binding site is located on the common β chain. The hypothesis is consistent with the highly effective blocking activity of soluble anti-β-chain mAbs and would explain the requirement that all three of the mAb directed to specific α chains must be employed simultaneously to fully inhibit binding of Hc. Of interest is the observation that the binding site for C3bi appears to be on the α chain of CR3 since LFA-1 and p150,95 do not recognize C3bi. In addition, anti-α chain mAb OKM 10 directly blocks the binding of C3bi to CR3.[8] However, OKM 10 has no blocking effect on MO attachment to Hc yeasts. Thus, CR3 may well express two binding sites, one for Hc on the β chain and one for C3bi on the α chain. This hypothesis is consistent with studies of Ross et al.[18] who suggest that CR3 contains a lectin-like binding site which is separate from the C3bi binding site. Another explanation for our findings is that Hc yeasts express several surface structures of which some may be recognized by the α chain of CR3, and others by the α chains of LFA-1 and p150,95, respectively.

Based on the present evidence, we postulate that the pathogenic yeast form of H. capsulatum gains entry to the phagocytic mononuclear cells of the lung principally by attachment to the CR3/LFA-1/p150,95 adhesion molecules. Thus, it is within phagocytes that infection is established successfully prior to development of specific cell mediated immune responses that enable these cells to restrict yeast replication effectively. It should be emphasized that, in nature, one of the first populations of cells presumed to encounter Hc yeasts is the pulmonary macrophage. Of importance, therefore are studies currently in progress to determine if Hc are bound to human alveolar MO by receptors that are similar in structure and avidity to those displayed by MO derived from peripheral blood monocytes.

Recently, it has become apparent that the CR3/LFA-1/p150,95 family of leukocyte adherence promoting proteins mediate opsonin independent binding of other microbes as well. These include the rough strains of Pseudomonas aeruginosa, Salmonella typhimurium and Escherischia coli.[7] The ligand on E. coli that is recognized by this adherence protein family lies within the lipid A region of the lipopolysaccharide molecule. Although the actual ligand(s) of Hc that bind to CR3/LFA-1/p150,95 is unknown at present, it may lie within one of the novel phosphoinositol-sphingolipids of Hc yeasts that have identical inositol phosphoceramide cores but differ in glycosyl substitutions of the polar head groups.[19]

It is tempting to speculate that the CR3/LFA-1/p150,95 proteins also may mediate opsonin independent binding of other pathogenic fungi by phagocytic cells. For example, it is possible that the well-described binding of both polymorphonuclear leukocytes and of monocytes to the surfaces of *Candida albicans* hyphae in the absence of serum[20,23] may be subserved by these receptor proteins. Consistent with this hypothesis are the findings that: 1) there is an absolute requirement for both Ca^{++} and Mg^{++} ions for attachment of neutrophils to hyphae of *C. albicans*;[20] 2), preincubation of neutrophils with trypsin or chymotrypsin severely inhibits attachment to hyphae; and 3), except at extremely high concentrations, mannose and mannan fail to reverse binding.[21] The latter finding is consistent with the fact that both polymorphonuclear leukocytes and monocytes lack the M/F receptor. Of interest is the observation that both neutrophils and monocytes bind poorly to yeast forms of *C. albicans* under serum free conditions.[20] (Diamond, R., Personal communication). Therefore, the yeasts of *C. albicans* may either fail to produce the surface ligand that is recognized on hyphae by adherence molecules that are common to both neutrophils and monocytes or they may produce it in quantities too small to permit stable binding by phagocytes.

Currently, little is known concerning the mechanisms of opsonin-independent attachment and phagocytosis of other dimorphic, zoopathogenic fungi including *Blastomyces dermatitidis* and *Coccidoides immitis*. However, the elucidation of these mechanisms can be expected to provide considerable insight into differing patterns of inflammatory response that may be evoked by the mycelial and yeast forms of the respective fungi. Likewise, it will be possible to better define the relationship between specific surface receptor-ligand interactions and the triggering of antifungal mechanisms intracellularly.

REFERENCES

1. R. A. Goodwin, J. E. Loyd, R. M. Des Prez. Histoplasmosis in normal hosts. *Medicine*. 60:231 (1981).
2. J. J. Procknow, M. I. Page, C. G. Loosli. Early pathogenesis of experimental histoplasmosis. *Arch. Pathol*. 69:413 (1960).
3. R. P. Baughman, C. K. Kim, A. Vinegar, D. E. Hendricks, P. J. Schmidt, and W. E. Bullock. The pathogenesis of experimental pulmonary histoplasmosis: correlative studies of histopathology, bronchoalveolar lavage, and respiratory function. *Amer. Rev. Resp. Dis.* (in press).
4. D. H. Howard. Intracellular growth of Histoplasma capsulatum. *J. Bacteriol*. 89:518 (1965).
5. W. E. Bullock, and S. D. Wright. The Role of the adherence-promoting receptors, CR3, LFA-1, and P150,95 in binding of *Histoplasma capsulatum* by human macrophages. *J. Exp. Med*.165:195 (1987).
6. S. D. Wright, and S. C. Silverstein. Tumor-promoting phorbol esters stimulate C3b and C3b' receptor-mediated phagocytosis in cultured human monocytes. *J. Exp. Med*. 156:1149 (1982).
7. S. D. Wright, and M. T. C. Jong. Adhesion-promoting receptors on human macrophages recognize Escherichia coli by binding to lipopolysaccharide. *J. Exp. Med* 164:1876-1888 (1986).
8. S. D. Wright, P. E. Rao, W. C. Van Voorhis, L. S. Craigmyle, K. Iida, M. A. Talle, E. F. Westberg, G. Goldstein, and S. C. Silverstein. Identification of the C3bi receptor of human monocytes and macrophages by using mononuclear antibodies. *Proc. Natl. Acad. Sci. USA* 80:569 (1983).
9. G. Strassman, T. A. Springer, D. D. Somers, and D. O. Adams. Mechanisms of tumor cell capture by activated macrophages: evidence for involvement of lymphocyte function-associated (LFA)-1 antigen. *J. Immunol*. 136:4329 (1986)
10. J. M. Harlan, P. D. Killen, F. M. Senecal, B. R. Schwartz, E. K. Yee, F. R. Taylor, P. G. Beatty, T. H. Price, and H. D. Ochs. The role of neutrophil membrane glycoprotein GP-150 in neutrophil adhesion to endothelium in vitro. *Blood* 66:167 (1985).

11. H. J. Muller-Eberhard, and R. D. Schreiber. Molecular biology and chemistry of the alternative pathway of complement. Adv. Immunol. 29:1 (1980).
12. J.K. Czop, and K. F. Austen. A β-glucan inhibitable receptor of human monocytes: Its identity with the phagocytic receptor for particulate activators of the alternative complement pathway. J. Immunol. 134:2588 (1985).
13. W. D. Ratnoff, J. M. Pepple, and J. A. Winkelstein. Activation of the alternate complement pathway by Histoplasma capsulatum. Infect. Immun. 30:147 (1980).
14. D. P. Speert, and S. C. Silverstein. Phagocytosis of unopsonized zymosan by human monocyte-derived macrophages: maturation and inhibition by mannan. J. Leukocyte Biol. 38:655 (1985).
15. G. A. Warr. A macrophage receptor for (mannose/glucosamine)-glycoproteins of potential importance in phagocytic activity. Biochem. Biophys. Res. Commun. 93:737 (1980).
16. M. E. Wilson, and R. D. Pearson. Evidence that Leishmania donovani utilizes a mannose receptor on human mononuclear phagocytes to establish intracellular parasitism. J. Immunol. 1386:4681-4688 (1986).
17. T. Mokoena, and S. Gordon. Human macrophage activation, modulation of mannosyl, fucosyl receptor activity in vitro by lymphokines, gamma dna alpha interferons, and dexamethasone. J. Clin. Invest. 73:624 (1985).
18. G. D. Ross, J. A. Cain, P. J. Lachmann. Membrane complement receptor type three (CR_3) has lectin-like properties analogous to bovine conglutinin and functions as a receptor for zymosan and rabbit erythrocytes as well as a receptor for iC3b. J. Immunol. 134:3307 (1985).
19. K. Barr, R. A. Laine, and R. L. Lester. Carbohydrate structures of three novel phosphoinosital-containing sphingolipids from the yeast Histoplasma capsulatum. Biochemistry 23:5589 (1984).
20. R. D. Diamond, R. Krzesicki, and W. Jao. Damage to Pseudohyphal forms of Candida albicans by neutrophils in the absence of serum in vitro. J. Clin. Invest. 61:349 (1978).
21. R. D. Diamond, and R. Krzesicki. Mechanisms of attachment of neutrophils to Candida albicans Pseudohyphae in the absence of serum, and of subsequent damage to pseudohyphae by microbicidal processes of neutrophils in vitro. J. Clin. Invest. 61:360 (1978).
22. R. D. Diamond and C.C. Haudenschild. Monocyte-mediated serum-independent damage to hyphal and pseudohyphal forms of Candida albicans in vitro. J. Clin. Invest. 67:173 (1981).

FUSION OF LYSOSOMES WITH PHAGOSOMES CONTAINING HISTOPLASMA CAPSULATUM: USE OF FLUORESCEINATED DEXTRAN

Linda Groppe Eissenberg and William E. Goldman

Department of Microbiology and Immunology
Washington University School of Medicine
St. Louis, Missouri 63110

The yeast form of *Histoplasma capsulatum* is able to survive and proliferate inside macrophages (1), the primary target cells for this dimorphic fungal pathogen. Rather than clearing these yeasts from the lung, the macrophages instead harbor the organism and promote the development of a severe pulmonary or disseminated disease. We now believe that the lack of an oxidative burst by macrophages which encounter *H. capsulatum* (2, 3) may permit the yeasts to enter host cells undamaged. However, the subsequent fate of the phagocytized *H. capsulatum* yeasts is unclear.

Like all intracellular organisms, *H. capsulatum* must evade destruction by lysosomal killing mechanisms. Several microbes are now known to circumvent phagosome-lysosome fusion (*Mycobacterium tuberculosis* [4, 5, 6], *Toxoplasma gondii* [7], *Chlamydia psittaci* [8, 9], and *Legionella pneumophila* [10, 11]); others appear to resist or inactivate lysosomal killing mechanisms, since they survive inside phagolysosomes (*Yersinia pestis* [12], *Salmonella typhimurium* [13], *Coxiella burnetii* [14], *Mycobacterium lepraemurium* [15, 16, 17], and various *Leishmania* spp. [see 18 for references]). A few organisms (*Trypanosoma cruzi* [19] and *Rickettsia tsutsugamushi* [20, 21]) actually escape into the cytoplasm. Since electron microscopy reveals the presence of a membrane surrounding ingested *H. capsulatum* yeasts, there is no evidence to suggest that this pathogen escapes its phagosome (22, 23). However, conflicting conclusions have arisen among investigators who have attempted to determine whether the phagosome containing *H. capsulatum* fuses with lysosomes (23, 24, 25).

Difficulties inherent in the assays chosen by these groups may have contributed to the disparate results that they obtained. Traditionally, electron microscopy or acridine orange have been used to monitor the fusion of lysosomes and phagosomes. To be accurate, the former technique requires that lysosomes be identified either by electron-dense tracers or by localization of lysosomal enzymes through immunoreactivity or cytochemistry. Numerous phagosomes must be surveyed to make a statistically significant conclusion. The fact that an individual phagosome may contain no lysosomal marker in one section, but large amounts in another section, makes examination of large numbers of phagosomes by electron microscopy even more cumbersome. While use of the fluorescent dye, acridine orange, avoids these statistical problems, it less clearly identifies vesicles as lysosomes than does the use of electron microscopy and lysosomal markers. This is because acridine orange permeates membranes until it becomes protonated and entrapped within an acidic vesicle such as a lysosome, an endosome, or even an acidified phagosome.

Other factors may also explain why the results with H. capsulatum have varied between laboratories. It is not known at this time whether the species or strain of host animal influences the intracellular fate of this fungus, so perhaps it is not valid to compare the results in macrophages obtained from hamsters (23) with those obtained from mice of unspecified strains (24, 25). The outcome might be similarly affected by the choice of H. capsulatum strain or the ratio of yeasts to macrophages, neither of which were reported in the abbreviated reports by Edwards (24) or von Behren et al. (25). The work by Dumont and Robert (23) is further complicated by the experimental protocol used. These investigators injected H. capsulatum intraperitoneally into hamsters, then recovered and examined macrophages from the peritoneal exudate at various times after inoculation. This poorly defined system makes it difficult to determine the contribution of the many cell types in the peritoneal exudate (macrophages, lymphocytes, polymorphonuclear leukocytes, etc.), since over the 48-hour period studied, considerable variation would be expected in their relative numbers, interactions, and fungicidal activities. It is known, for example, that lymphokines activate macrophages such that they inhibit H. capsulatum growth (26) and also that these yeasts are killed within polymorphonuclear leukocytes (27).

The in vivo study by Dumont and Robert (23), which is the only full-length published report on this issue, used electron microscopy to show that acid phosphatase was found in phagosomes containing H. capsulatum yeasts at early times (5 min to 1 hour post-inoculation), but not at 24 to 48 hours after inoculation. This result is surprising because one would expect more phagolysosome fusion at later times, especially since the continued recruitment of inflammatory cells should result in increasing numbers of activated macrophages over the course of the experiment. Once again, the lack of statistical considerations makes these results difficult to interpret.

We decided to re-evaluate the issue of whether lysosomes fuse with phagosomes containing H. capsulatum using fluorescein isothiocyanate-labeled dextran (FITC-dextran) as a convenient probe to monitor the fusion of lysosomes with phagosomes. The advantages of this method over the aforementioned techniques are (a) it allows rapid screening of large numbers of phagosomes; and (b) since it is not membrane-permeable, this molecule can only enter a vesicle through membrane fusion events. Using subcellular fractionation techniques, previous investigators have shown that FITC-dextran begins to accumulate within lysosomes 15 minutes after cells are exposed to it (28). By allowing uptake of 10 mg FITC-dextran/ml for 4 hours, and following this with an overnight chase in unlabeled medium, concentration of the dye within the lysosomes is encouraged.

Lysosomes labeled with FITC-dextran were initially visible as punctate yellow-green fluorescence on a dark cytoplasmic background. Subsequently, they migrated to and surrounded phagosomes containing ingested yeasts, forming a beaded ring of fluorescence. In similar studies using mouse peritoneal macrophages, Goren et al. (29) reported low levels of fusion of FITC-labeled lysosomes with phagosomes containing Saccharomyces cerevisiae even 6 hours after addition of the yeasts. However, in the P388D1 macrophage-like cell line, we observed phagolysosomes at the earliest time examined (15 min), regardless of whether the inoculum was live S. cerevisiae or live H. capsulatum (Figs. 1 and 2). By 3 hours post-inoculation, greater than 85% of the phagosomes containing yeasts of either species had fused with lysosomes (Figs. 3 and 4). The amount of phagolysosome fusion was unaffected by the inoculum dose, using ratios of yeasts to macrophages between 5:1 and 50:1.

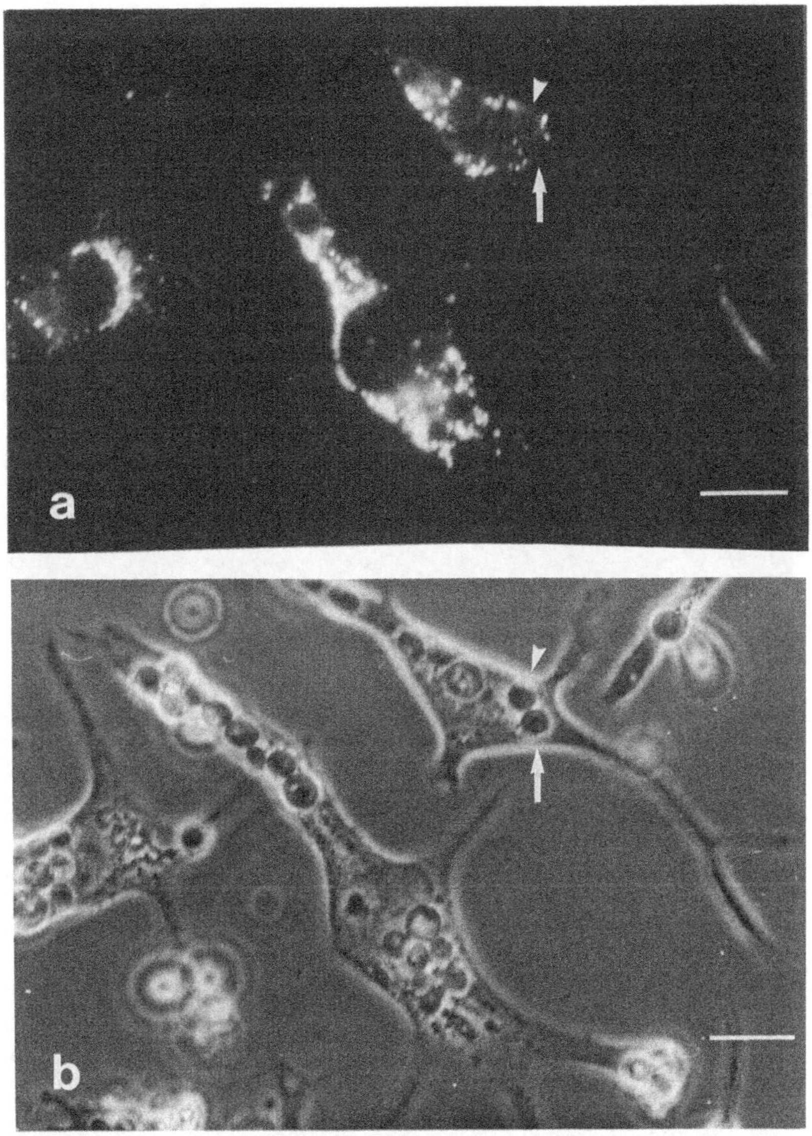

FIGURE 1. (a) P388D1 cells pretreated for 4 hours with FITC-dextran and chased overnight in fresh medium. The cells were then inoculated with S. cerevisiae and examined 15 min. later by fluorescence microscopy. Many yeast-laden phagosomes were either surrounded by lysosomes (visible as discrete spots of fluorescence around a dark yeast [arrow]) or had fused with them so that the yeasts appeared to be "rimmed" with fluorescence [arrowhead]. (b) Same field examined by phase-contrast microscopy, revealing intracellular phase-dark yeasts. Extracellular organisms were phase bright. Bar in all figures represents 10 μm.

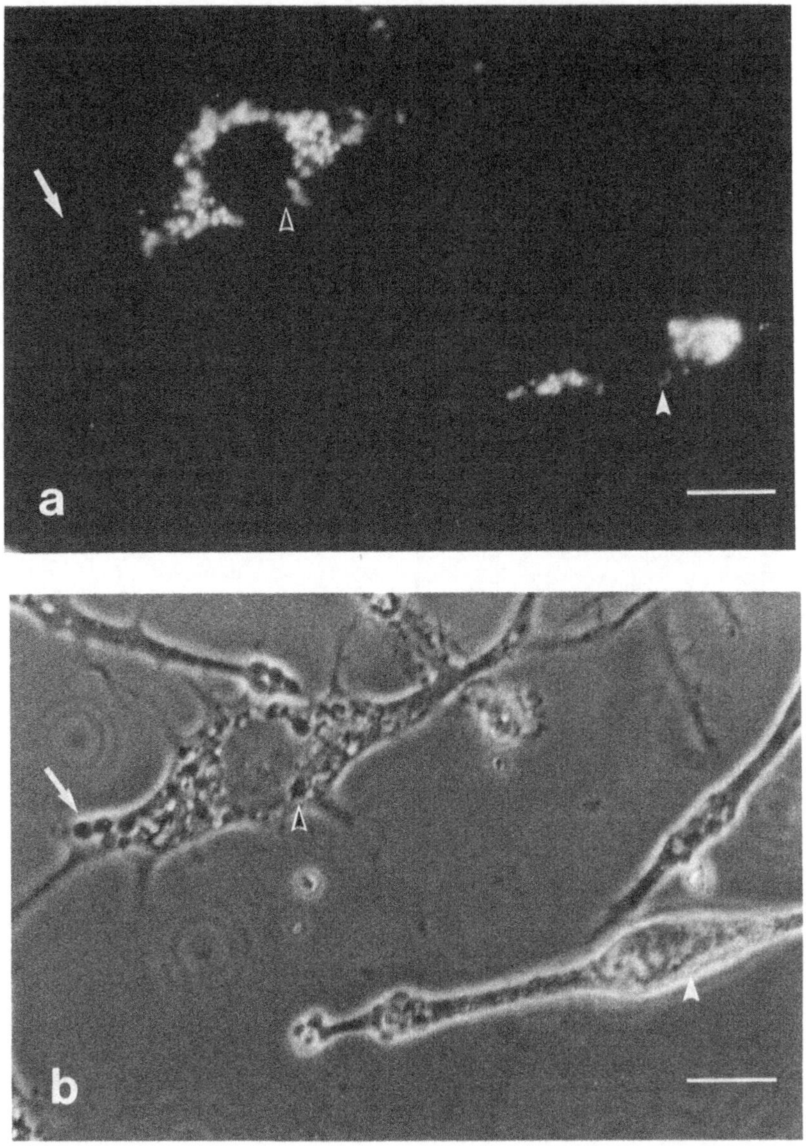

FIGURE 2. Same as Figure 1, but the inoculum was H. capsulatum strain G217B. Note examples in which lysosomes had not yet migrated to phagosomes containing yeasts [arrow] as well those in which the phagosomes and lysosomes had fused [arrowhead]. At this early time fusion is sometimes barely detectable [open arrowhead]. Similar images were obtained for all H. capsulatum strains examined.

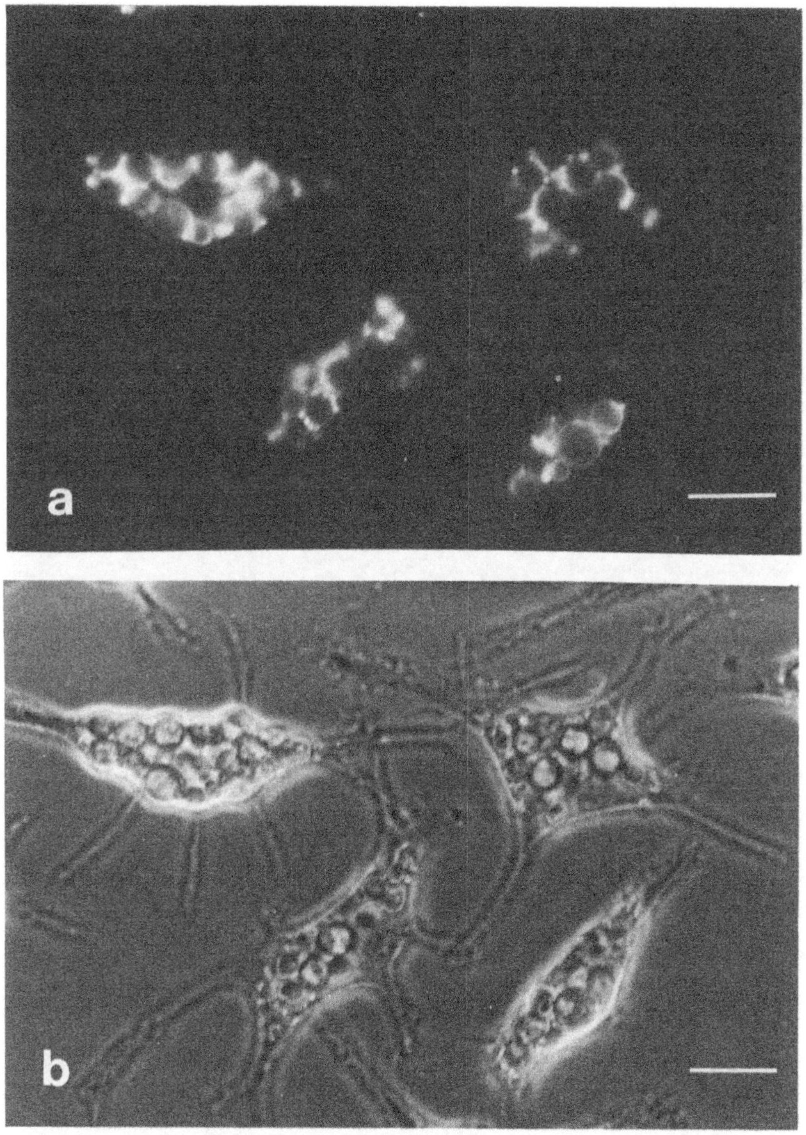

FIGURE 3. (a) At 3 hours after inoculation of P388D1 cells with S. cerevisiae, the vast majority of yeasts were detected in phagolysosomes by fluorescence microscopy. Few discrete lysosomes remained. (b) Same field observed by phase-contrast microscopy.

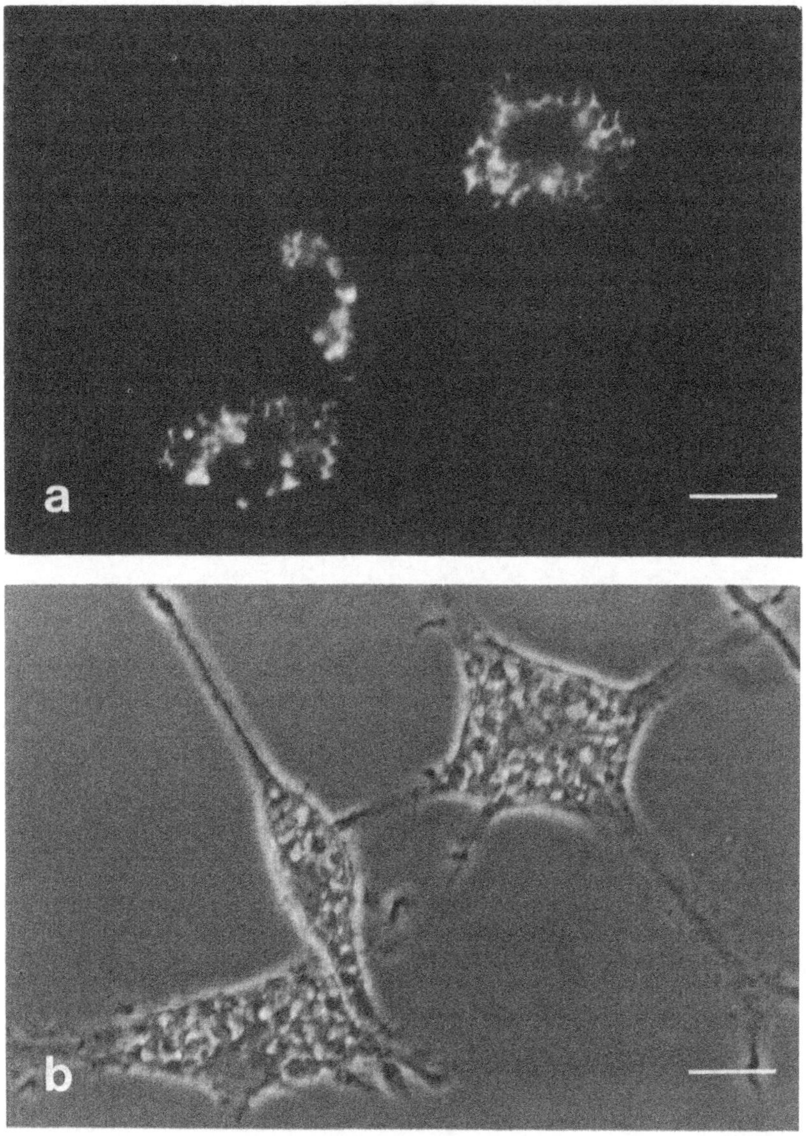

FIGURE 4. Same as Figure 3, but using cells inoculated with _H_. _capsulatum_ strain G217B.

Phagolysosome formation was independent of the strain of H. capsulatum used. Both North American (G217B) and South American (G186A and G184A) isolates were tested. These strains are not only of diverse geographic origins, but also fall into distinct evolutionary classes based on restriction endonuclease analysis of their mitochondrial and ribosomal DNAs: G217B has class 2 restriction patterns, while G184A and G186A have class 3 patterns (30). From the South American strains, our laboratory has isolated a series of spontaneous avirulent variants (31). Lysosomes also fused with phagosomes containing these organisms.

We believe that FITC-dextran is a valuable probe for studying phagosome-lysosome fusion. In our experiments, we obtained similar results using either FITC-dextran or acridine orange. However, there are certain instances in which we predict that acridine orange would give erroneous results, while FITC-dextran should not: (a) when an organism which avoids phagosome-lysosome fusion nonetheless resides in a vesicle which acidifies, or (b) when a microorganism survives in a phagolysosome, but inactivates lysosomal enzymes by preventing acidification.

Our results to date indicate that lysosomes fuse with Histoplasma capsulatum in a macrophage-like cell line. The large proportion of yeasts which were located in phagolysosomes (>85%) excludes the possibility that it is only those phagosomes containing dead or damaged yeasts which undergo fusion. Since H. capsulatum continues to multiply within and eventually destroy these cells, this organism probably resists or inactivates the lysosomal killing mechanisms. Using FITC-dextran, it is now feasible to evaluate the reasons for the discrepancies in the previous reports on H. capsulatum, and we are presently comparing the results obtained in our cell line with corresponding experiments using freshly harvested macrophages.

ACKNOWLEDGMENTS

FITC-dextran was a generous gift from Dr. Paul Schlesinger, Washington University School of Dental Medicine, St. Louis, Missouri.

REFERENCES

1. D. H. Howard, Intracellular behavior of Histoplasma capsulatum, J. Bacteriol. 87:33 (1964).
2. L. G. Eissenberg and W. E. Goldman, Histoplasma capsulatum fails to trigger release of superoxide from macrophages, Infect. Immun. 55: in press (1987).
3. J. E. Wolf, V. Kerchberger, G. S. Kobayashi, and J. R. Little, Modulation of the macrophage oxidative burst by Histoplasma capsulatum, J. Immunol. 138: in press (1987).
4. J. A. Armstrong and P. D. Hart, Response of cultured macrophages to Mycobacterium tuberculosis, with observations on fusion of lysosomes with phagosomes, J. Exp. Med. 134:713 (1971).
5. M. B. Goren, P. D. Hart, M. R. Young, and J. A. Armstrong, Prevention of phagosome-lysosome fusion in cultured macrophages by sulfatides of Mycobacterium tuberculosis, Proc. Natl. Acad. Sci. U.S.A. 73:2510 (1976).
6. P. D. Hart and M. R. Young, Interference with normal phagosome-lysosome fusion in macrophages, using ingested yeast cells and suramin, Nature 256:47 (1975).
7. T. C. Jones and J. G. Hirsch, The interaction between Toxoplasma gondii and mammalian cells. II. The absence of lysosomal fusion with phagocytic vacuoles containing living parasites, J. Exp. Med. 136:1172 (1972).

8. R. Friis, Interaction of L-cells and Chlamydia psittaci: Entry of the parasite and host responses to its development, J. Bacteriol. 110:706 (1972).
9. P. B. Wyrick and E. A. Brownridge, Growth of Chlamydia psittaci in macrophages, Infect. Immun. 19:1054 (1978).
10. M. A. Horwitz and F. R. Maxfield, Legionella pneumophila inhibits acidification of its phagosome in human monocytes, J. Cell Biol. 99:1936 (1984).
11. M. A. Horwitz, The Legionnaires' disease bacterium (Legionella pneumophila) inhibits phagosome-lysosome fusion in human monocytes, J. Exp. Med. 158:2108 (1983).
12. S. C. Straley and P. A. Harmon, Yersinia pestis grows within phagolysosomes in mouse peritoneal macrophages, Infect. Immun. 45:655 (1984).
13. M. E. W. Carrol, P. S. Jackett, V. R. Aber, and D. B. Lowrie, Phagolysosome formation, cyclic adenosine 3':5'-monophosphate and the fate of Salmonella typhimurium within mouse peritoneal macrophages, J. Gen. Microbiol. 110:421 (1979).
14. E. T. Akporiaye, J. D. Rowatt, A. A. Aragon, and O. G. Baca, Lysosomal response of a murine macrophage-like cell line persistently infected with Coxiella burnetii, Infect. Immun. 40:1155 (1983).
15. C. A. Brown and P. Draper, An electron-microscope study of rat fibroblasts infected with Mycobacterium lepraemurium, J. Pathol. 102:21 (1970).
16. I. N. Brown and P. Draper, Growth of Mycobacterium lepraemurium in the mouse bone marrow: An ultrastructural study, Infect. Immun. 13:1199 (1976).
17. P. D. Hart, J. A. Armstrong, C. A. Brown, and P. Draper, Ultrastructural study of the behavior of macrophages toward parasitic mycobacteria, Infect. Immun. 5:803 (1972).
18. K.-P. Chang, Cellular and molecular mechanisms of intracellular symbiosis in Leishmaniasis, Int. Rev. Cytol. 14S:267 (1983).
19. N. Nogueira and Z. Cohn, Trypansoma cruzi: Mechanism of entry and intracellular fate in mammalian cells", J. Exp. Med. 143:1402. (1976).
20. E. P. Ewing, A. Takeuchi, A. Shirai, and J. V. Osterman, Experimental infection of mouse peritoneal mesothelium with scrub typhus rickettsiae: An ultrastructural study, Infect. Immun. 19:1068 (1978).
21. Y. Rikihisa and S. Ito, Intracellular localization of Rickettsia tsutsugamushi in polymorphonuclear leukocytes, J. Exp. Med. 150:703 (1979).
22. A. Dumont and C. Piche, Electron microscopic study of human histoplasmosis, Arch. Pathol. 87:168 (1969).
23. A. Dumont and A. Robert, Electron microscopic study of phagocytosis of Histoplasma capsulatum by hamster peritoneal macrophages, Lab. Invest. 23:278 (1970).
24. M. R. Edwards, Intracellular fate of Histoplasma capsulatum phagocytosed by murine peritoneal macrophages, Fed. Proc. 41:963 (1982).
25. L. A. Von Behren, S. Chaudhary, S. Rabinovitch, and R. P. Tewari, Electron microscopic study of phagosome-lysosome (P-L) fusion in normal mouse peritoneal macrophages after exposure to yeast cells of Histoplasma capsulatum (HC), Abstr. Annu. Meet. Am. Soc. Microbiol. 1983:388 (1983).
26. B. Wu-Hsieh and D. H. Howard, Inhibition of growth of Histoplasma capsulatum by lymphokine-stimulated macrophages, J. Immunol. 132:2593 (1984).
27. D. H. Howard, Fate of Histoplasma capsulatum in guinea pig polymorphonuclear leukocytes, Infect. Immun. 8:412 (1973).
28. M. Merion, P. Schlesinger, R. M. Brooks, J. M. Moehring, T. J. Moehring, and W. S. Sly, Defective acidification of endosomes in

Chinese hamster ovary cell mutants "cross-resistant" to toxins and viruses, Proc. Natl. Acad. Sci. U.S.A. 80:5313 (1983).
29. M. B. Goren, C. L. Swendsen, J. Fiscus, and C. Miranti, Fluorescent markers for studying phagosome-lysosome fusion, J. Leuk. Biol. 36:273 (1984).
30. R. D. Vincent, R. Goewert, W. E. Goldman, G. S. Kobayashi, A. M. Lambowitz, and G. Medoff, Classification of Histoplasma capsulatum isolates by restriction fragment polymorphisms, J. Bacteriol. 165:813 (1986).
31. K. R. Klimpel and W. E. Goldman, Isolation and characterization of spontaneous avirulent variants of Histoplasma capsulatum, Infect. Immun. 55: in press (1987).

THE RESPIRATORY BURST IN ACTIVATED MACROPHAGES: STUDIES OF ITS MOLECULAR BASIS AND EVIDENCE FOR DOWNREGULATION IN CHRONIC INFECTION

Richard B. Johnston, Jr., Seiichi Kitagawa, Carl K. Edwards, III, Jacqueline Y. Channon, Hitoshi Suzuki and Michael J. Pabst

Department of Pediatrics, University of Pennsylvania School of Medicine and The Children's Hospital of Philadelphia, Philadelphia, PA 19104,
and Department of Pediatrics, National Jewish Center for Immunology and Respiratory Medicine, Denver, CO 80206

INTRODUCTION

Macrophages (Mø) elicited by injection of inflammatory agents or obtained from animals infected with intracellular parasites are primed so that they respond to phagocytosis or exposure to phorbol myristate acetate (PMA) with a marked increase in the respiratory burst (1). Unstimulated Mø release little if any reactive oxygen metabolites; stimulation is required to demonstrate the primed state. This capacity for an increased stimulated release of reactive oxygen metabolites appears to play an essential role in the increased microbicidal capacity of activated Mø (2-4). Priming is a manifestation of Mø activation, but it is not the same as activation; i.e., priming may not always reflect the fully activated state (5).

The molecular basis for this priming is not understood (3). Possibilities include an increase in the number or affinity of plasma membrane receptors, a change in the function of the enzyme or enzyme system responsible for the respiratory burst (the NADPH oxidase), and modification of one or more of the steps in stimulus-response coupling involved in the respiratory burst.

It appears that modification of membrane receptors cannot explain the enhanced respiratory burst. The number and affinity of receptors for phorbol ester, which most effectively demonstrates the primed state, are equivalent in resident (nonactivated) and activated Mø (reviewed in 6). Expression of receptors for other ligands (studied mostly as extent of binding) varies in activated compared to resident Mø. In particular, receptors for the Fc piece of IgG2b and for mannose-terminated glycoconjugates are decreased and those for the Fc of IgG2a are increased in activated Mø (7,8).

In regard to possible modification of the NADPH oxidase, results to date indicate that catalytic efficiency of the oxidase is increased in activated Mø. Specifically, the NADPH oxidase has a decreased K_m for NADPH when it it is studied in membrane-rich fractions from PMA-stimulated activated Mø, compared to results with fractions from stimulated resident

Table 1. Lag Time and Initial Rate of O_2^- Release in Resident Mø, LPS-Mø, and BCG-Mø[a]

Mø Type	Lag Time (sec)	Initial rate (nmol/min/mg)
Resident	107 ± 10(4)	3.7 ± 0.2
LPS-elicited	86 ± 11(4)	32.1 ± 2.1[b]
BCG-activated	77 ± 3(2)[b]	35.2 ± 2.1[b]

[a]The initial rate of O_2^- release was calculated from the initial linear portion of the tracing, and the lag time was calculated from extrapolation of the initial linear portion to the base-line absorbance. Data are expressed as means ± SEM; the number of experiments, each done in triplicate, is given in parentheses beside the value for the lag time. PMA was the stimulus.

[b]Value is significantly different from that with resident Mø, $p < 0.01$.

cells (9-11). The V_{max} is not greatly modified. It appears that cytochrome b, a proposed component of the oxidase system, is not modified in activated Mø (10,11).

This change in efficiency of the NADPH oxidase could be due, at least in part, to enhanced transduction of the activating signal from the receptor to the oxidase (9). In fact, priming as we have defined it here might be the result of a fundamental change (or changes) in one or more of the relevant transduction events (3). We describe here functional and biochemical studies that support the concept that priming of Mø, and also Mø activation, are associated with alteration of certain components of the transduction pathway. We also present evidence suggesting that the primed state in Mø can be downregulated in vivo during chronic mycobacterial infection in mice.

ALTERED TIME COURSE OF SUPEROXIDE ANION (O_2^-) RELEASE IN ACTIVATED MACROPHAGES

The capacity to cultivate mouse Mø for 1 to 3 days in reproducible numbers on coverslips permitted us to measure release of O_2^- continuously (12). The coverslips were placed in cuvettes, PMA was added to begin the reaction, and the extent of superoxide dismutase - inhibitable reduction of cytochrome c was recorded continuously. The results (Table 1, from reference 12) indicate that the lag time is reduced in activated Mø, a change most likely due to altered transduction, and that the initial rate is markedly increased.

ACCENTUATED CHANGES IN MEMBRANE POTENTIAL IN STIMULATED ACTIVATED MACROPHAGES

We used adherent Mø to study membrane potential changes because Mø functions, including the respiratory burst, have been studied primarily in the adherent state. Changes in trans-membrane potential were measured continuously using the fluorescent carbocyanine dye, di-O-C_5(3), which was preloaded into the cells in a physiologic NaCl buffer (12). Pre-loading in KCl buffer markedly reduced the extent of fluorescence. Addition of PMA to the cells in the cuvette induced depolarization within 20 sec of addition, which was the time required for mixing.

Figure 1 shows the time courses of changes in membrane potential in Mø stimulated by PMA. The initial rate and maximum response of the changes in membrane potential in LPS-Mø and BCG-Mø were greater than those in resident Mø (Fig. 1), and there was greater release of O_2^- by the elicited and activated Mø on exposure to PMA (Table 1). Membrane potential changes began 60 to 90 sec before release of O_2^- could be detected in each cell type. The dose-response curves for triggering of membrane potential changes and O_2^- release by PMA were identical. The magnitude of membrane potential changes and of O_2^- release in LPS-Mø and BCG-Mø declined progressively during in vitro culture, and values on day 3 approached those in resident Mø. Extracellular glucose was required for effective stimulated change in membrane potential and O_2^- release. These findings indicate that membrane potential changes are closely associated with O_2^- releasing capacity in Mø, and that the systems that mediate membrane potential changes and production of O_2^- develop or decline concomitantly during activation or deactivation of the cells.

DEACTIVATION OF THE RESPIRATORY BURST IN ACTIVATED MACROPHAGES

Activated Mø undergo a decline in their capacity to release O_2^- (a deactivation) when placed in culture. We explored the mechanisms underlying deactivation of activated mouse peritoneal macrophages (6). Deactivation was observed when the assay was performed in a physiologic Na^+ buffer, and by day 3 of culture, release of O_2^- from activated Mø stimulated with PMA was almost identical to that in resident Mø. In contrast, when the assay was performed in a buffer in which Na^+ was replaced by K^+, release of O_2^- from activated Mø on day 3 was equal to or greater than that on day 0, suggesting that the enzyme responsible for the respiratory burst was not altered during culture. The number and affinity of PMA receptors were not changed during culture and were not affected by high external K^+. Continuous assay of O_2^- release by coverslip-adherent macrophages in a cuvette indicated that the lag time between addition of stimulus and release of O_2^- was reduced, and the initial rate of O_2^- release was enhanced in K^+ buffer. The potency of monovalent cations to support O_2^- release was $K^+ > Rb^+ >$ choline$^+ > Cs^+ = Na^+ > Li^+$, suggesting that characteristics such as ionic radius or molecular size influence this effect, and the effect is not due simply to absence of Na^+. Extracellular Ca^{2+} or Mg^{2+} was required for the maximal effect of high external K^+, and enhancement by high K^+ and divalent cations increased progressively during culture.

These findings suggest that deactivation is caused primarily by changes in signal transduction from PMA receptors to the respiratory burst enzyme, rather than by changes in these receptors or the enzyme itself, and that signal transduction can differ in different Mø populations (6).

PRIMING OF MACROPHAGES BY EXPOSURE TO THE CALCIUM IONOPHORE IONOMYCIN

We explored the possible involvement of intracellular Ca^{2+} in priming by exposing resident mouse peritoneal Mø to the calcium ionophore, ionomycin (13). Concentrations of the ionophore up to 4μM did not stimulate release of O_2^- by Mø. However, preincubation of the Mø with ionomycin, 1-2 μM, for 2-5 min primed them so that release of O_2^- was more than doubled when the cells were stimulated by PMA over a broad range of concentrations. Similar studies with neutrophils indicated that ionomycin priming was associated with a decrease in the lag time between addition of the stimulus and onset

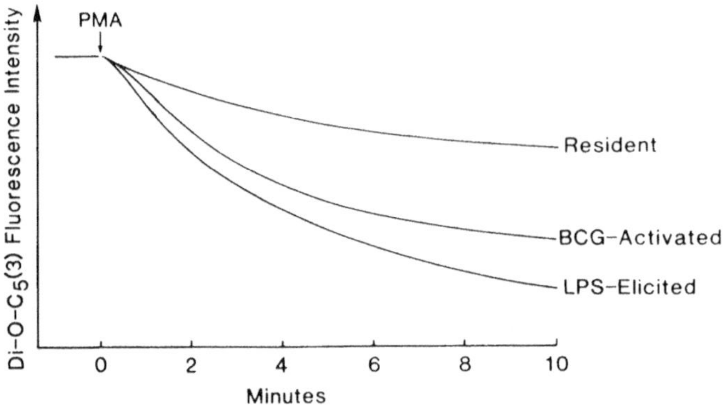

Fig. 1. Time course of changes in membrane potential in resident Mø, LPS-Mø, and BCG-Mø stimulated by PMA. Adherent Mø on a coverslip were preincubated with di-O-C_5(3) for 50 min at 37°C before PMA (100 ng/ml) was added. The tracings are simulated from actual recordings and have been drawn with the same starting point (baseline). The results shown are representative of three experiments with BCG-Mø and six experiments each with resident Mø and LPS-Mø. (Reproduced from 12, with permission)

of detectable release of O_2^-. These results are compatible with the concept that the "charge" assumed by phagocytes in the process of priming includes an increase in or rearrangement of (or both) the intracellular pools of Ca^{2+}.

STUDIES OF THE RELATIONSHIP BETWEEN MEMBRANE PHOSPHOLIPID REMODELING AND THE RESPIRATORY BURST IN MACROPHAGES

In several cell types, a major pathway of signal transduction involves turnover of the inositol lipids to produce the second messengers, diacylglyceride and inositol trisphosphate (14). A correlation between phosphatidylinositol (PI) turnover and O_2^- production has been suggested in neutrophils (15) and alveolar Mø (16) stimulated with soluble chemotactic peptide. The accumulation of phosphatidic acid (PA) has been used as a measure of PI turnover in lymphocytes (17), although a recent report with neutrophils has suggested that PA may also be produced from phosphatidylcholine (PC) (18).

We examined the relationship between phospholipid turnover and O_2^- production in cultured Mø exposed to a particulate stimulus, unopsonized zymosan (19). Zymosan-stimulated Mø produced increased amounts of PA; the increase was first detected at 1.5 min and continued prominently for 10 min of incubation. Production of O_2^- was not detected until between 2 to 4 min after stimulation, and continued to increase through 60 min. Inhibition experiments suggested that these two processes were linked. Theophylline (theo)/dibutyrylcylic AMP (dbcAMP) and theo/prostaglandin E_2 (PGE_2) inhibited O_2^- production at every time point (79% and 80% inhibition, respectively, at 4 min). Corresponding inhibition of PA production was also achieved at every time point (85% by theo/dbcAMP; 67% by theo/PGE_2 at

4 min). These results are compatible with a role for phospholipid remodeling in the transduction process associated with the respiratory burst in Mø. Preliminary results suggested that the phospholipid species could be PC as well as PI (19).

REGULATION OF THE RESPIRATORY BURST IN VIVO DURING CHRONIC MYCOBACTERIAL INFECTION IN MICE

A variety of substances that have the capability of activating Mø or interfering with Mø activation through suppression of lymphokine release are produced by spleen cells from mice infected with mycobacteria (reviewed in reference 20). These substances are not well characterized. Investigators studying other host-parasite interactions have described several mediators thought to be involved in modulating Mø function, including IFN-γ and prostaglandins (PG) (reviewed in reference 21). That PG can modulate the host response to mycobacterial infection is suggested by the observation that indomethacin, a PG synthetase inhibitor, can correct the defective mitogenic response of lymphocytes from patients with atypical mycobacteriosis (22).

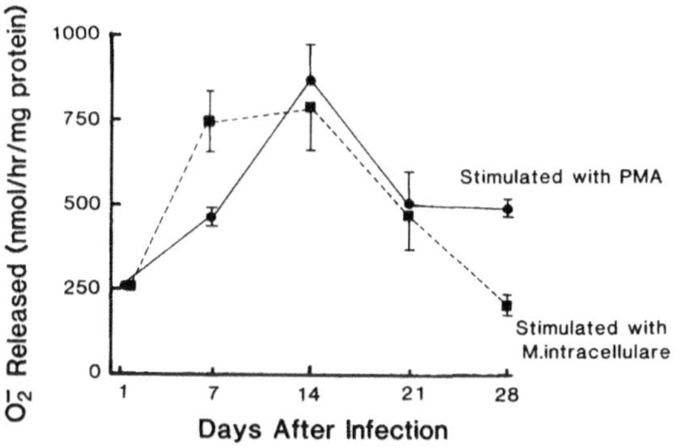

Fig. 2. Release of O_2^- by peritoneal Mø from mice injected i.v. with viable M intracellulare. At day 1 and at weekly intervals after injection, peritoneal Mø were isolated and were assayed for release of O_2^- in response to PMA or a suspension of live bacteria. Values shown are means ± SE from experiments performed in duplicate or triplicate with cells from 10 mice at each point (n = 10). Unstimulated Mø from infected mice release <50 nmol of O_2^-/hr/mg at all time points. Mø from uninfected animals released 60 ± 18 nmol of O_2^-/hr/mg in response to PMA (n = 4). For comparison, Mø from uninfected animals that were exposed overnight in vitro to LPS (10 ng/ml) or MDP (10 μg/ml) released 431 ± 35 and 227 ± 10 nmol O_2^-/hr/mg, respectively, n = 6, in response to stimulation with PMA. (From reference 20, with permission)

As a model for the study of human atypical mycobacterial disease, we explored the basis for the prolonged mycobacteriosis in mice infected with M intracellulare (20). Two weeks after i.v. injection of mycobacteria, peritoneal Mø were found to be activated, as indicated by their capacity to produce large amounts of O_2^- in response to PMA or viable M intracellulare. However, as shown in Figure 2, 4 wk after infection, despite the continued presence of large numbers of mycobacteria in the spleen, macrophages from infected animals produced low amounts of O_2^-.

As shown in Figure 3, the decline in O_2^- production was not the result of clearing of the infection. On the contrary, large numbers of viable bacteria remained in the spleen during the 8-wk study period.

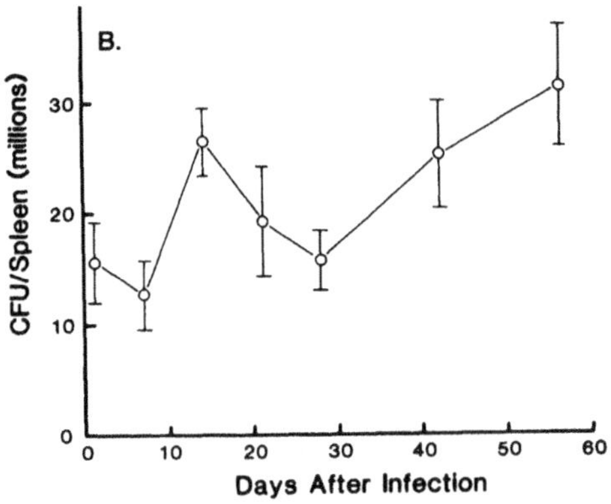

Fig. 3. Time course of infection with M intracellulare. CFU of bacteria were determined at weekly intervals after i.v. injection of 10^8 viable bacteria. Values are from experiments performed with four mice at each point. (From reference 20, with permission)

In an attempt to understand the basis for this decline in O_2^- release at 3 and 4 wk after infection, we studied cultured spleen cells from infected mice. Unfractionated spleen cells from mice infected 4 wk earlier produced increased amounts of interleukin 2 and interferon (IFN) when stimulated with the mitogen concanavalin A, but less of these lymphokines than unstimulated cells when exposed to antigens derived from M intracellulare, suggesting production of an inhibitory factor. Spleen cells from infected mice were not stimulated to incorporate (^{3}H) thymidine by exposure to mycobacterial antigens; but this unresponsiveness could be reversed by addition of indomethacin to the cultures.

Additional investigation, summarized in Figure 4, showed that Mø from infected animals produced large amounts of PGE_2 when stimulated by mycobacterial antigens. In vitro, such concentrations of PGE_2 inhibited uptake of [^{3}H]thymidine by stimulated spleen lymphocytes from infected animals. Thus, it seemed likely that in infected animals, macrophage-derived PG suppressed production of IFN-γ by lymphocytes, which in turn prevented activation of the macrophages to full microbicidal activity.

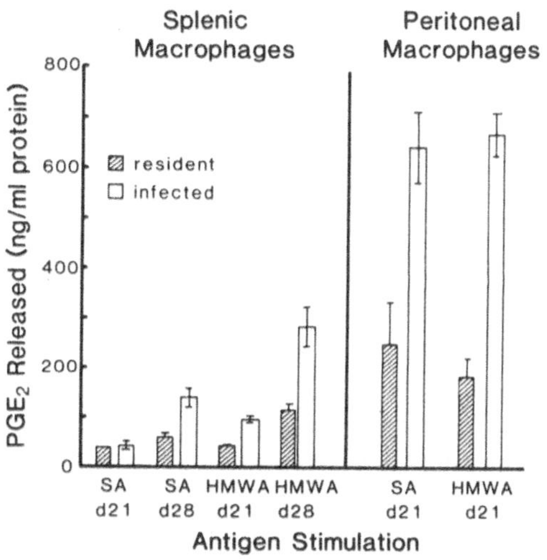

Fig. 4. Production of PGE_2 by uninfected (resident) and M intracellulare infected splenic and peritoneal Mø after stimulation for 48 hr with HMWA (10 μg/ml) or SA (15 μg/ml), high molecular weight and soluble antigens from the infecting organism. The antigen used and the day (d) after infection at which the Mø were cultured are shown beneath each pair of columns. Supernatants were prepared, and the concentration of PGE_2 in each supernatant was determined by radioimmunoassay. The results are expressed as ng of PGE_2 produced per mg of adherent Mø protein. A value of 300 ng/mg protein corresponds to approximately 10 nM PGE_2 in the supernatant. Values are mean ± SE, n = 2, in triplicate. Unstimulated values for splenic macrophages were 1 to 4 ng PGE_2/mg protein for infected or uninfected cells on days 21 or 28; unstimulated values for peritoneal Mø were 46 ± 8 ng/mg for uninfected cells and 48 ± 19 ng/mg for infected cells. (From reference 20, with permission)

To test this hypothesis, we administered either indomethacin, IFN-γ, or muramyl dipeptide (MDP) to infected mice. The results are shown in Table 2.

Mice treated with each of these agents showed decreased spleen and lung weights (not shown) and decreased numbers of viable myobacteria in these organs (Table 2). These results support the concept that interaction between the host and M intracellulare is modulated profoundly by PG and suggest that administration of agents that directly promote macrophage activation can enhance resistance to infection by this organism.

Table 2. Treatment of Mice Infected with M intracellulare with Agents that Promote Macrophage Activation[a]

Treatment	CFU/Spleen (millions)	CFU/Lungs (millions)
Saline	13.3 ± 1.3(12)	4.3 ± 0.3(9)
MDP (50 μg)	0.45 ± 0.01(12)	0.03 ± 0.01(9)
Indomethacin (600 μg)	2.0 ± 0.4 (9)	0.45 ± 0.01(9)
IFN-γ (500 U)	0.21 ± 0.02(11)	0.02 ± 0.01(6)
IFN-γ (2500 U)	0.30 ± 0.01(15)	0.03 ± 0.01(6)
MDP (50 μg) + IFN-γ (500 U)	0.5 ± 0.02(6)	0.03 ± 0.01(6)

[a]Mice were injected with 10^8 viable bacteria into the tail vein. Four weeks after infection, 6 to 15 mice were treated with each of the indicated agents given daily for 7 days by i.v. injection; studies were performed on day 8. Four different groups of infected mice were used for the total experiments. The results represent the mean ± SE. The number of mice studied in each group is given in parentheses. CFU were determined with plating in triplicate. In infected mice given no treatment, CFU/spleen ($15.7 \pm 2.8 \times 10^6$, n = 11) were equivalent to values obtained with mice given saline. (Adapted from reference 20)

CONCLUSIONS

Activation of macrophages is the end result of cell-mediated immunity, and priming for an enhanced respiratory burst is an essential component of that process. Some knowledge of the molecular basis of priming has been acquired. However, greater understanding probably will be needed before priming of macrophages can be achieved pharmacologically in order to increase resistance to infection, or suppressed to avoid oxidative tissue damage. In addition, knowledge of how priming is achieved during activation should lead to a better understanding of how activation itself is induced.

ACKNOWLEDGEMENTS

The authors' research described here was supported by USPHS grants AI 24782 and DE 05494 from the National Institutes of Health.

REFERENCES

1. Johnston, R.B., Jr., 1981, Enhancement of phagocytosis-associated oxidative metabolism as a manifestation of macrophage activation, Lymphokines, 3:33.

2. Sasada, M., and Johnston, R.B., Jr, 1980, Macrophage microbicidal activity: correlation between phagocytosis-assoicated oxidative metabolism and the killing of candida by macrophages, J. Exp. Med., 152:85.

3. Johnston, R.B., Jr., and Kitagawa, S., 1985, Molecular basis for the enhanced respiratory burst of activated macrophages, Fed. Proc., 44:2927.

4. Nathan, C.F., 1983, Mechanisms of macrophage antimicrobial activity, Trans. R. Soc. Trop. Med. Hyg., 77:620.

5. Harris, L.K., Pabst, M.J., and Johnston, R.B., Jr., 1984, Inreased transglutaminase activity in elicited and activated macrophages: relationship to production of superoxide anion, J. Leukocyte Biol., 36:719.

6. Kitagawa, S., and Johnston, R.B., Jr., 1986, Deactivation of the respiratory burst in activated macrophages: evidence for alteration of signal transduction, J. Immunol., 136:2605.

7. Ezekowitz, R.A.B., Bampton, M., and Gordon, S., 1983, Macrophage activation selectively enhances expression of Fc receptors for IgG2a, J. Exp. Med., 157:807.

8. Stahl, P., and Gordon, S., 1982, Expression of a mannosyl-fucosyl receptor for endocytosis on cultured primary macrophages and their hybrids, J. Cell. Biol., 93:49.

9. Sadada, M., Pabst, M.J., and Johnston, R.B., Jr., 1983, Activation of mouse peritoneal macrophages by lipopolysaccharide alters the kinetic parameters of the superoxide-producing NADPH oxidase, J. Biol. Chem., 258:9631.

10. Tsunawaki, S., and Nathan, C.F., 1984, Enzymatic basis of macrophage activation: kinetic analysis of superoxide production in lysates of resident and activated mouse peritoneal macrophages and granulocytes. J. Biol. Chem., 259:4305.

11. Berton, G.M., Cassatella, M., Cabrini, G., and Rossi, F., 1985, Activation of mouse macrophages causes no change in expression and function of phorbol diesters' receptors, but is accompanied by alterations in the activity and kinetic parameters of NADPH oxidase, Immunology, 54:371.

12. Kitagawa, S., and Johnston, R.B., Jr., 1985, Relationship between membrane potential changes and superoxide-releasing capacity in resident and activated mouse peritoneal macrophages, J. Immunol., 135:3417.

13. Finkel, T.H., Suzuki, H., Guthrie, L.A., Forehand, J.R., Phillips, W.A., Pabst, M.J., and Johnston, R.B., Jr., Priming of neutrophils and macrophages for enhanced release of superoxide anion by the calcium ionophore ionomycin: implications for activation of the respiratory burst, Manuscript submitted.

14. Berridge, M.J., 1984, Inositol trisphosphate and diacylglycerol as second messengers, Biochem. J., 220:345.

15. Holian, A.J., and Stickle, D.F., 1985, Calcium regulation of phosphatidylinositol turnover in macrophage activation by formyl peptides, J. Cell. Physiol., 123:39.

16. DeTogni, P., Della Bianca, V., Grzeskowiak, M., DiVirgilio, F., and Rossi, F., 1985, Mechanism of desensitization of neutrophil response to N-formylmethionylleucylphenylalanine by slow rate of receptor occupany: studies on changes in Ca^{2+} concentration and phosphatidylinositol turnover, Biochem. Biophys. Acta 838:23.

17. Coggeshall, K.M., and Cambier, J.C., 1984, B cell activation. VIII. Membrane immunoglobulins transduce signals via activation of phosphatidylinositol hydrolysis, J. Immunol., 133:3382.

18. Agwu, D.E., McPhail, L.C., Daniel, L.W., Bass, D.A., and McCall, C.E., 1986, Activation of phospholipase C in human neutrophils by phorbol myristate actate, Fed. Proc., 45:4049A.

19. Channon, J.Y., Leslie, C.C., and Johnston, R.B., Jr., Zymosan-stimulated production of phosphatidic acid by macrophages: relationship to release of superoxide anion and inhibition by agents that increase intracellular cyclic AMP, J. Leukocyte Biol., in press

20. Edwards, C.K., III, Hedegaard, H.B., Zlotnik, A., Gangadharam, P.R., Johnston, R.B., Jr., and Pabst, M.J., 1986, Chronic infection due to Mycobacterium intracellulare in mice: association with macrophage release of prostaglandin E_2 and reversal by injection of indomethacin, muramyl dipeptide, or interferon-γ, J. Immunol., 136:1820.

21. Allison, A.C., 1984, Role of macrophage activation in the pathogenesis of chronic inflammation and its pharmacological control, Adv. Inflam. Res., 7:201.

22. Mason, U.G., III, Greenberg, L.E., Yen, S.Y., and Kirkpatrick, C.H., 1982, Indomethacin-responsive mononuclear cell dysfunction in "atypical" mycobacteriosis. Cell. Immunol., 71:54.

FLOW CYTOMETRIC ANALYSIS OF OXIDASE ACTIVITY OF NEUTROPHILS FROM CHRONIC GRANULOMATOUS DISEASE PATIENTS

Nassef F. Hassan[1], Donald E. Campbell[2], and Steven D. Douglas[1]

[1]Division of Allergy-Immunology, Department of Pediatrics, University of Pennsylvania School of Medicine, The Joseph Stokes, Jr. Research Institute and the [2]Clinical Immunology Laboratory, Children's Hospital of Philadelphia, Philadelphia, PA 19104

INTRODUCTION

Phagocyte cells, neutrophils and macrophages constitute the main defense mechanisms of the human body against invading microorganisms. The bactericidal activity of polymorphonuclear leukocytes (PMNs) involves the activation of a cell membrane associated NADPH oxidase enzyme[1]. Following activation of the NADPH oxidase enzyme, a cascade of oxidation/reduction reactions occurs, with the generation of several oxygen radicals. Superoxide (O_2^-) hydrogen peroxide (H_2O_2), hydroxyl radical (HO) singlet oxygen ($\dot{O}$) are the main oxygen by-products of the respiratory burst of PMNs[2] and have an important role in killing of bacteria. The enzyme NADPH oxidase has a major function in the generation of O_2^- radical while other enzymes including superoxide dismutase[3], myeloperoxidase[4], catalase and glutathione peroxidase[5] serve a regulatory activity in the respiratory burst. NADPH oxidase differs from other cellular oxidase enzymes (i.e., mitochondrial), since it is a cyanide insensitive enzyme[6]. The activation of the NADPH oxidase enzyme with different soluble stimulants as phorbol esters[7], formyl-methionyl-leucyl-phenylalanine[8] and γ-hexachlorocyclohexane[9] results in the generation of active oxygen radicals and mimics the biochemical events which occur during phagocytosis _in vivo_.

Several diseases have been described with a partial or complete defect in respiratory burst. Chronic granulomatous disease (CGD)[10,11] described 30 years ago is a disorder with an aberrant NADPH oxidase enzyme in phagocyte cells. The most common form of CGD inheritance is the X-linked form; however, autosomal inheritance has also been described[10]. Chronic granulomatous disease is usually characterized clinically by recurrent, life-threatening infections, granuloma formation, hepatosplenomegaly, generalized lymphadenopathy, anemia and hypergammaglobulinemia. Neutrophils from CGD patients do not generate any detectable O_2^- or H_2O_2 or show any bactericidal activity.

Recently, Bass, et.al.[12,13] developed a sensitive assay for evaluation of the oxidase burst of PMNs using single cell analysis by flow cytometry in the presence of dichlorofluorescin diacetate (DCFH-DA). 2'-7'-dichlorofluorescin diacetate is a non-fluorescent, stable, non-polar compound that can diffuse through PMNs cell membranes. Intracellularly, the acetyl groups are cleaved from the compound by cytosolic enzymes and the polar DCFH is trapped within the cell. DCFH (non-fluorescent) is rapidly oxidized to the highly fluorescent 2',7'-dichlorofluorescein by hydrogen peroxide upon the stimulation of the respiratory burst. Using single cell analysis by flow cytometry to monitor intracellular DCFH oxidation in PMNs, a quantitative assessment of the respiratory burst in individual cells was performed. DCFH oxidation by stimulated PMNs from a heterozygous and a CGD patient were evaluated. Furthermore, the effect of the metabolic inhibitor, potassium cyanide on shunt activity was studied.

MATERIALS

Reagents

Phorbol myristate acetate (PMA), formyl methionyl leucyl phenylalanine (FMLP), nitroblue tetrazolium dye and γ-hexachlorocyclohexane (HCCH) were obtained from Sigma Chemicals (St. Louis, MO). Sodium cyanide was purchased from Fisher Scientific (Fair Lawn, NJ). Phosphate-buffered saline (PBS) was obtained from GIBCO (Grand Island, NY) and RBC lysing reagent was obtained from Ortho Diagnostic Systems (Raritan, NJ). 2'7-dichlorofluorescin diacetate (DCFH-DA) was purchased from Eastman Kodak (Rochester, NY).

DCFH-DA and PMA were dissolved in ethanol and acetone concentrations of 10mM and 1 mg/ml, while FMLP and HCCH were dissolved in dimethyl sulfoxide and dimethyl formamide at 10mM and 20mM, respectively.

Flow cytometric assay of dichlorofluorescin (DCFH) oxidation by PMNs

Blood was collected in EDTA from normal volunteers and patients with CGD. Evaluations were performed on whole blood, a technique performed in our study in order to minimize preactivation of PMNs that occurs with the more time consuming and complex purification techniques. To a 100μl aliquot of blood 2 ml lysing buffer was added. Cells were then washed with PBS and resuspended in 100μl PBS, followed by the addition of 100μl of DCFH-DA in PBS (final concentrations 5μM), and incubated for 15 min. at 37°C. PBS or potassium cyanide (final concentration 1 mM) were then added to the reaction mixture to yield a volume of 0.9 ml. After temperature equilibration, 100μl of PMA (100ng), FMLP (10^{-7}M), HCCH (200μM) or PBS were added to reaction mixture. Cell preparations were then incubated for 15 minutes at 37°C, and evaluated immediately by flow cytometric analysis (EPICS C, Coulter Inc.). Individual PMNs were identified by the combination of forward and right angle light scatter and aggregated cells and other cell types (lymphocytes, monocytes and erythrocytes) were excluded from analysis. Fluorescence intensity data was expressed as the mean of the logarithm of green fluorescence (LGFL).

Table 1. Intracellular DCFH Oxidation by Neutrophils from a Normal Donor and a Patient with CGD which were stimulated with Phorbol myristate acetate, N-formyl methionyl leucyl phenylalanine and γ-hexachlorocyclohexane in the Presence and Absence of Cyanide (1mM)

	Mean Fluorescence Intensity*						
	Resting	Resting(CN)	PMA	PMA(CN)	FMLP	FMLP(CN)	HCCH
Cells							
PMNs(control)	12.30	29.94	93.60	132.12	52.85	121.15	113.39
PMNs(patient)	20.58	29.00	29.57	63.44	38.33	71.33	60.77

*mean fluorescence intensity values presented are representative of individual experiment.

DCFH oxidation by stimulated CGD PMNs

PMNs from a CGD patient (previously shown to lack bactericidal activity, NBT[14] and ferricytochrome C reduction) and normal adults were analyzed in the presence or absence of KCN (1mM) (Table 1). CGD PMNs demonstrate significant intracellular DCFH oxidation (approximately 30% of control) upon stimulation. Furthermore, a significant increase in DCFH oxidation was achieved upon addition of CN for both patient and control. The oxidation of DCFH in CGD PMNs was also detected upon activation of cells with other soluble stimulants as FMLP or HCCH (Table I). A significant increase in DCFH oxidation by FMLP-stimulated PMNs, occurs in the presence of KCN (1mM).

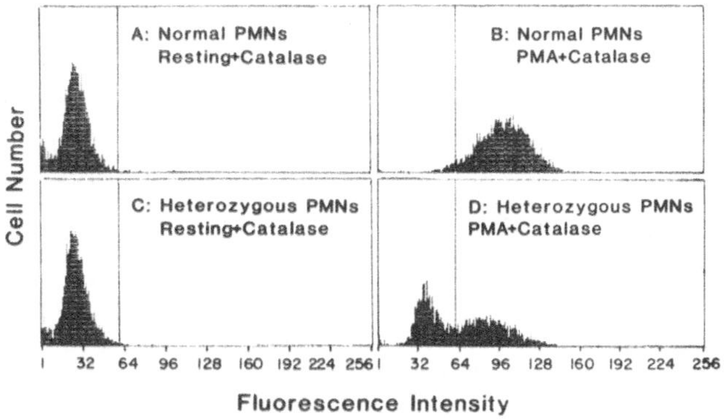

Figure 1. Flow cytometric fluorescence histogram of PMNS from a normal donor (A,B) and CGD carrier (C,D), in the presence of catalase (2.1mg/ml). Catalase was added to reaction mixtures (B,D) prior to PMA stimulation. Fluorescence intensity is plotted on the abscissa and cell number on the ordinate. All histograms illustrate a negative fluorescence cutoff at channel 60, which was established with resting control PMNs (A). Cells with fluorescence greater than channel 60 were recorded as positive fluorescence. PMA stimulation produced 96% positive cells for the control (B) and 50% positive cells for the heterozygous carrier (D).

DCFH oxidation by stimulated heterozygous CGD PMNs

PMNs from an X-linked obligate heterozygous carrier of CGD were analyzed by a qualitative NBT reduction test[15,16] and the DCFH oxidation test. Flow cytometric evaluation of PMA stimulated PMNs from a heterozygous mother of the CGD patient reveal two distinct populations of cells (Figure 1). One population, has a fluorescence intensity comparable to control PMNs, and represents 50% of the total PMN distribution. The second population is characterized by a level of fluorescence intensity similar to that obtained with CGD PMNs. The qualitative NBT test, which was performed in parallel, revealed NBT reduction in 52% of the PMNs. Thus, the DCFH oxidation test generates quantitative data which was previously restricted to the histochemical NBT test, in accurately identifying the carrier state in CGD.

DISCUSSION

Oxygen radicals generated from activated polymorphonuclear leukocytes have been thoroughly studied during the last decade. Several techniques have been used to measure different oxygen by-products, namely nitroblue tetrazolium reduction[17], superoxide dismutase inhibitable ferricytochrome C reduction[18] and O-phenylenediamine oxidation[19] for the assessment of O_2^- generation; scopoletin[20] and homovanilic acid[21] oxidation for the measurement of H_2O_2 generation. Bass, et.al.[12,13] recently described a more sensitive fluorescent test to assess intracellular H_2O_2 generation by activated PMNs. The technique offers several advantages over standard tests, the most obvious being the ability to quantitatively examine characteristics of large numbers of individual cells rather than measure mean responses of the total population which is achieved through the single cell analysis by flow cytometry.

Since only a small volume of blood is available for analysis from children, a modification in the DCFH fluorescent technique has been developed. The use of whole blood after lysis of RBCs offers advantages over standard PMN purification techniques. Beside the ability to analyze small aliquots of blood, the processing of blood samples in five minutes prevents preactivation of PMNs that occur with the more time consuming purification techniques.

Moreover, the specificity of DCFH oxidation of H_2O_2 generated from the respiratory burst was studied by including cyanide in reaction mixtures which produced an enhancement of DCFH oxidation[22] (Table I). It is likely that such enhancement is due to inhibition of cyanide sensitive scavengers of H_2O_2, namely, myeloperoxidase and catalase enzymes. Polymorphonuclear leukocytes from CGD patients oxidize DCFH upon its stimulation with phorbol myristate acetate, formyl methionyl leucyl phenylalanine and γ-hexachlorocyclohexane (Table I). The presence of cyanide (1mM) in the reaction mixtures enhancing DCFH oxidation indicates that cyanide sensitive mitochondrial oxidases are not involved in DCFH oxidation. Moreover, the uninduced hematopoietic cell line U-937, stimulated with PMA does not oxidize DCFH since the cell line lacks expression of the NADPH oxidase enzyme. With the induction of differentiation and expression of NADPH oxidase, however, PMA stimulated U937 cells oxidize DCFH with an increase in fluorescence intensity in the presence of cyanide[22].

Moreover, flow cytometric analysis of PMA stimulated PMNs from a CGD heterozygote demonstrate two populations of cells (Figure 1). One population (50%) is similar to PMA stimulated CGD cells while the other (50%) are comparable to PMA stimulated control PMNs.

Our study has shown that DCFH oxidation in stimulated CGD PMNs is mediated by a cyanide insensitive oxidase enzyme. The activation of this enzyme through three different soluble stimulants leads to hydrogen peroxide generation. The nature of this oxidase enzyme and its possible functional role in bactericidal activity in CGD neutrophils is not known.

ACKNOWLEDGEMENT

We thank Shree Lighty for her expert secretarial assistance. This work was supported in part by Grants HL-27068 and NS-17752 from the National Institutes of Health.

REFERENCES

1. B.M. Babior, J.T. Curnutte, and R.S. Kipnes, Pyridine nucleotide-dependent superoxide production by a cell-free system from human granulocytes, J. Clin. Invest., 56:1035, 1975.
2. D.P. Clifford and J.E. Repine, Measurement of oxidizing radicals by polymorphonuclear leukocytes, Meth. in Enzymol., 105:393, 1984.
3. I. Fridovich, Superoxide radical and superoxide dismutase, Accts. Chem. Res., 5:321, 1972.
4. S.J. Klebanoff and C.B. Hamon, Role of myeloperoxidase-mediated antimicrobial systems in intact leukocytes, J. Reticuloendothel. Soc., 12:170, 1972.
5. P.C. Hinkle, R.A. Butow, E. Racker, and B. Chance, Partial resolution of the enzymes catalyzing oxidative phosphorylation, J. Biol. Chem., 242:5169, 1967.
6. A.J. Sbarra and M.L. Karnovsky, The biochemical basis of phagocytosis. I: Metabolic changes during the ingestion of particles by polymorphonuclear leukocytes, J. Biol. Chem., 234:1355, 1959.
7. J.E. Repine, J.G. White, and C.C. Clanson, and B.M. Holmes, The influence of phorbol myristate acetate on oxygen consumption by polymorphonuclear leukocyte, J. Lab. Clin. Med., 83:911, 1974.
8. C.E. McCall, D.A. Bass, L.R. DeChatelet, A.R. Link, Jr., and M. Mann, In vitro responses of human neutrophils to N-formyl-methionyl-leucyl-phenylalanine: correlation with effects of acute bacterial infection, J. Infect. Dis., 140:277, 1979.
9. D.B. Kuhns, S.S. Kaplan, and R.E. Basford, Hexachlorocyclohexanes, potent stimuli of O_2^- production and calcium release in human polymorphonuclear leukocytes, Blood, 68:535, 1986.
10. A.I Tauber, N. Borregaard, E. Simons, and J. Wright, Chronic granulomatous disease: a syndrome of phagocyte oxidase deficiencies, Medicine, 62:286, 1983.
11. J.I. Gallin, E.S. Buescher, B.E. Seligmann, J. Nath, T. Gaither, and P. Katz, Recent advances in chronic granulomatous disease, Ann. Int. Med., 99:657, 1983.
12. D.A. Bass, J.W. Parce, L.R. DeChatelet, P. Szejda, M.C. Seeds, and M. Thomas, Flow cytometric studies of oxidative product formation by neutrophils: A graded response to membrane stimulation, J. Immunol., 130:1910, 1983.
13. D.A. Bass, P. Olbrantz, P. Szejda, M.C. Seeds, and C.E. McCall, Subpopulations of neutrophils with increased oxidative product formation in blood of patients with infection, J. Immunol., 136:860, 1986.
14. S.D. Douglas, Metabolic and immunologic studies of phagocytes with abnormal bactericidal function, 1973, pp. 392-398, in: Erythrocytes Thrombocytes Leukocytes, E. Gerlach, K. Moser, E. Deutsch, W. Wilmanns, ed., Georg Thieme, Stuttgart.
15. H.D. Ochs and R.P. Igo, The NBT slide test: a simple screening method for detecting chronic granulomatous disease and female carriers, J. Pediatrics, 83:77, 1973.
16. R.B. Johnston III, R.J. Harbeck, and R.B. Johnston, Jr., Recurrent severe infections in a girl with apparently variable expression of mosaicism for chronic granulomatous disease, J. Pediatrics, 106:50 1985.
17. R.L. Baehner and D.G. Nathan, Quantitative nitroblue tetrazolium test in chronic granulomatous disease, N. Engl. J. Med., 278:971, 1968.
18. M.L. Salin and J.M. McCord, Superoxide dismutase in polymorphonuclear leukocytes, J. Clin. Invest., 54:1005, 1974.
19. N.F. Hassan, D.E. Campbell, and S.D. Douglas, O-phenylenediamine oxidation by phorbol myristate acetate stimulated human polymorphonuclear leukocytes: Characterization of two distinct oxidative mechanisms, Clin. Imm. Immunopathol, In press.

20. R.K. Root, J. Metcalf, N. Oshino, and B. Chance, H_2O_2 release from human granulocytes during phagocytosis, J. Clin. Invest., 55:945, 1975.
21. W. Ruch, P.H. Cooper, and M. Gaggiolini, Assay of H_2O_2 production by macrophages and neutrophils with homovanilic acid and horse radish peroxidase, J. Immunol. Meth., 63:347, 1983.
22. N.F. Hassan, D.E. Campbell, and S.D. Douglas, Phorbol myristate acetate induced oxidation of 2'7-dichlorofluorescin by neutrophils from patients with chronic granulomatous disease (submitted).

A MUTATION IN SALMONELLA TYPHIMURIUM THAT ENHANCES RESISTANCE TO OXYGEN-INDEPENDENT ANTIMICROBAL NEUTROPHIL PROTEIN

John K. Spitznagel

Department of Microbiology and Immunology
Emory University
Atlanta, Georgia 30322 USA

INTRODUCTION

Our experience with the cationic antimicrobial proteins (CAPs) of human neutrophil leukocytes and the experiences of other investigators have led us to believe that resistance to them in *Salmonella typhimurium* is under the control of at least two distinct genes or clusters of genes. We think the matter of importance for, although these bacteria can survive intracellularly in neutrophils, the basis for their capacity to survive is poorly understood. Perhaps enhanced understanding of the *in vitro* resistance of *Salmonella* to the CAPs will shed light on *Salmonella* strategies for intracellular survival.

It is known that *Salmonella* at risk of being killed by neutrophils potentially have two defensive strategies. They can avoid being phagocytized or they can foil neutrophil microbicidal mechanisms after being phagocytized. To a substantial degree the *Salmonella* O antigen serves both purposes. It is antiphagocytic, but it also inhibits intracellular killing (Okamura and Spitznagel, 1982).

What is responsible for the complex process of intracellular killing (Table 1) (Spitznagel, 1984)? We now recognize two mechanisms, each involving several mediators. One of these, the oxygen-independent killing mechanism, functions whether oxygen is present in the neutrophil or not. The other mechanism, the oxygen-dependent mechanism, only functions in the presence of molecular oxygen and essential reducing enzymes. This paper focuses on mechanisms of oxygen-independent killing. Then we will consider genetic controls of microbial resistance to them, controls with which bacterial cells might resist killing after being phagocytized by neutrophils.

Table 1. Intraphagosomal Killing Systems

O_2 Independent
O_2 Dependent

Table 2
Antimicrobial Mechanisms of PMN
Independent of O_2

Hydrogen ion shift
Organic acids
Lysozyme
Lactoferrin
Cationic proteins

Oxygen-independent antimicrobial action (Spitznagel, 1984) is mediated by several things (Table 2): low pH, low molecular weight fatty acids, and several antimicrobial proteins distinctly different from each other and yet associated with the granules of the neutrophil. Convincing evidence for the importance of the cationic proteins in this process is steadily growing (Hirsch, 1956a; Hovde and Gray, 1986; Modzrakowski et al, 1979; Odeberg and Olsson, 1975; Shafer et al, 1984; Skarnes and Watson, 1956; Spitznagel and Chi, 1963; Weiss et al, 1978; Zeya and Spitznagel, 1963; Zeya and Spitznagel, 1968). Clearly, Salmonella that find themselves in the phagolysosomes of neutrophils would need to be

Table 3
The 57KD cationic antimicrobial protein
CAP57 has a defined range of activity

Resistance or sensitivity of gram-negative bacteria	%[a] Survival at pH	
	5.5	7.5
Sensitive		
Acinetobacter lwoffii	34	80
Escherichia coli	4	60
Neisseria gonorrhoeae	38	53
Pseudomonas aeruginosa	36	100
Pseudomonas cepacia	39	72
Salmonella typhi	14	40
Salmonella typhimurium (LT-2)	42	93
Shigella sonnei	29	82
Resistant		
Proteus mirabilis	100	95
Proteus vulgaris	100	99
Serratia marcescens	100	100
Bacillus subtilis	100	100
Staphylococcus aureus (Wood)	100	100
Staphylococcus epidermidis	100	92
Streptoococcus pneumoniae	98	98
Streptococcus pyogenes	100	98

a % bacteria surviving after one hour of 5 ug CAP57/ml.

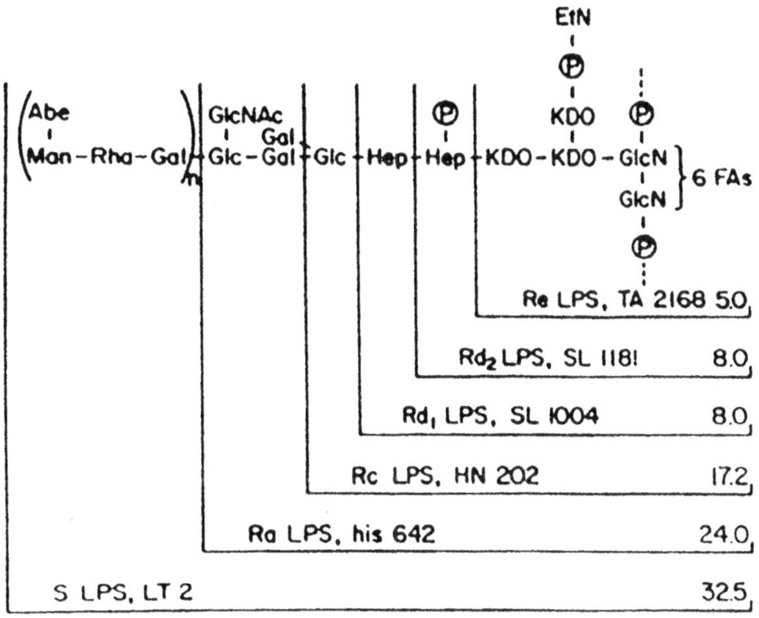

Fig. 1. Relation of LPS chemotype to resistance to CAP. LPS chemotypes (Ra, Rc, Rd_1, Rd_2, Re) of Salmonella typhimurium LT2 and its OM mutants (his642, HN202, SL1004, SL1181, TA2168) were used in these experiments. The numbers to the right of the figure indicate the concentration per milliliter of azurophil granule protein required to kill 50% of a standard inoculum of Salmonella typhimurium and several OM mutants in 60 min. Abe, Abequose; Man, mannose; Rha, rhamnose; Gal, galactose; GlcNac, N-acetylglucosamine; Glc, glucose; Hep, heptose; EtN, ethanolamine; KDO, ketodeoxyoctonate; GlcN, glucosamine; P, phosphate.

able to deal with many of these mediators. Since our own work on antimicrobial resistance mechanisms has been greatly concerned with one such protein, which we call CAP57, this is what I shall discuss here.

CAP57 is bactericidal for a considerable spectrum of gram-negative bacteria (Table 3): Salmonella, Escherichia coli, Neisseria, Pseudomonas, etc. However, CAP57 has different minimal inhibitory concentrations for different species and for different strains of the same species. What are the determinants of resistance?

It has long been known that smooth Salmonella and related species lose their resistance to CAPs as these bacteria mutate to roughness. In Figure 1 you can see the relationship of the percent of bacteria killed by various concentrations of crude granule protein in relation to the chemotype of the Salmonella lipopolysaccharide (from Okamura and Spitznagel, 1982). As the bacteria lose first their O-side chains and then their core polysaccharides, they become less and less able to resist CAP. This phenotypic behavior defines certain gene clusters as influential in this form of antimicrobial resistance. They include the rfa and rfb gene clusters, which map at 79 and 42 minutes, respectively.

Since they direct the synthesis of these outer membrane polysaccharide antigens, they control one form of resistance to CAPs. The mutant alleles are rough and have lower antimicrobial resistance. They would not be expected to enhance the survival of Salmonella in neutrophils. Reversion to smooth chemotypes tends to increase antimicrobial resistance in the rough mutants.

Are there any mutations that can increase the resistance of Salmonella to CAP57? Recently, Bill Shafer (1983) discovered that the pmrA mutation, described and mapped by Makela et al. (1978) at 94 minutes, increases resistance of the pmrA mutant to polymyxin B in rough Salmonella. The pmrA allele also enables these rough forms, which are usually less resistant to CAP57 than the wild-type parents, to gain substantial resistance to it. In other words, Shafer found the pmrA strains were cross resistant to CAP57 and polymyxin B (Shafer et al, 1983). Figure 2 shows the kinetics of killing of SH9178, a normally resistant strain of Salmonella, and SH7426, a pmrA mutant hyperresistant to polymyxin B. The abscissa shows the concentrations of CAP57 used and the ordinate shows the percentage of bacteria killed. The 50% effective concentration is higher with the pmrA mutant.

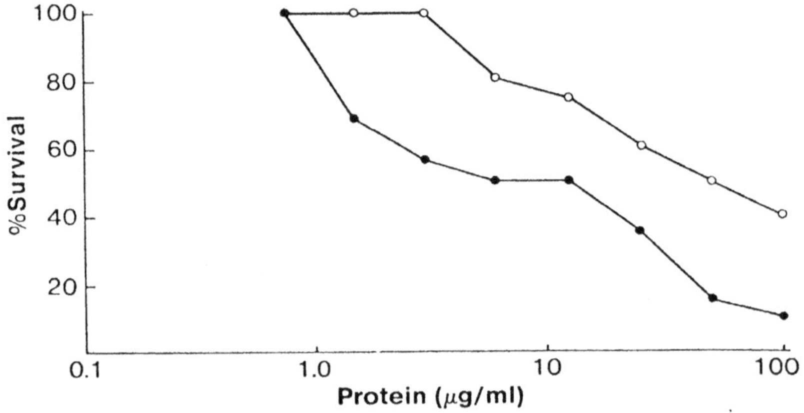

Fig. 2. Salmonella typhimurium resistance to CAP57 is enhanced by the pmrA mutation. O---O depicts concentration dependence for killing SH7426 rfaJ pmrA 163 (R471a); LD_{50}, ca. 10 ug/ml. ●---● depicts concentration dependence for killing SH9178 rfaJ4041(R471a); LD_{50}, ca. 3 ug/ml.

To better understand the effects of the mutation, we studied the binding of iodinated (but still biologically active) CAP57 to the pmrA mutant SH7426 and to the parent SH9178. Constant amounts of iodinated CAP57 were added in the presence of increasing excess of cold CAP57. The results (not shown) revealed that the pmrA mutant bound substantially less iodinated protein. Moreover, the binding with both organisms was saturable, suggesting that it was specific. Degree of binding correlated with killing capacity of CAP57 for the bacteria.

These results raised several questions. Could a mutation to CAP resistance appear spontaneously in Salmonella? What might be the frequency of the spontaneous mutations? Would the mutation be expressed in smooth organisms? Where would the mutation map? We thought that if such events could happen with fair frequency they might have some bearing on pathogenesis. At the very least, we might find out something more about how CAP kill Salmonella. Because polymyxin is readily available and cheap we decided to select for spontaneous mutations to resistance to polymyxin B. Then, we planned to examine such mutants for their resistance to CAPs. Mutations with cross resistance to CAPs were to be mapped and then the nature of the genes characterized.

We found that spontaneous mutants appeared in populations of LT-2 with a frequency of about 10^{-7} (see Table 4). We then proceeded to characterize several of these mutants (Table 5). As you can see, the MIC for polymyxin B increased two- to fourfold for several of the mutants, compared to the MIC for LT-2. It increased from four- to almost sixtyfold when compared with the Rb chemotype 9178. Comparable increases were found in the MICs for CAP 57 (not shown). The sensitivity of all of the mutants to phage P22 showed that the mutants were still fully smooth. The electrophoretic behavior of their LPS was identical with the LPS of LT-2 (not shown). In addition, Monica Farley also compared saturable binding of CAP57 with the mutant JKS5 and the parent LT-2. The mutation to resistance resulted in a definite reduction in

Table 4
Frequency of Spontaneous Mutation to Pb^r

	Polymyxin b[a] (ug/ml)					
Cells Plated	0	1	2	4	8	16
3×10^7	--	CG[b]	CG	1.1[c]	.28	.15
3×10^6	--	CG	29	1.5	.33	.15
3×10^5	--	CG	30	0	1.5	0
3×10^2	289	--	--	--	--	--

[a] ug/ml of LB agar
[b] Confluent growth
[c] Colonies X 10^{-6} cells

The spontaneous mutation rate to Pb^r was 3×10^{-7}. An overnight culture of S. typhimurium LT-2 was plated on LB agar. The number of cells plated is shown in the first column. Resistance to polymyxin B was defined as the capacity to grow on $\geq$ 8 ug of polymyxin B per ml LB agar.

binding. The binding was saturable (data not shown). We found that overall the smooth Salmonella bound less protein than the rough ones. However, even in LT-2 the mutation to polymyxin B resistance and CAP57 resistance correlated with a decrease in binding.

We have begun experiments with mapping. For this purpose we have constructed two generalized transducing phages F4 and D7 with P22(HT) int^-. These bacteriophage were prepared with standard techniques (Davis et al., 1980). F4 transduces a Tn10 transposon inserted near the mutation of interest, which we tentatively call gapA (granule antibacterial protein). It cotransduces LT-2 to Tet^rPb^r at a rate of 48%. D7 has the Tn10 inserted near $gapA^+$. It cotranduces JKS5 (Table 5) to Tet^rPb^r with a frequency of 90%.

Table 5
Properties of Spontaneous Mutants with Pb^r Phenotype

Strain	Polymyxin B (ug/ml)	MIC Granule Protein (ug/ml)	P22 Sensitive	Remarks
JKS0001	50	95	Yes	Spon taneous mutant of LT-2
JKS0002	50	80	Yes	"
JKS0003	12.5	52	Yes	"
JKS0004	25.0	57	Yes	"
JKS0005	50.0	>100	Yes	"
JKS0007	50	40	Yes	"
LT-2 WT	12	25	Yes	---
SH9178	3	5	No	Rb chemo-type LPS LT-2 mutant

We have transduced several Hfrs (obtained from Dr. Kenneth Sanderson) and performed both interrupted and uninterrupted matings (Figure 3). Interrupted and uninterrupted matings were done as described in Miller (1972). The figure shows the results of interrupted matings done with HfrKA and HfrK17. The recombinants were selected on tetracycline and counterselection was done against the auxotrophy of the donor. HfrKA inserts clockwise and HfrK15 inserts counterclockwise. As shown in Figure 3, the Tn10 entered the recipient at 98 minutes from HfrKA and at 3 minutes from HfrK17. We are making further efforts to refine this mapping so we can proceed to characterize the gene.

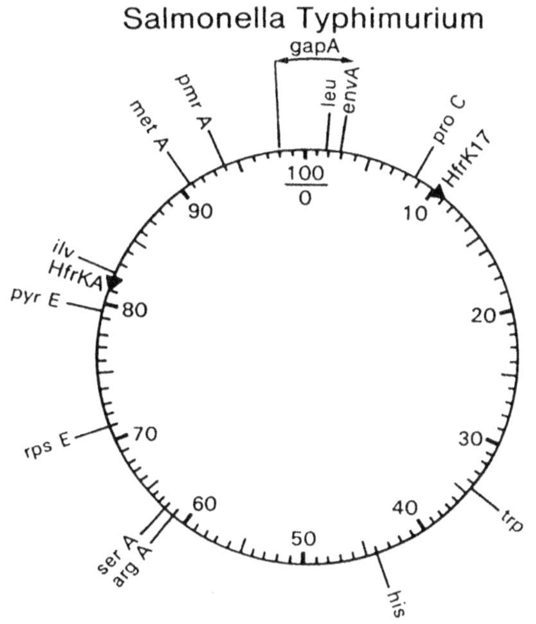

Fig. 3. The tentative location of gapA on the Salmonella chromosome lies within a region, represented here as an arc, extending clockwise from 98 min to 3 min. We use gapA to signify the locus for a mutant allele with phenotype Pb^r and $CAP57^r$ because the locus maps away from the pmrA locus established by Makela (1978). Shown by arrowheads are the points of origin and direction of transfer of two Hfr strains transduced to Tet^rPb^r with phage F4 and used for conjugal mapping. The markers for envA and pmrA are shown, as are the auxotrophic mutations of F^- strain SA1145, which we used as recipient in these crosses. Recombinants were selected on LB agar with tetracycline and streptomycin. Uninterrupted matings (gradient of transfer) led to similar results.

DISCUSSION

What are the possible explanations for the Pb^rCAP57^r phenotypes of these mutants? Polymyxin B is cationic, as shown in Figure 4, and it has a hydrophobic tail. CAP57 has a relatively high concentration of basic amino acids, suggesting it is also cationic (Table 6). It is also relatively hydrophobic due to its hydrophobic amino acids. It is reasonable to suppose the cationic groups of Pb or CAP57 bind to anionic substituents on the microbial outer surface, bringing the hydrophobic parts of Pb or CAP57 close enough to intercalate into the hydrophobic domains of the outer membrane.

What might these anionic substituents be on microbial surfaces? They could be the 4' phosphates of the lipid A or they could be the phosphates in the 1' position.

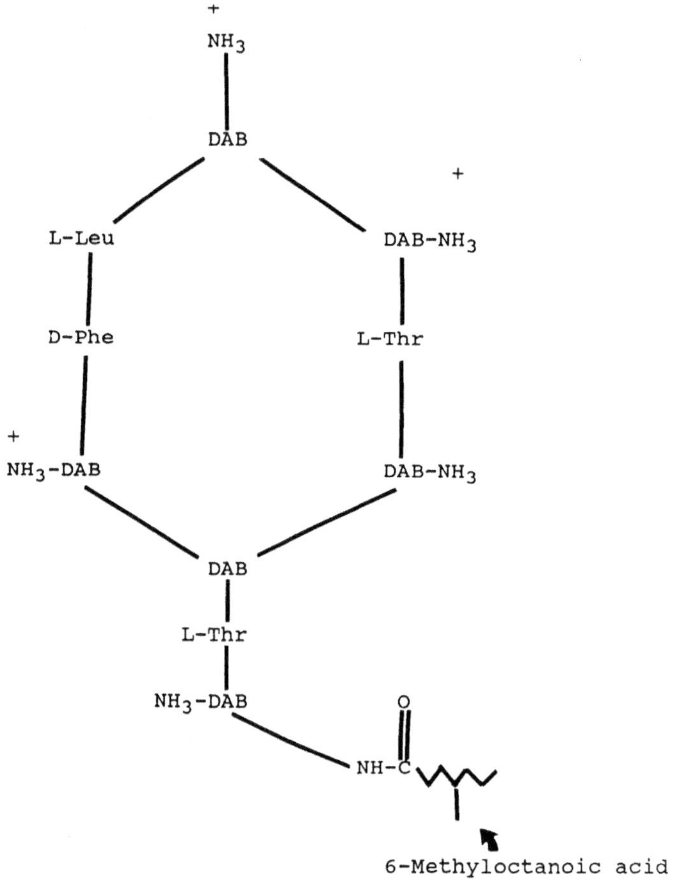

Fig. 4. Structure of polymyxin B. The molecule comprises a hydrophilic, strongly cationic head group that is a cyclic peptide of L-leucine (L-Leu), L-threonine (L-thr), and diaminobutyric acid (DAB), and a hydrophobic tail (indicated by the wavy line) that is 6-methyl octanoic acid. The other polymyxins have different hydrophobic tail groups (not shown).

Table 6. Amino acid compositions of CAPs[a] from human neutrophil granules compared with those of human lysozyme[b] and cathepsin G[b].

	Amino Acids of Antimicrobial Proteins			
	57 Kd CAP	37 Kd CAP	Lysozyme	Cathepsin G
Nonpolar	51%	50%	35%	37%
Positively charged	15.8%	15.2%	13.9%	18%

a We have studied two CAPs in detail. CAP57 is the subject of this paper. However, CAP37, also a potent antimicrobial agent, is shown here for comparison.

b These are also components of neutrophil granules.

This notion was suggested by the work of Vaara and his colleagues (1981) who found that polymyxin B-sensitive strains of Salmonella typhimurium have less than 20% of their lipid A 4' phosphates blocked with 4-amino-arabinose. Thus, 80% or more of these phosphates bear two negative charges. Substitution with 4-amino-arabinose converts the $PO_4^{=}$ groups to Zwitterions, resulting in fewer negative charges. In contrast to the Pb-sensitive strains, the polymyxin B-resistant pmrA mutants have 100% of their lipid A 4' phosphates blocked. It is also important that the 1' phosphates of lipid A tend to show more extensive substitution with ethanolanine in the pmrA mutants. This would also tend to reduce the anionic charges due to these phosphates. Clearly, the biochemistry of our gapA mutants must be compared with that of their gapA$^+$ isogenic parents before we can do more than speculate on these interactions.

CONCLUSIONS

Smooth Salmonella do mutate to cross resistance to polymyxin B and CAP57. They do this with a frequency of 10^{-7}. The mutation in JKS5 is tentatively mapped between 98 and 3 minutes. Resistance is associated with reduced binding of the CAP57 protein, compared to the binding of the pmrA$^+$ parent. The binding is, however, saturable with both strains.

REFERENCES

Davis RW, Botstein D, Roth JR (1980) Advanced Bacterial Genetics. Cold Spring Harbor Laboratory, Cold Spring Harbor, New York

Ganz T, Selsted ME, Szklarek D, Harwig SS, Daher D, Bainton DF, Lehrer RI (1985) J Clin Invest 76:1427-1435

Hirsch JG (1956a) Phagocytin: A bactericidal substance from polymorphonuclear leukocytes. J Exp Med 103:589-611

Hovde CJ, Gray BH (1986) Characterization of a protein from normal human polymorphonuclear leukocytes with bactericidal activity against Pseudomonas aeroginosa. Infect Immun 54:142-148

Makela PH, Sarvas M, Calcagno S, Lounatmaa K (1978) Isolation and genetic characterization of polymyxin-resistant mutants of Salmonella. FEMS Microbiol Letters 3:323-326
Makela PH, Stocker BAD (1984) Genetics of lipopolysaccharide, in Handbook of Endotoxin VI, Chemistry of Endotoxin. Rietschel ET (ed) Elsevier Amsterdam, pp 59-119
Miller JH (1972) Experiments in Molecular Genetics. Cold Spring Harbor Laboratory, Cold Spring Harbor, New York
Modzrakowski MC, Cooney MH, Martin LE, Spitznagel JK (1979) Bactericidal activity of fractionated granule contents from human polymorphonuclear leukocytes. Infect Immun 23:587-590
Odeberg H, Olsson I (1975) Antibacterial activity of cationic proteins from human granulocytes. J Clin Invest 56:1118-1124
Okamura N, Spitznagel JK (1982) Outer membrane mutants of Salmonella typhimurium LT2 have lipopolysaccharide-dependent resistance to the bactericidal activity of an aerobic human neutrophils. Infect Immun 36:1086-1095
Sanderson KE, Ross H, Ziegler L, Makela PH (1972) F^+, Hfr, and F' strains of Salmonella typhimurium and Salmonella abony Bact Rev 36:608-637
Shafer WM, Casey SJ, Spitznagel JK (1983) Lipid A and resistance of Salmonella typhimurium to antimicrobial granule protein of human neutrophil granulocytes. Infect Immun 43:834-838
Shafer WM, Martin LE, Spitznagel JK (1984) Cationic antimicrobial proteins isolated from human neutrophil granulocytes in the presence of diisopropyl fluorophosphate. Infect Immun 45:29-35
Skarnes RC, Watson DW (1956) Characterization of leukin: An antimicrobial factor from leukocytes active against gram-positive pathogens. J Exp Med 104:829-845
Spitznagel JK (1984) Nonoxidative Antimicrobial Reactions of Leukocytes, in Regulation of Leukocyte Function, Snyderman R (ed) Plenum New York and London, pp 284-343
Spitznagel JK, Chi H-Y (1963) Cationic proteins and antibacterial properties of infected tissues and leukocytes. Am J Pathol 43:697-711
Vaara M, Vaara T, Jensen M, Helander I, Nurminen M, Rietschel ET, Makela PH (1981) Characterization of the lipopolysaccharide from the polymyxin-resistant pmrA mutants of Salmonella typhimurium. FEBS Letters 129:145-149
Weiss J, Elsbach P, Olsson I, Odeberg H (1978) Purification and characterization of a potent bactericidal and membrane active protein from the granules of human polymorphonuclear leukocytes. J Biol Chem 253:2664-2672
Zeya HI, Spitznagel JK (1963) Antibacterial and enzymatic basic proteins from leukocyte lysosomes: Separation and identification. Science 142:1085-1087
Zeya HI, Spitznagel JK (1968) Arginine-rich proteins of polymorphonuclear leukocyte lysosomes. Antimicrobial specificity and biochemical heterogeneity. J Exp Med 127:927-941

ACKNOWLEDGMENTS

This work was supported by NIH Grant # AI17662 to JKS and an NIH Training Grant # AI07265. We wish to thank Joy Royer for the preparation of this manuscript.

INTERACTION OF LEGIONELLA PNEUMOPHILA WITH PERITONEAL MACROPHAGES FROM VARIOUS MOUSE STRAINS

Yoshimasa Yamamoto, Thomas W. Klein, Catherine A. Newton, and Herman Friedman

University of South Florida, College of Medicine
Tampa, FL 33612

INTRODUCTION

Legionella pneumophila (Lp) is a facultative intracellular bacterium which causes legionellosis in humans. This bacterium replicates well in cultures of human and guinea pig mononuclear phagocytes (1,2), and infections caused by these organisms appear to correlate with the host's cellular immune system (3). In this regard, the importance of mononuclear phagocytes in legionellosis has been suggested by a number of investigators (4,5,6). Guinea pigs are susceptible to infection with Lp and have been widely used as an animal model for legionellosis (7). Although the mouse has been found highly useful for studying infection and immunity to a variety of bacteria, this animal species appears to be relatively resistant to Lp infection (7). Moreover, it has been reported that Lp is markedly restricted in peritoneal macrophages obtained from most inbred mouse strains, even at relatively high infectivity ratios (8). Recently, we observed that macrophages from the A/J inbred mouse strain supported the intracellular growth of Lp. In the present study, we report on the permissive nature of A/J macrophages for Lp growth and the possible involvement of permissive cells in host resistance to infection.

MATERIALS AND METHODS

Animal - Inbred female mice, BDF_1, A/J, DBA/2, C3H/HeN, C3H/HeJ, C57BL/6 and BALB/c, were obtained from Jackson Laboratories, Bar Harbor, ME and were 6-8 weeks of age at the initiation of each experiments. All of the animals were housed and cared for according to NIH guidelines.

Bacteria - A virulent strain of Legionella pneumophila, serogroup 1, was obtained at autopsy from a case of fatal legionellosis at Tampa General Hospital and cultured on buffered charcoal yeast extract agar (BCYE), Gibco Laboratories, Madison, WI, exactly as described previously (9). Listeria monocytogenes (Lm) strain EGD and Staphylococcus epidermidis (Se) were cultured on trypticase soy agar (BBL, Cockeysville, MD) for 18 hrs at 37°C. These bacteria were adjusted to a working concentration with a spectrophotometer (620 nm).

Macrophages - Resident macrophages (MPs) were obtained by peritoneal lavage with Hanks' balanced salt solution (HBSS, Gibco) supplemented with 5 units/ml sodium heparin (Wyeth Laboratories, Philadelphia, PA). Elicited peritoneal MPs were obtained 4 days after intraperitoneal (i.p.) injection of thioglycollate broth (TGC, Difco Laboratories, Detroit, MI). Resident and elicited MPs were suspended in RPMI 1640 medium (Gibco) supplemented with 15% heat inactivated fetal calf serum (FCS, Hyclone Laboratories, Logan, UT). MPs were identified by microscopic examination and viability of the cells was determined by the trypan blue dye exclusion method. Elicited populations were 69 to 85% MPs and more than 95% viable. The MP suspensions (10^6 morphologically distinct macrophages per ml) were allowed to adhere to 24-well tissue culture plates (Mark II, Costar, Cambridge, MA) for 2 hrs in 5% CO_2 at 37°C. The resulting cell monolayers were washed with HBSS and then used for experiments.

Infection and Enumeration of Bacteria - For in vitro experiments, MP monolayers (approximately 10^6 cells/well) were infected with $2x10^4$ - $2x10^6$ bacteria for 30 min at 37°C, washed three times with HBSS to remove non-phagocytized bacteria, treated with 1 ml medium (RPMI 1640 supplemented with 15% FCS) and then incubated for various times at 37°C in 5% CO_2. In the cases of Lm and Se, the culture medium was changed several times for the duration of the experiment. The starting point of this incubation represented 0 time. The number of viable bacteria in either MPs lysed (intracellular) with sterile distilled water or in combined MP lysates and culture supernatants, was determined by plate counts. The plates (trypticase soy agar plates or BCYE plates) were incubated at 37°C for 24 hrs in the cases of Lm and Se or 72 hrs in the case of Lp and then counted for colony forming units (CFU). For in vivo experiments, mice were injected i.p. with 3 ml TGC 4 days prior to an i.p. infection with $2.5x10^6$ bacteria. At various times after infection, peritoneal lavages were collected in 4 ml heparinized (5 u/ml) RPMI 1640 medium and allowed to adhere to 24-well tissue culture clusters (1 ml/well). The resulting adherent cell monolayers were washed three times with HBSS and then lysed with 1 ml sterile distilled water. Either a portion (0.2 ml) of lavage fluids combined with 1.8 ml of sterile distilled water or adherent cell lysates were appropriately diluted with HBSS and plated on BCYE plates for enumeration of CFU.

IL-1 Assay - Interleukin 1 (IL-1) content of culture supernatant of MP monolayers stimulated with Lp vaccine (10) or E. coli lipopolysaccharide (LPS, 0111:B4, phenol extract, Difco) was measured by the standard thymocyte proliferation assay using C3H/HeJ mice. Briefly, MP monolayers (10^6 cells/well) were incubated with or without either $3x10^8$ or $1x10^8$ cells of Lp vaccine or 10 ug of LPS for 24 hrs in 5% CO_2 at 37°C. Following incubation, all culture supernatants were filter sterilized and the IL-1 content was measured essentially as previously described (11).

RESULTS

Fate of Lp in elicited peritoneal MPs - Thioglycollate-elicited peritoneal MPs were obtained from BDF_1, A/J, DBA/2, C3H/HeN, C57BL/6, and BALB/c mice and assayed for the ability to promote the growth of Lp. MP monolayers were infected with $1\text{-}2x10^6$ bacteria (infectivity ratio of 1-2 bacteria per MP) and then the number of viable bacteria was measured in the total culture (MP lysates and culture supernatants combined) 2 days after incubation. With the exception of A/J, macrophage populations from all other mouse strains tested markedly restricted the growth of Lp. In MPs from A/J mice, the number of CFU was about 2 logs higher at 48 hrs than at the initiation of culture. However, the initial uptake of Lp by MPs from all inbred strains was about the same (Figure 1).

Figure 2 shows the data concerning the fate of Lp in elicted MP monolayers from A/J mice using different infectivity ratios. Different concentrations of bacteria were added to the MP monolayers resulting in infectivity ratios of 0.02, 0.2, and 2 bacteria per MP. After phagocytosis the cultures were washed and then incubated for 2 days at 37°C. At all infectivity ratios tested, A/J MPs readily supported the growth of Lp (Figure 2.)

Fate of Listeria and Staphylococci in A/J MPs in comparison with other mouse strains - Elicited peritoneal MPs from A/J mice were analyzed for intracellular killing activity of intra-and extracellular pathogens using Listeria monocytogenes and Staphyloccocus epidermidis respectively. The purpose of these experiments was to confirm that A/J MPs had a normal intracellular killing function using the same experimental conditions as for the Lp experiments. Thioglycollate

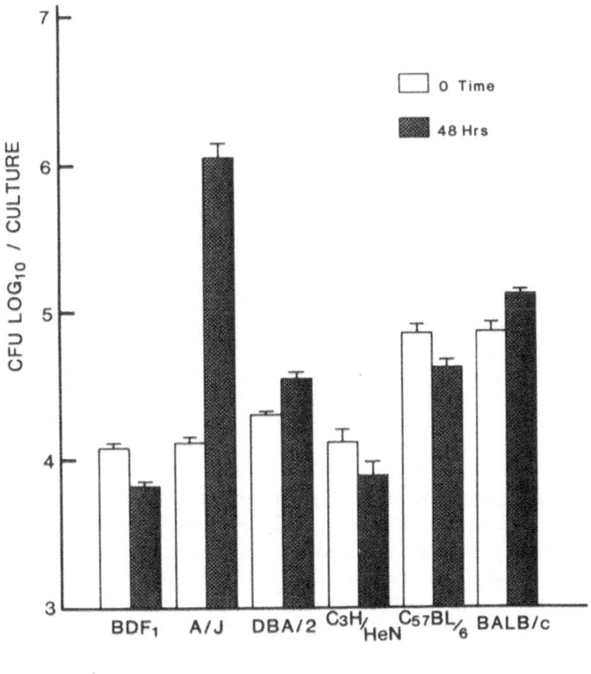

Fig. 1. Fate of Legionella in thiogylcollate-elicited peritoneal macrophage (PEC) cultures from various inbred mouse strains. Macrophage monolayers (approximately 1×10^6 cells/well) were infected with 2×10^6 bacteria for 30 min at 37°C, washed and then incubated for 48 hrs. Each bar represents the mean CFU $\pm$ S.D. of triplicate macrophage cultures.

elicited peritoneal MPs otained from A/J, BDF_1, DBA/2 and C3H/HeN were assessed in regard to their ability to support growth of Listeria, a typical intracellular bacterium. All tested MPs supported the intracellular growth of Listeria (Figure 3). Furthermore, intracellular killing activity of A/J MPs for S. epidermidis was also measured under the same conditions. It was observed (Figure 3) that A/J MPs markedly restricted the growth or killed this organism.

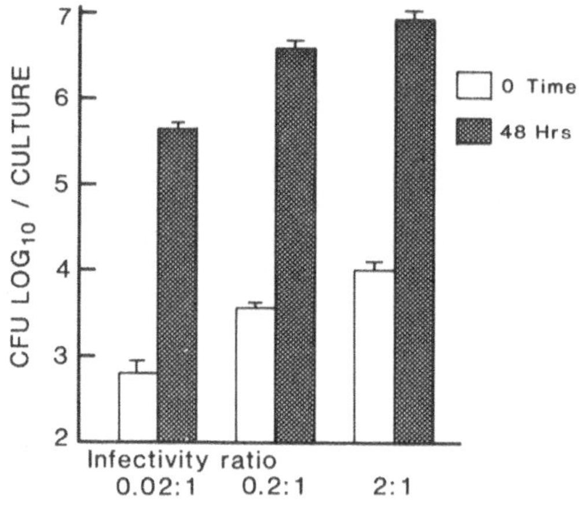

Fig. 2. Fate of Legionella in elicited peritoneal macrophage cultures from A/J mouse at different infectivity ratios. A/J mouse peritoneal eleicited macrophage monolayers (approximately $1x10^6$/well) were infected with $2x10^4$, $2x10^5$, and $2x10^6$ bacteria. Resulting infectivity ratios are 0.02:1, 0.2:1, and 2:1, respectively. Each bar represents the mean CFU $\pm$ S.D. of triplicate macrophage cultures.

IL-1 production by MPs stimulated with Lp vaccine - Elicited peritoneal MPs from four different inbred mouse strains, BALB/c, C57BL/6, A/J and BDF_1, were assessed for production of IL-1 when stimulated with Lp vaccine and E. coli LPS. All tested MPs stimulated with Lp vaccine or E. coli LPS produced in culture supernatants a high proliferation inducing activity (high ^{3}H-TIR uptake, IL-1) on thymocytes (Figure 4).

Growth of Lp in resident MPs - Resident MPs were obtained from eight mice of either A/J or BDF_1 strain. MPs were pulsed with $2x10^6$ bacteria, resulting in an infectivity ratio of 2 bacteria per MP. After 2 days incubation, the number of viable bacteria was measured in combined MP lysates and culture supernatants. Results of these experiments are shown in Fig. 5. Initial uptake of Lp by resident MPs obtained from both strains was almost the same. However, at 2 days after incubation, no viable bacteria were recovered from the cultures of BDF_1 resident MPs. In contrast, in the cultures of A/J resident MPs the number of viable bacteria decreased only slightly.

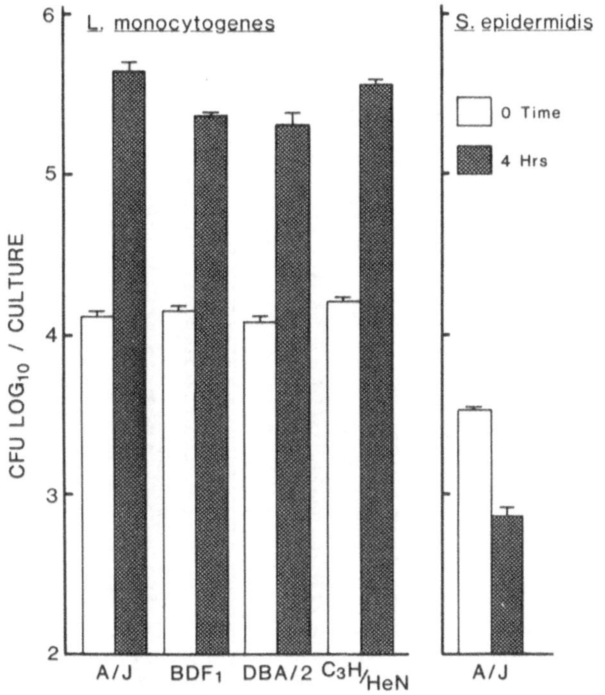

Fig. 3. Intracellular fate of Listeria and Staphylococcus in peritoneal elicited macrophages from various mouse strains. Macrophage monolayers (approximately $1x10^6$ cells/well) were infected with either $1x10^6$ (Listeria) or $2x10^5$ (Staphylococcus) for 30 min, washed and then incubated for 4 hrs at 37^oC in 5% CO_2. Each bar represents the mean CFU $\pm$ S.D. of triplicate macrophage cultures.

Fate of Legionella in peritoneal cavity - In in vivo experiments, A/J and BDF_1 mice were injected i.p. with 3 ml TGC 4 days prior to an i.p. infection with $2.5x10^6$ Lp. The mice were sacrificed at appropriate intervals (30 min, 6, 24 and 48 hrs after infection) and the peritoneal lavage fluids collected and individually analyzed for Legionella CFUs. CFUs in adherent cell lysates (with sterile distilled water) were also determined. Results are shown in Fig. 6. In mice not receiving a prior injection of TGC, there is an early decline in the number of CFUs isolated from the lavage fluids. This decline continues over the next several days in BDF_1 mice as does the decline in CFUs isolated from adherent cells. In A/J mice, however, the number of lavage CFUs appears to level off after the first day in culture and the number of CFUs isolated from A/J adherent cells stays relatively constant throughout the culture period. Fig. 6 also shows that pretreatment of A/J mice with TGC significantly changed the CFU recovery pattern of both lavage and adherent cell preparations to one suggestive of rapid growth and decline of Lp in the peritoneal environment. BDF_1 mice injected previously with TGC showed a much less change in CFU recovery patterns indicative of growth restriction of Lp (data not shown).

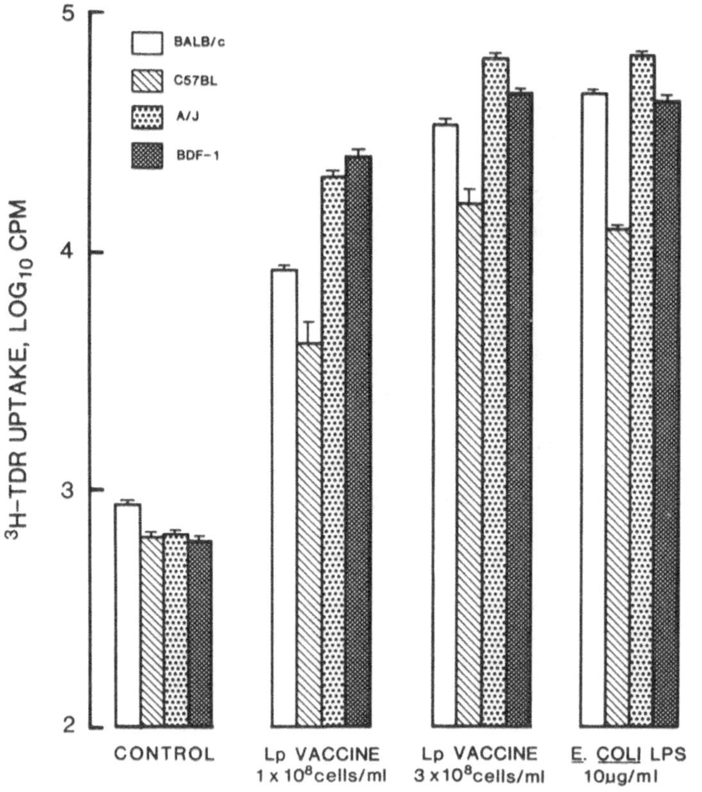

Fig. 4. IL-1 production by elicited peritoneal macrophages from various inbred mice. Thioglycollate induced peritoneal macrophage monolayers were stimulated with Lp vaccine or *E. coli* LPS for 24 hrs at 37°C. IL-1 content in culture supernatant of macrophage monolayers was measured by the standard thymocyte proliferation assay in C3H/HeJ mice. Each bar represents the mean ± S.D. of triplicate culture supernatants.

DISCUSSION

Legionella pneumophila has been reported to multiply *in vitro* in the presence of human peripheral blood monocytes, human alveolar macrophages, monkey alveolar macrophages, guinea pig macrophages and other cell lines (1,2,5,6,12). However, in order to better understand the mechanism involved in susceptibility, we examined the interaction of Lp with macrophages from susceptible and resistant species such as guinea pig and mouse. We (8) and others (13) reported that the permissive nature of guinea pig MP in culture correlated somewhat with susceptibility of the whole animal to infection. On the other hand, strain BDF_1 mouse macrophages restricted the growth of Lp in culture and the animals were relatively resistant to challenge with Lp.

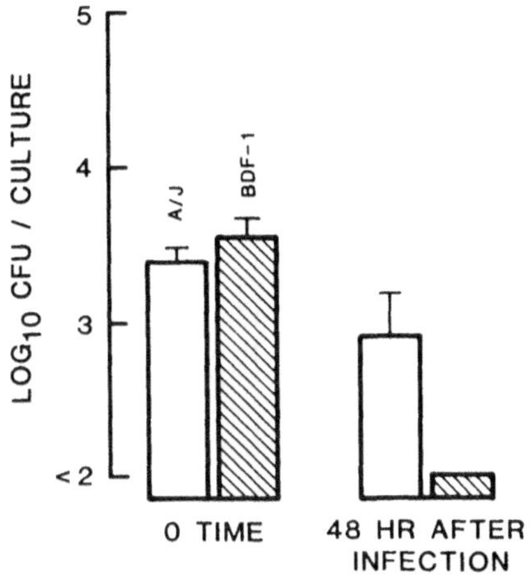

Fig. 5 Fate of Legionella in resident peritoneal macrophage cultures from A/J and BDF_1 mice. Resident peritoneal macrophages were cultured in monolayers (approximately $1x10^6$ cells/well) and infected with $2x10^6$ bacteria for 48 hrs at 37°C in 5% CO_2. Each bar represents the mean CFU + S.D. of triplicate macrophage cultures. The lower limit of detection for viable bacteria in macrophage culture is $1x10^2$ CFU/culture.

Although illustrative, these studies employed MPs from two different animal species, and we therefore examined for a mouse system permissive for Lp growth. Strain A/J mice have been reported to have immune abnormalities and to be susceptible to Listeria infection (14). We analyzed the growth restricting capacity of MPs from these mice as well as others. Of the strains tested, TGC elicited peritoneal MP from A/J mice supported the growth of Lp (Figures 1 & 2). The extent of growth was similar to that observed in guinea pigs (8). However, A/J MP cultures did restrict the growth of S. epidermidis (Figure 3) suggesting that these cells were not devoid of bactericidal capacity.

Also, A/J MPs responded to Lp antigens like cells from other strains in the production of IL 1-like activity (Figure 4). Furthermore, unlike the growth of Lp, the growth of Listeria organisms was not restricted to only MPs from A/J mice but occurred in MP cultures from all strains tested (Figure 3). These observations suggest the possibility that A/J MP have a selective bactericidal deficit in response to Lp antigens and

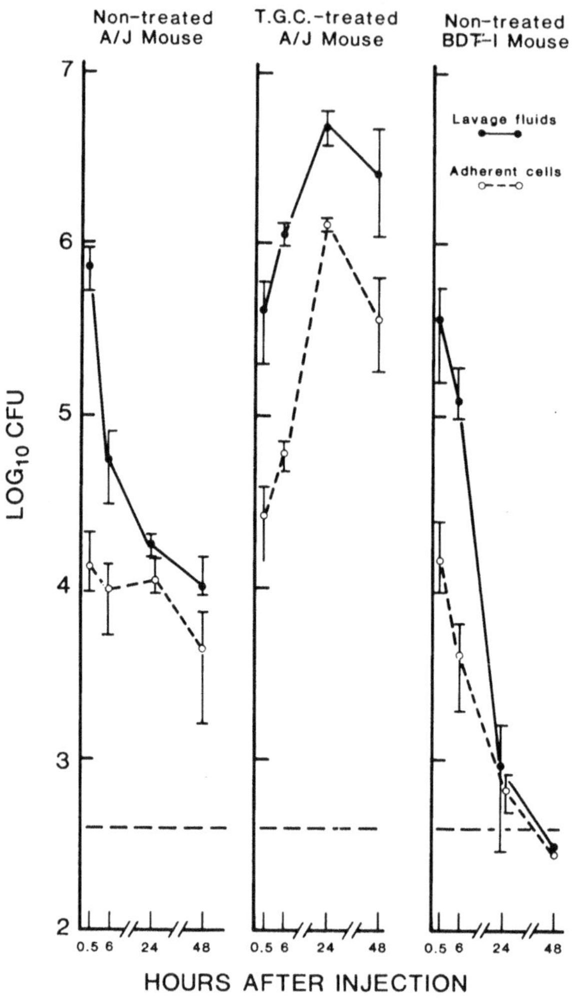

Fig. 6 Fate of Legionella ($2.5x10^6$) injected into the peritoneal cavity of A/J and BDF_1 mice previously injected i.p. (4 days) with TGC. At various times after infection, peritoneal lavage material was collected in RPMI medium containing heparin. Lavaged peritoneal leukocytes were allowed to adhere to tissue culture plates (24 wells) for 90 min at 37°C. Resulting adherent cells were washed with HBSS and lysed with sterilie distilled water. The number of viable bacteria in peritoneal lavage fluids and adherent cell lysates was determined by plate counts. Each point represents the mean CFU ± S.D. of three mice. Horizontal borken line indicates the detection limit of viable bacteria (CFU).

that these cells might therefore provide a unique murine model for studying cellular mechanisms permissive for Lp growth.

The growth of Lp in cultures of resident macrophages obtained from A/J mice was also examined. In contrast to TGC elicited cells, resident macrophages were not as permissive as elicited cells. However, A/J macrophages did not totally eliminate Lp in 48 hrs as did macrophages from BDF_1 mice (Fig. 5). These results suggest that resident macrophages are less permissive for Lp growth and that as previously reported (17) thioglycollate elicited cells display a reduced bactericidal capacity. These *in vitro* findings were extended to *in vivo* experiments, wherein it was observed that prior injection of mice with TGC resulted in an enhanced recovery of viable Lp from the peritoneal environment following an i.p. infection (Fig. 6). Together, our data suggest that the permissive nature of peritoneal macrophages might account for the growth of Lp in the peritoneal cavity at an early phase after infection. However, because the LD_{50} of A/J mice pretreated with thioglycollate did not change substantially from non-TGC pretreated mice (unpublished observation), it would appear that this early growth of Lp in macrophages can be subsequently restricted by other resistance mechanisms. Indeed, we have shown that mouse lymphocytes generally respond strongly to Lp antigens in the production of cytokines (11) and proliferation (9) and this responsiveness extends to cells from A/J mice which proliferate and respond with the production of cytokines in response to Lp antigens (unpublished observations). It would appear, therefore, that although macrophages from A/J mice tend to initially support the growth of Lp the animals are able to eventually resist Lp infection because of lymphocyte mediated mechanisms and possibly other host resistance factors.

REFERENCES

1. Horwitz, M.A. and S.C. Silverstein. 1980. The Legionnaire's disease bacterium (*Legionella pneumophila*) multiplies intracellulary in human monocytes. J. Clin. Invest. 66:441-450.
2. Kishimoto, R.A., J.D. White, F.G. Shirey, V.G. MacGann, R.F. Berendt, E.W. Larson and K.W. Hedlund. 1981. *In vitro* response of guinea pig peritoneal macrophages to *Legionella pneumophila*. Infect. Immun. 31:1209-1213.
3. Eisenstein, T.K. and H. Friedman. 1985. Immunity to *Legionella*. *In*: Legionellosis Vol. II. (ed. Katz, S.M.) p. 159-169. CRC Press. Boca Raton, Florida.
4. Horwitz, M.A. 1985. Host resistance to *Legionella pneumophila*: Interactions of *L. pneumophila* with leukocytes. *In*: Legionellosis Vol. II. (ed. Katz, S.W.) p. 143-157. CRC Press, Boca Raton, Florida.
5. Horwitz, M.A. and S.C. Silverstein. 1981. Activated human monocytes inhibit the intracellular multiplication of Legionnaires' disease bacteria. J. Exp. Med. 154:1618-1635.
6. Kishimoto, R.A., M.D. Kastello, J.D. White, F.G. Shirey, V.G. McGann, E.W. Larson and K.W. Hedlund. 1979. *In vitro* interaction between normal cynomolgus monkey alveolar macrophages and Legionnaires' disease bacteria. Infect. Immun. 25:761-763.
7. Katz, S.M. and J.P. Matus. 1985. Animal models of legionellosis. *In*: Legionellosis Vol. II (ed. Katz, S.M.) p. 119-132. CRC Press. Boca Raton, Florida.

8. Yamamoto, Y., T.W. Klein, C.A. Newton, R. Widen and H. Friedman. 1986. Differential growth of Legionella pneumophila in guinea pig vs mouse macrophage cultures. Infect. Immun. Accepted.
9. Friedman, H., R. Widen, T. Klein, L. Searls and K. Cabrian. 1984. Legionella pneumophila-induced blastogenesis of murine lymphoid cells in vitro. Infect. Immun. 43:314-319.
10. Friedman, F., R. Widen, T. Klein, and H. Friedman. 1984. Lymphoid cell blastogenesis as an in vitro indicator of cellular immunity to Legionella pneumophila antigens. J. Clin. Microbiol. 19:834-837.
11. Klein, T.W., C.A. Newton, D.K. Blanchard, R. Widen and H. Friedman. 1987. Induction of interleukin 1 by Legionella pneumophila antigens in mouse macrophage and human mononuclear leukocyte cultures. Zbl.Bakt.Hyg. A262. in press.
12. Wong, M.C., E.P. Ewing, C.S. Callaway and W.L. Peacock, Jr. 1980. Intracellular replication of Legionella pneumophila in cultured human embryonic lung fibroblasts. Infect. Immun. 28:1014-1018.
13. Yoshida, S. and Y. Mizuguchi. 1986. Multiplication of Legionella pneumophila Philadelphia-1 in cultured peritoneal macrophages and its correlation to susceptibility of animals. Can. J. Microbiol. 32:438-442.
14. Gervais, F., A. Morris-Hooke, T.A. Tran and E. Skamene. 1986. Analysis of macrophage bactericidal function in genetically resistant and susceptible mice by using the temperature-sensitive mutant of Listeria monocytogenes. Infect. Immun. 54:315-321.
15. Horwitz, M.A. and S.C. Silverstein. 1981. Interaction of the Legionnaires' disease bacterium (Legionella pneumophila) with human phagocytes I. L. pneumophila resists killing by polymorphonuclear leukocytes, antibody, and complement. J. Exp. Med. 153:386-397.
16. Horwitz, M.A. and S.C. Silverstein. 1981. Interaction of the Legionnaires' disease bacterium (Legionella pneumophila) with human phagocytes II. Antibody promotes binding of L. pneumophila to monocytes but does not inhibit intracellular multiplications. J. Exp. Med. 153:398-406.
17. Baker, L.A. and P.A. Campbell. 1980. Thiglycollate medium decreases resistance to bacterial infection in mive. Infect. Immun. 27:455-460.

THE PROTECTIVE ROLE OF T CELLS IN IMMUNITY TO MALARIA

William P. Weidanz, David A. Brake, Lisa A. Cavacini, and Carole A. Long

The Malaria Research Group
Department of Microbiology and Immunology
Hahnemann University School of Medicine
Philadelphia, PA 19102

Members of the genus Plasmodium have a complex life cycle which involves both vertebrate and invertebrate hosts. In the former, they parasitize the erythron, causing malaria, a disease characterized by high morbidity and mortality worldwide. In an effort to develop an effective vaccine to combat this disease, research has focused primarily on extracellular stages of the parasite presumably because they should be more accessible to antibody-dependent resistance mechanisms than intracellular parasites. Target stages include sporozoites, gametes, and merozoites. In addition, plasmodial antigens expressed on the membranes of infected erythrocytes are being studied as potential targets of protective antibodies.[1] Certain of the stage specific antigens which have been identified and expressed by recombinant DNA technology or synthesized biochemically in the laboratory are currently being investigated in experimental animals and humans as candidate vaccines.[2-4] In contrast, other data suggest that plasmodia can be destroyed during intracellular development by immune mechanisms apart from or in addition to those mediated by antibodies.[5] While efforts to define these immune mechanisms and to identify and characterize parasite antigens responsible for their activation have only recently begun, it is possible that they will provide a basis for the design of additional immunizing agents to be tested against malaria. In this article, we will review certain evidence that T cells, in addition to their function as helper cells in the production of protective antibodies, play an essential though as yet undefined role in antibody-independent immunity to malaria, and we will speculate on mechanisms by which protection is achieved.

Antibody-Independent Immunity to Malaria

Several lines of evidence suggest that acquired immunity to malaria may be mediated by antibody-independent mechanisms and have been reviewed by ourselves and others.[5-8] Briefly, these include: a) the existence of heterologous immunity wherein infection with one species of plasmodia subsequently protects against another despite low levels of cross-reacting antibody; b) the ability of assorted immunomodulating agents, i.e. BCG, *Propionibacterium parvum*, etc. to protect mice against experimental malaria; c) the correlation between T-cell responses such as delayed-type hypersensitivity and protection against infection with assorted plasmodia; d) the failure to uniformly correlate resistance to infection with antibody specificity or titer; and e) the induction of immunity to plasmodia in B-cell deficient hosts.

During the past 15 years, our laboratory has been actively engaged in studying malaria in B-cell deficient hosts. Accordingly, we will focus our discussion on these models and the information we have gained.

Experimental Malaria in B-cell Deficient Hosts

Initial studies in bursectomized chickens and anti-IgM suppressed mice with *P. gallinaceum* and *P. yoelii* strongly supported the concept that antibodies were required for protection against acute infection with blood stage plasmodia. These B-cell deficient animals usually died when infected with avirulent plasmodia.[9-11] However, when such infections were suppressed by means of chemotherapy, B-cell deficient hosts controlled their remaining parasites at low levels and resisted exogenous challenge infection with homologous parasites.[9,12,13] On the basis of these findings, we concluded that antibodies were required for resolving acute blood-stage infections but that resistance to recurring malaria depended upon antibody-independent mechanisms of immunity.

Subsequently, we observed that acute infection with the murine malarial parasite *P. chabaudi adami* in B-cell deficient mice resolved spontaneously without chemotherapy.[14] Nude mice infected with the same parasite developed unremitting malaria and eventually died (Fig. 1). Together, these findings suggested that acute malarial infections could be controlled by either antibody-dependent or antibody-independent mechanisms of immunity relative to the infecting species of parasite. While antibodies play a dominant role in protecting mice against acute blood-stage infection with P. yoelii, a contention supported by passive immunization studies utilizing both polyclonal and monoclonal antibodies,[15-17] they make little, if any, contribution to resistance against acute P. chabaudi adami malaria. Recent unpublished studies with other hemosporidia including Babesia microti, P. vinckei petteri, and possibly P. chabaudi chabaudi demonstrate that resistance to acute blood-stage infections by antibody-independent mechanisms of immunity against malaria may be more commonplace than originally surmised. B-cell deficient mice infected with these parasites terminated their acute infection in the absence of chemotherapy. Such mice lacked detectable IgM and antibodies reactive with the infecting species of plasmodia in their sera. In contrast, acute P. vinckei petteri and B. microti infections were fatal in nude mice.

It is also possible that resistance to particular stages of a single species of plasmodia may be mediated by different mechanisms. For example, we have already cited evidence that antibodies mediate protection against intra-erythrocytic parasites of P. yoelii; however, Chen et al.[18] observed that the immunization of B-cell, but not T-cell, deficient mice with irradiated P. yoelii sporozoites protected the animals against viable sporozoite challenge. Recent findings suggest that IFN- and alpha tumor necrosis factor inhibit the normal development of the parasite within hepatocytes following sporozoite invasion.[19,20]

3. The Role of T-cells in Antibody-Independent Immunity to Plasmodia

Early studies using T-cell defective rodents demonstrated that immunity to either blood stage or sporozoite infection with plasmodia required the presence of T-cells, i.e., infection of T-cell deficient hosts with normally avirulent plasmodia resulted in death.[21,22] Whether T-cells functioned as helper cells in the production of protective antibodies or participated in protective cellular immune reactions was not determined at that time. It would now appear that T cells function

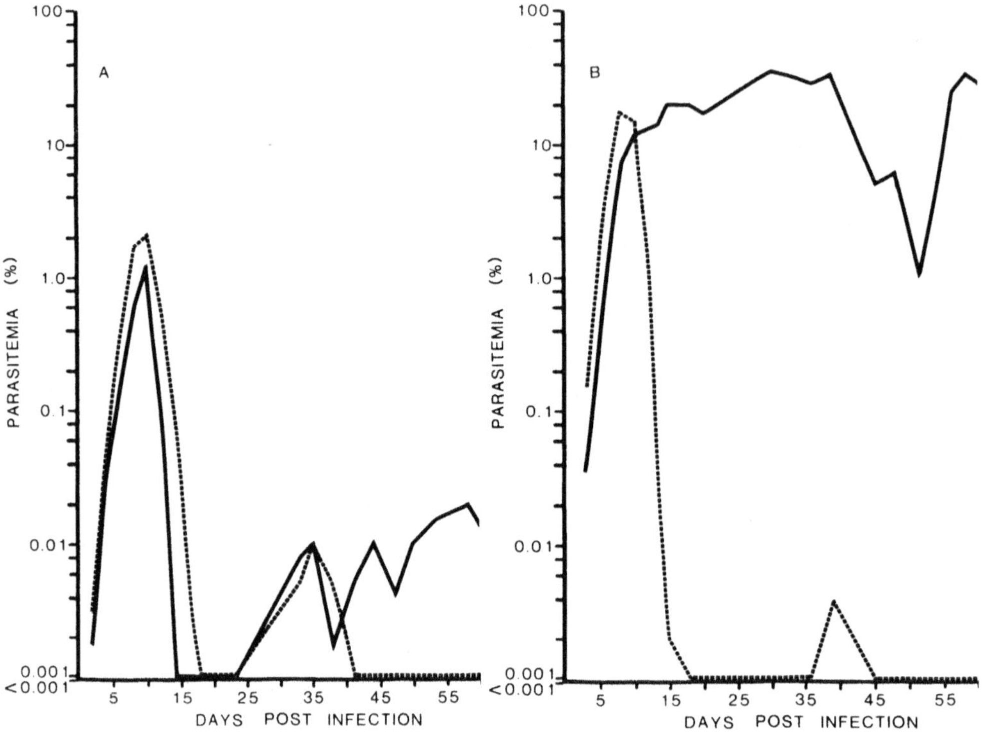

Fig. 1A. The course of P. chabaudi adami malaria in B-cell deficient (▬) and in immunologically intact (▪▪) (C57BL/6xCBA)F1 mice infected i.v. with $1x10^5$ parasitized erythrocytes. B. P. chabaudi infections in athymic nude mice (▬) and in euthymic littermates (▪▪). Data adapted with permission from Grun and Weidanz, 1981.

in both capacities, i.e., they are required for the production of protective antibodies in P. yoelii infection and are intimately involved in antibody-independent immune mechanisms capable of protecting B-cell deficient mice against P. chabaudi adami as well as other murine malarial parasites.

Additional evidence that T cells are required for the expression of antibody-independent mechanisms of immunity has been obtained from adoptive transfer studies in which the transfer of splenic lymphocytes from either nonimmune mice or mice immune to P. chabaudi adami allowed nude mice to suppress otherwise lethal challenge infections with the homologous parasite.[22] Nude mice grafted with either normal or immune splenocytes developed patent parasitemia upon challenge with homologous

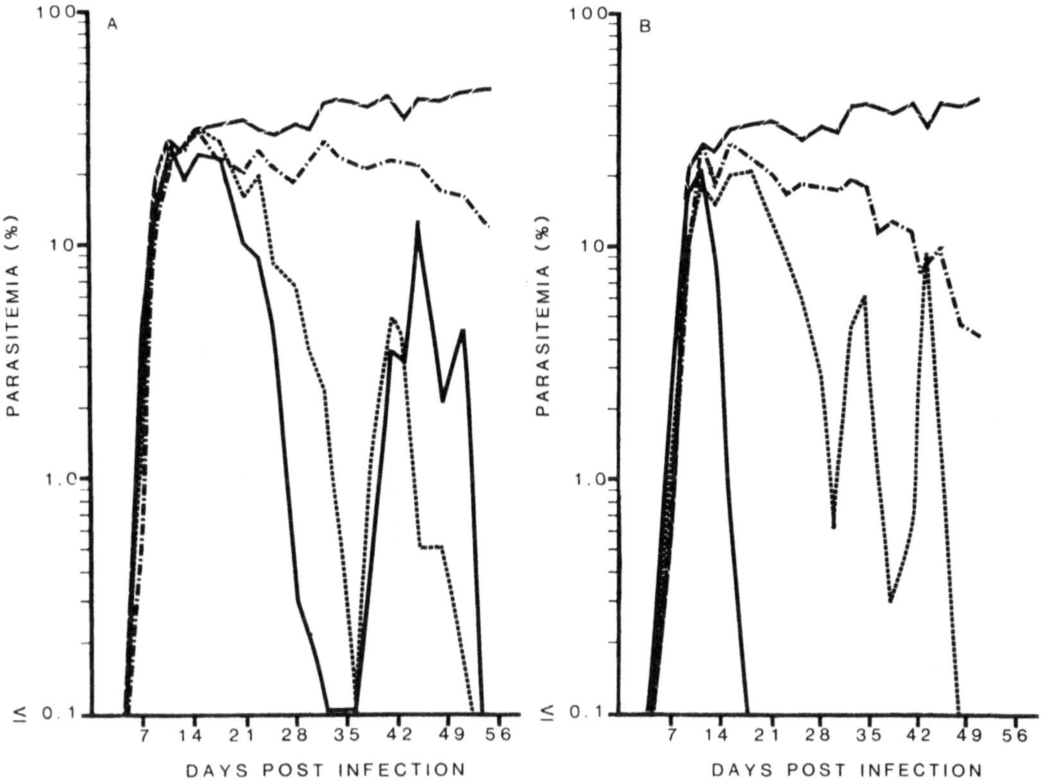

Fig. 2. Protection against P. chabaudi adami malaria in nude mice reconstituted with spleen cells from nonimmune (A) and immunized (B) congenic mice. Recipient mice received $1x10^7$ (▬), $1x10^6$ (▬), or $1x10^5$ (▬) spleen cells. Control mice were not grafted (▬). All mice were challenged i.p. with $1x10^5$ P. chabaudi adami on the day of transfer. Data adapted with permission from Cavacini et al. 1986.

parasites but parasitemias were of lesser magnitude and of shorter duration in mice receiving immune cells versus equivalent numbers of normal cells (Fig. 2). When sufficient numbers of immune cells were grafted into nude mice, they prevented the second wave of parasitemia characteristic of this infection in euthymic mice. Equivalent numbers of splenocytes from nonimmune animals failed to suppress the second wave of parasitemia. Additional adoptive transfer experiments utilizing populations of normal or immune splenocytes enriched for either T cells or B cells showed that T cells but not B cells conferred resistance to recipient mice (Fig. 3). Once again, T cells from immune mice appeared to be more protective than equivalent numbers of cells derived from

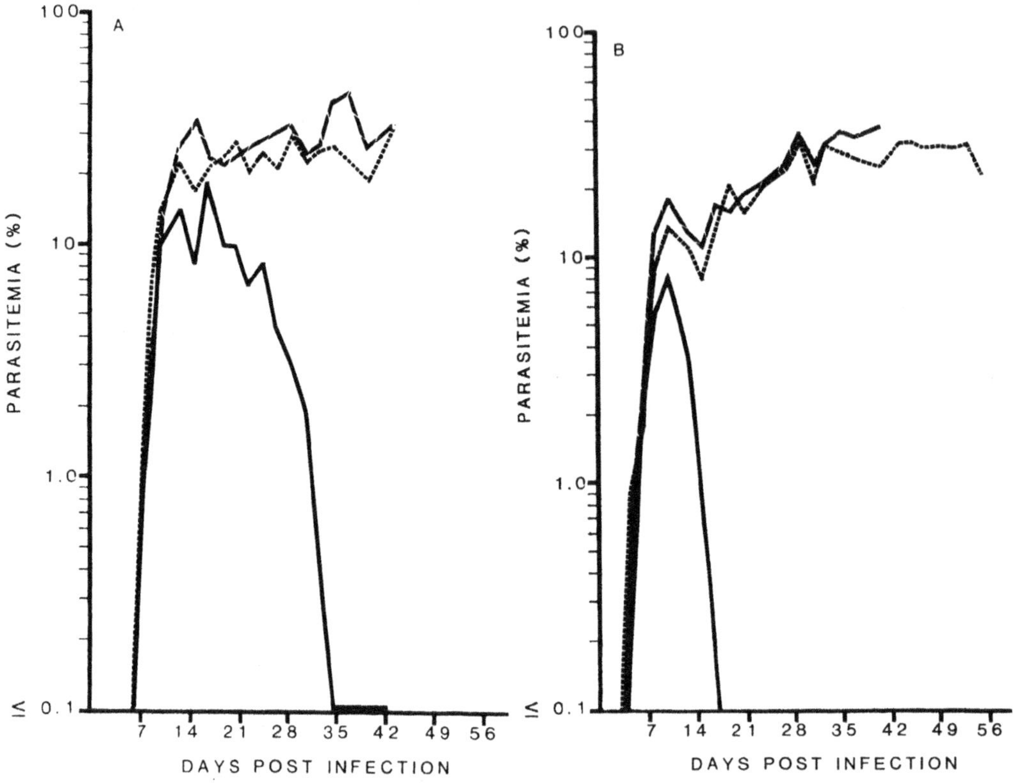

Fig. 3. Adoptive transfer of immunity to P. chabaudi adami with lymphocytes from normal (A) and immune (B) mice. In panel A, nude mice were reconstituted with $7x10^6$ T-cell enriched spleen cells (▬) or an equivalent number of B-cell enriched spleen cells (▪▪) from nonimmune nu/+ congenic mice or remained untreated (▬). In panel B, nude mice were grafted with $1x10^7$ T-cell enriched spleen cells (▬) or an equivalent nunmber of B-cell enriched spleen cells (▪▪) obtained from immune donor mice or remained untreated (▬). All mice were challenged intraperitoneally with $1x10^5$ P. chabaudi adami on the day of cell transfer. Data adapted with permission from Cavacini et al. 1986.

normal mice, and immune T cells bearing the L3T4$^+$ Lyt 2$^-$ phenotype were more protective than L3T4$^-$ Lyt 2$^+$ spleen cells. It is noteworthy that both T-cell grafted mice and nongrafted mice developed patent parasitemia. In fact, the kinetics of the initial ascending parasitemia curves in both types of mice were similar; however, the subsequent suppression of parasitemia to subpatent levels occurred only in nude mice grafted with a sufficient number of T cells. We will discuss the significance of this observation later.

Protective T Cell Lines and Clones

Having shown that immunity to P. chabaudi adami malaria was activated through the adoptive transfer of CD4 T cells, we developed T-cell lines from spleen cells obtained from P. chabaudi adami immune mice.[23] Splenic cells from mice immunized by infection were enriched for T cells by panning on anti-immunoglobulin coated plates, cultured in the presence of IL-2, and subjected to antigenic stimulation with solubilized P. chabaudi adami antigen at periodic intervals. Such cells bore the Thy 1^+, $L3T4^+$, Lyt 2^- phenotype and proliferated in response to stimulation with homologus antigen. Proliferation was MHC restricted, and required antigen presenting cells of the correct haplotype. These T cells did not respond to soluble antigens derived from uninfected erythrocytes.

The adoptive transfer of T-cell lines into nude mice allowed the mice to resolve their infections (Fig. 4). As indicated earlier, non-grafted nude mice infected with P. chabaudi adami developed unremitting malaria and eventually died when infected with this parasite. The protection afforded by these propagated T-lymphocytes was specific in that immune mice failed to resist challenge infection with the heterologous parasite P. yoelii.

More recently, cell lines exhibiting protective activity in vivo against P. chabaudi adami have been cloned by limiting dilution (Brake, Long, Weidanz, unpublished observations). Of the nine resulting clones tested, only one, designated CTR 2.1, provided protection against P. chabaudi adami infection upon adoptive transfer into nude mice (Fig. 5). Whereas nude mice grafted with splenic T-cells derived from normal mice resolved their infections, mice reconstituted with the remaining clones of T-cells developed unremitting malaria and died as did nongrafted nude mice infected with P. chabaudi adami. This finding suggests the limited clonality of the cell lines tested. Additional evidence supporting the limited heterogeneity of CTR 2.1 was obtained from several experiments in which grafted mice immune to P. chabaudi adami failed to develop allergic contact dermatitis following sensitization and challenge with dinitrofluorobenzene. Similarly, such grafted mice failed to make antibodies in response to immunization with keyhole limpet hemocyanin administered with complete Freund's adjuvant. Subclones derived from cloned line CTR 2.1 by limiting dilution also proved to be protective in

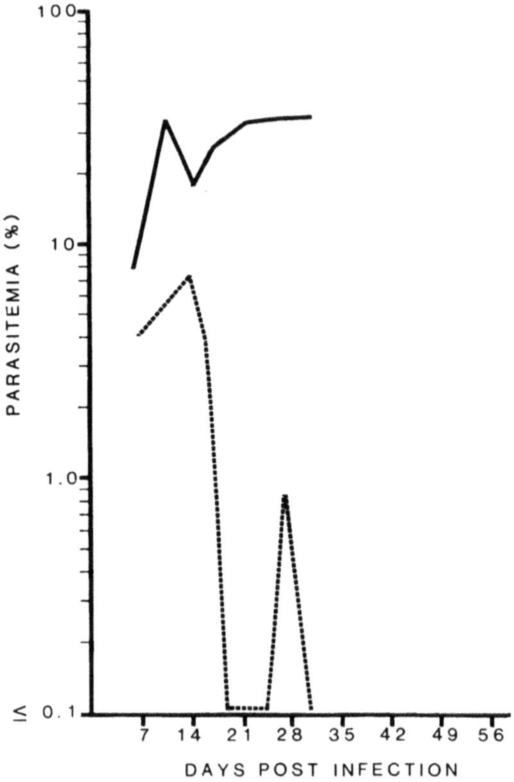

Fig. 4. Protection against P. chabaudi adami in nude mice reconstituted with $2x10^6$ IL-2 dependent antigen-specific T lymphocytes which had been stimulated twice with malarial antigen during a 16-day culture period prior to transfer (▪▪▪). Control nude mice were not grafted (▬). All mice were challenged i.v. with $1x10^5$ P. chabaudi adami on the day of cell transfer. Data adapted with permission from Brake et al. 1986.

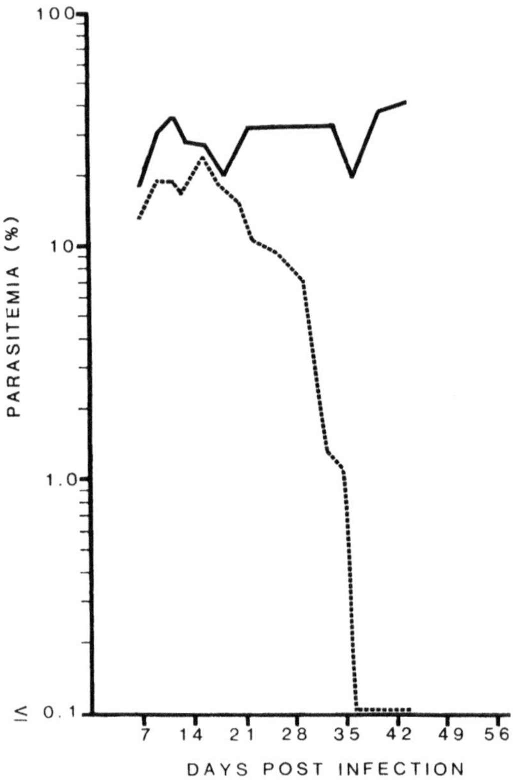

Fig. 5. Protection against P. chabaudi adami in nude mice reconstituted with $1x10^6$ IL-2 dependent antigen-specific cloned T cells (▪▪▪). Control nude mice were not grafted (▬). All mice were challenged with P. chabaudi adami as in Fig. 4. Data adapted with permission from Weidanz and Long 1987.

adoptive transfer studies. Cells of the CTR 2.1 cloned line bore the Thy 1^+, $L3T4^+$ Lyt 2^- phenotype and secreted both IFN- and IL-2 following stimulation *in vitro* with soluble *P. chabaudi adami* antigen, suggesting that these cells belong to the T1 subset of T-cells as defined by Cher and Mossman.[24] We suspect that these cells do not secrete IL-4 nor IL-5.

DISCUSSION

There is no doubt that T cells play an essential role in immunity to malaria.[5] In addition to their role as helper cells in the production of protective antibody, they appear to function in ill-defined cellular immune mechanisms which cause intra-erythrocytic parasite death with a resultant suppression of parasitemia. Previous studies in our laboratory had shown that resistance to P. chabaudi adami was achieved by such antibody-independent mechanisms of immunity.[14] Accordingly, we have utilized this experimental model to identify and characterize the T cells involved as an initial step in effort to understand how cellular immune mechanisms effect parasite destruction. The data show P. chabaudi adami infections were unremitting and lethal in nude mice; however, when nude mice were grafted with sufficient numbers of either normal or immune T cells, they developed acute malarial infections which resolved spontaneously.[22] In contrast, the transfer of B lymphocytes had no effect on the outcome of infection. Similar findings were obtained with grafts of antigen-propagated T-cell lines and antigen-reactive T-cell clones derived from splenic T cells of P. chabaudi adami immune mice.[23] In all instances, the infected mice developed parasitemia which subsequently decreased only in mice grafted with polyclonal or antigen-specific T cells. Of interest was the fact that the time at which parasites first appeared in the blood of infected mice was the same regardless of whether or not the animals had been grafted with T cells. Since the length of the prepatent period is inversely proportional to the number of viable parasites injected, the data suggest that the grafted T cells act to suppress parasitemia by some means other than direct cytotoxicity, a finding in keeping with the observations of others.[25]

The T cells mediating resistance against acute P. chabaudi adami infections appear to be CD4 cells, T cells displaying the $L3T4^{+}$ $Lyt\ 2^{-}$ phenotype. Moreover, they proliferate in response to stimulation with P. chabaudi adami antigen and respond with the production of IL-2 and IFN- (Brake et al., unpublished observations). It is possible that these cells effect resistance by altering the behavior of other cells which bring about parasite destruction. For example, it has been proposed [26,27] that the production of toxic species of oxygen by macrophages chemotactically attracted to the spleen and activated by lymphokines such as monocyte chemotactic factor and IFN- respectively may kill intraerythrocytic plasmodia. Plasmodia have been shown to be killed by such agents both in vitro and in vivo[28-30]. It is also possible that the grafted cells responding to plasmodial antigens or the cells which they activate may produce other antiplasmodial substances, i.e., Jayawardena [31] indicated that lymphotoxin had antiplasmodial activity, and Jensen et al.[32] suggested that "crisis-form factor" found in the sera of individuals in areas where malaria was endemic caused the intracellular death of *P. falciparum*. Thus far, attempts to show that recombinant cytotoxins including IFN- , TNF, and lymphotoxin could kill intracellular parasites in vitro have been unsuccessful.[33-35]

We believe that the development of a cloned T cell line capable of protecting mice against *P. chabaudi adami* is especially noteworthy. This suggests that the activation of cellular immune mechanisms capable of protecting the host against malaria is highly specific and not the result of the known mitogenic activity of plasmodia. Moreover, it indicates that the number of T-cell epitopes responsible for activation of these cells is also limited. We plan to use these cells to identify plasmodial antigens which are the targets of such protective immune responses. By cloning and sequencing the genes responsible for the expression of protective antigens, it should be possible to identify the T-cell epitopes involved and to evaluate their immunizing potential. Similar epitopes might be found in cross-reacting species of plasmodia and possibly in the plasmodia which infect man. Finally, we believe that the use of these cells in in vivo and in vitro experiments may aid us in understanding the complex immune mechanisms leading to parasite destruction.

ACKNOWLEDGMENTS

We thank Alice Smith for her excellent secretarial assistance and Lydia Parke for preparing the figures. This work was supported by Public Health Service grant AI12710 from the National Institute for Allergy and Infectious Diseases.

REFERENCES

1. L.H. Miller, R.J. Howard, R. Carter, M.F. Good, V. Nussenzweig, and R.S. Nussenzweig, Research toward malaria vaccines. Science, 234:1349 (1986).
2. J.E. Egan, J.L. Weber, W.R. Ballou, W. Majarian, D.M. Gordon, S.L. Hoffman, R.A. Wirtz, S. Schneider, G. Woollett, M.R. Hollingdale, J.F. Young, and W.T. Hockmeyer, Efficacy of murine malaria sporozoite vaccines: Implications for human vaccine development. Science, 236:453 (1987).
3. W.R. Ballou, J.A. Sherwood, F.A. Neva, D.M. Gordon, R.A. Wirtz, G.F. Wasserman, C.L. Diggs, S.L. Hoffman, M.R. Hollingdale, W.T. Hockmeyer, I. Schneider, J.F. Young, P. Reeve, and J.D. Chulay, Safety and efficacy of a recombinant DNA Plasmodium falciparum sporozoite vaccine, Lancet, 1:1278 (1987).
4. D.A. Herrington, D.F. Clyde, G. Losonsky, M. Cortesia, J.R. Murphy, J. Davis, S. Bagar, A.M. Felix, E.P. Heimer, D. Gillessen, E. Nardin, R.S. Nussenzweig, V. Nussenzweig, M.R. Hollingdale, and M.M. Levine, Safety and immunogenicity in man of a synthetic peptide vaccine against Plasmodium falciparum sporozoites, Nature, 328:257 (1987).
5. A.C. Allison and E.M. Eugui, The role of cell-mediated immune responses in resistance to malaria with special reference to oxidant stress, Ann. Rev. Immunol. 1:361 (1983).
6. J.H.L. Playfair, Immunity to malaria, Brit. Med. Bull. 38:167 (1982).
7. W.P. Weidanz and J.L. Grun, Antibody-independent mechanisms in the development of acquired immunity to malaria, in: "Host defenses to intracellular pathogens," T.K. Eisenstein, P. Actor, and H. Friedman, eds., Plenum Press, New York (1983).
8. W.P. Weidanz and C.A. Long, The role of T cells in immunity to malaria, in: "Malaria Immunology," Progress in Allergy, P. Perlmann and H. Wigzell, eds., S. Karger, Basel (in press).
9. R.G. Rank and W.P. Weidanz, Nonsterilizing immunity in avian malaria: an antibody-independent phenomenon, Proc. Soc. Exp. Biol. Med. 151:257 (1976).
10. F.I. Weinbaum, C.B. Evans, R.E. Tigelaar, Immunity to Plasmodium berghei yoelii in mice. I. The course of infection in T cell and B cell deficient mice, J. Immunol. 117:1999 (1976).
11. D.W. Roberts, R.G. Rank, W.P. Weidanz, and J.F. Finerty, Prevention

of recrudescent malaria in nude mice by thymic grafting or by treatment with hyperimmune serum, Infect. Immun. 16:321 (1977).

12. D.W. Roberts and W.P. Weidanz, T-cell immunity to malaria in the B-cell deficient mouse, Amer. J. Trop. Med. Hyg. 28:1 (1979).

13. J.L. Grun and W.P. Weidanz, Antibody-independent immunity to reinfection malaria in B-cell deficient mice, Infect. Immun. 41:1197 (1983).

14. J.L. Grun and W.P. Weidanz, Immunity to Plasmodium chabaudi adami in the B-cell deficient mouse, Nature 290:143 (1981).

15. A.N. Jayawardena, G.A.T. Targett, E. Leuchars, and A.J.S. Davies, The immunological response of CBA mice to P. yoelii. II. The passive transfer of immunity with serum and cells, Immunol. 34:157 (1978).

16. R.R. Freeman, A.J. Trejdosiewicz, and G.A.M. Cross, Protective monoclonal antibodies recognizing stage-specific merozoite antigens of a rodent malaria parasite, Nature 284:366 (1980).

17. W.M. Majarian, T.M. Daly, W.P. Weidanz, and C.A. Long, Passive immunization against murine malaria with an IgG3 monoclonal antibody, J. Immunol. 132:3131 (1984).

18. D.H. Chen, R.E. Tigelaar, F.I. Weinbaum, Immunity to sporozoite-induced malaria infection in mice. I. The effect of immunization of T and B cell-deficient mice, J. Immunol. 118:1322 (1977).

19. A. Ferreira, L. Schofield, V. Enea, H. Schellekens, P. Van der Meide, W.E. Collins, R.S. Nussenzweig, and V. Nussenzweig, Inhibition of development of exoerythrocytic forms of malaria parasites by gamma-interferon, Science 232:881 (1986).

20. L. Schofield, A. Ferreira, V. Nussenzweig, and R.S. Nussenzweig, Antimalarial activity of alpha tumor necrosis factor and gamma interferon, Fed. Proc. 46:7560 (1987).

21. I.N. Brown, A.C. Allison, and R.B. Taylor, Plasmodium berghei infections in thymectomized rats, Nature 219:292 (1968).

22. L.A. Cavacini, C.A. Long, and W.P. Weidanz, T-cell immunity in murine malaria: adoptive transfer of resistance to Plasmodium chabaudi adami in nude mice with splenic T cells, Infect. Immun. 52:637 (1986).

23. D.A. Brake, W.P. Weidanz, and C.A. Long, Antigen-specific, interleukin 2-propagated T lymphocytes confer resistance to a murine malaria parasite, Plasmodium chabaudi adami, J. Immunol. 137:347 (1986).

24. D.J. Cher and T.R. Mossmann, Two types of murine helper T-cell clone. II. Delayed-type hypersensitivity is mediated by T_H1 clones, J. Immunol. 138:3688.

25. S. Cohen and P.H. Lambert, Malaria, in: "Immunology of Parasitic Infections," S. Cohen and K.S. Warren, Eds., Blackwell Scientific Publications, Oxford (1982).

26. A.C. Allison and E.M. Eugui, A radical interpretation of immunity to malaria parasites, Lancet 2:1431 (1982).

27. I.A. Clark and N.H. Hunt, Evidence for reactive oxygen intermediates causing hemolysis and parasite death in malaria, Infect. Immun. 39:1 (1983).

28. I.A. Clark, W.B. Cowden, and G.A. Butcher, Free oxygen generators as antimalarial drugs, Lancet 1:234 (1983).

29. C.F. Ockenhouse and H.L. Shear, Oxidative killing of intraerythrocytic malaria parasite Plasmodium yoelii by activated macrophages, J. Immunol. 132:424 (1984).

30. H.M. Dockrell and J.H.L. Playfair, Killing of blood-stage malaria parasites by hydrogen peroxide. Infect. Immun. 39:456 (1983).

31. A.N. Jayawardena, Immune responses in malaria, in: "Parasitic Diseases," J. Mansfield, ed., Marcel Dekker, New York (1981).

32. J.B. Jensen, M.T. Boland, J.S. Allan, J.M. Carlin, J.A. Vande Waa, A.A. Divo, and M.A. Akood, Association between human serum-induced crisis forms in cultured Plasmodium falciparum and clinical immunity to malaria in Sudan, Infect. Immun. 41:1302 (1983).

33. J.M. Carlin, J.B. Jensen, and T.G. Geary, Comparison of inducers of crisis forms in Plasmodium falciparum in vitro, Am. J. Trop. Med. Hyg. 34:668 (1985).

34. J.B. Jensen, Crisis forms in falciparum malaria. J. Cell. Biochem. Suppl. 10A:121 (1986)

CHANGES IN SIZE AND CELL POPULATIONS IN LYMPHOID ORGANS DURING PLASMODIUM CHABAUDI INFECTION IN RESISTANT AND SUSCEPTIBLE MICE

Darlene Rae and Mary M. Stevenson

Department of Physiology, McGill University and
The Montreal General Hospital Research Institute
1650 Cedar Avenue, Montreal, Quebec H3G 1A4

The level of host resistance to *Plasmodium chabaudi* is genetically determined by a major, dominant, autosomal, non H-2 linked gene which has been designated *Pchr* (for resistance to *P. chabaudi*). The genetic control was defined by our laboratory by analysis of hybrid and backcross progeny derived from the strain combination of resistant C57BL/6J (B) and susceptible A/J (A) mice and was confirmed by analysis of the AXB/BXA series of recombinant inbred (RI) strains (1,2). The RI strain analysis showed, furthermore, that resistance and, consequently, survival are genetically linked with marked splenomegaly while susceptibility and death are linked with minimal splenomegaly.

P. chabaudi is unique among the malaria species infecting mice because control and elimination of this parasite is by a B-cell independent, cell mediated immune mechanism (3). This observation was described for the *P. chabaudi adami* strain and has now been extended to other *P. chabaudi* strains (W.P. Weidanz, Personal Communication). The expression of this immunity is dependent on the presence of an architecturally intact spleen (4). It is of interest to point out that the development of splenomegaly, a characteristic feature of malaria, is thymus dependent; in addition, as described above, the magnitude of splenomegaly has been found to be genetically linked to the level of resistance to *P. chabaudi* (2,5).

The cellular basis of the intraerythrocytic parasite destruction is most likely the release of anti-Plasmodia mediators from macrophages activated by specifically sensitized T cells during infection. The T cells mediating resistance have recently been shown to be splenic cells of the L3T4 phenotype (helper/inducer subset) (6,7). Their proliferation *in vitro* was demonstrated to be interleukin-2 dependent, antigen specific and H-2 restricted. *In vivo*, these cells are able to transfer resistance to *P. chabaudi adami* infection to both nude and sublethally irradiated receipients.

Since the T cells of the spleen have been demonstrated to be of prime importance in resistance to *P. chabaudi*, we were interested to determine if a quantitative difference in this population of T cells is related to the difference in the magnitude of splenomegaly and, thus, to the outcome of infection in genetically resistant B and susceptible A mice. In order to examine this possibility, organ weight, total nucleated cell number and the percentage and number of Thy 1.2+ cells were determined on spleens of malaria infected B and A mice at various times after infection.

When the genetic studies (1,2) were performed, the parasite was maintained by weekly passage in inbred, susceptible A mice. Intraperitoneal infection with 1 x 10^6 parasitized erythrocytes (P-RBC) of this parasite preparation produced infection in susceptible A and resistant B mice which was characterized by a significant difference between the strains in the level of peak parasitemia (< 40% P-RBC for resistant B versus > 50% P-RBC for susceptible A mice) apparent at day 10 of infection (Figure 1A). Resistant B mice were able to control and eliminate the parasite by 3 weeks after infection; 100% of susceptible A mice succumbed to infection. The mean survival time of A mice was < 10 days (1).

For the studies presented here, the parasite was maintained by weekly passage in outbred CD-1 mice. Infection with 1 x 10^6 P-RBC of this parasite preparation produced infection in susceptible A and resistant B mice which was characterized by an equal level of peak parasitemia of approximately 45% P-RBC (Figure 1B). The peak parasitemia level was apparent at day 7. Despite the similarity in parasitemia levels, A mice succumbed to the infection while B mice survived and were able to eliminate the parasite. Thus, the genetic difference, as defined by death, was maintained in spite of the change in virulence of the P. chabaudi. We have previously observed a similar course and outcome of infection in A and B mice following infection with a dose of 1 x 10^8 P-RBC of the A strain passaged P. chabaudi (1). The use of an inoculum of 1 x 10^6 P-RBC of the CD-1 passaged P. chabaudi, thus, alleviated the possibility of any differences in host response being due to a difference in parasite load.

Within the first 5 days after P. chabaudi infection, spleen weights were increased significantly in both A and B mice (Figure 2A). There was a significant difference in spleen weight between the strains at day 7 which became even more apparent at day 9 ($P \leq 0.005$). In each case, the maximum spleen weight was at day 9. The spleen weight of resistant B mice was still significantly increased in comparison to that of normal, uninfected B mice through 28 days after infection but, at this time, it was returning to normal size. In spite of a significant difference in the magnitude of splenomegaly following P. chabaudi infection, the number of total nucleated cells increased equally within the first 7 days in both resistant B and susceptible A mice (Figure 2B). Thus, these results indicate that hyperplasia due to proliferation and expansion of the splenic, nucleated cell population, which accompanies the splenomegaly of malaria and is composed of leukocytes and immature erythrocyte precursors, occurs equally well in P. chabaudi resistant B and susceptible A mice (8-10).

To determine the contribution of T cells to splenomegaly during malaria in resistant and susceptible mice, the percentage of Thy 1.2+ splenocytes was determined at various times through 7 days after P. chabaudi infection by a standard cytotoxicity assay using anti-Thy 1.2 monoclonal antibody followed by rabbit complement (Table 1). We also calculated the number of T cells per organ using the number of total, viable nucleated cells and the percentage cytotoxicity. Although there was an overall decrease in the percentage of splenic Thy 1.2+ cells within the first 7 days after P. chabaudi infection in both B and A mice, the absolute number of T cells increased significantly in each strain. As we observed with the number of total nucleated, spleen cells, the increase in the number of splenic T cells was not

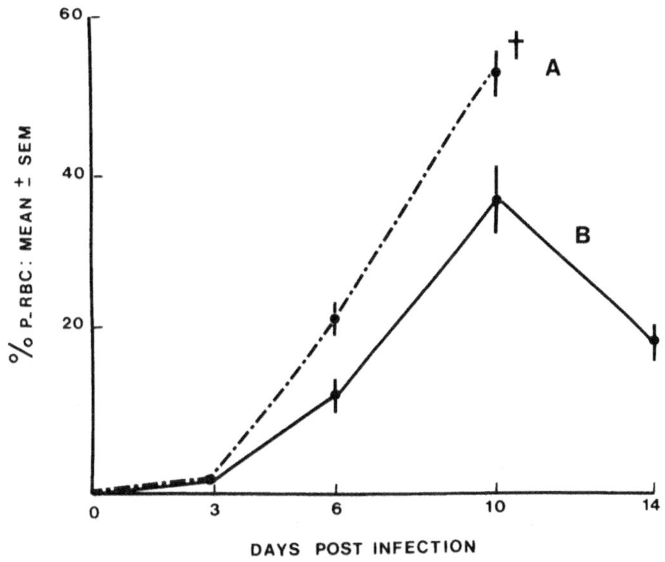

A. Mice infected IP with 1 x 10^6 P-RBC of A-passaged *P. chabaudi*.

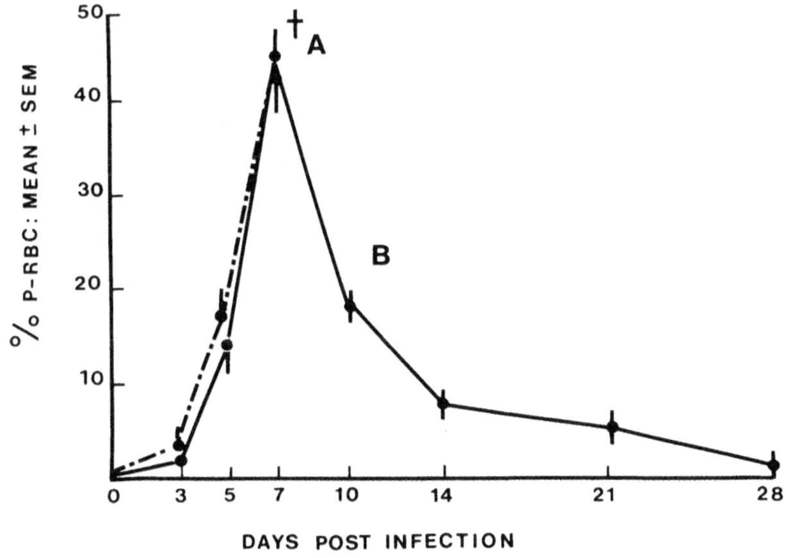

B. Mice infected IP with 1 x 10^6 P-RBC of CD-1-passaged *P. chabaudi*.

Figure 1. Course of *P. chabaudi* Infection in Resistant B and Susceptible A Mice.

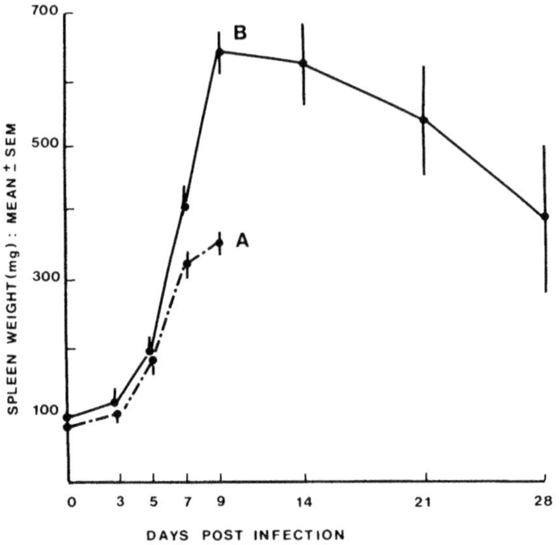

A. Spleen weight (in mg) following IP infection with 1 x 10^6 P. chabaudi P-RBC.

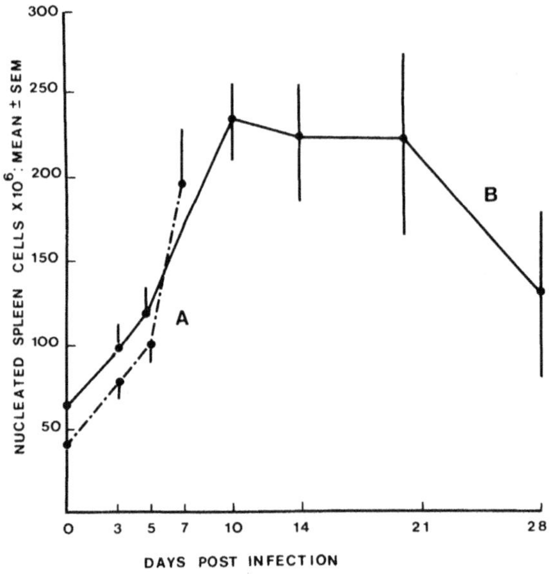

B. Total nucleated cells per spleen following IP infection with 1 x 10^6 P. chabaudi P-RBC.

Figure 2. Development of Splenomegaly During P. chabaudi Infection in Resistant B and Susceptible A Mice.

Table 1. Percentage and Number of Thy 1.2+ Spleen Cells During *P. chabaudi* Infection in Resistant B and Susceptible A Mice

Days After IP Infection with 1 x 10^6 P-RBC	Resistant B Mice		Susceptible A Mice	
	Cytotoxicity Index[a,b]	Thy 1.2+ Cells x 10^6 Per Spleen[a,c]	Cytotoxicity Index[a,b]	Thy 1.2+ Cells x 10^6 Per Spleen[a,c]
Normal	20.2 ± 1.3	12.0 ± 1.3	19.7 ± 3.6	4.9 ± 0.7
Day 3	16.7 ± 2.9	14.6 ± 1.9	22.5 ± 6.0	11.2 ± 1.4[d]
Day 5	17.7 ± 2.2	20.2 ± 2.3[d]	15.2 ± 2.3	14.0 ± 2.6[d]
Day 7	15.6 ± 2.3	28.9 ± 3.2[d]	10.3 ± 2.4	17.1 ± 5.3[d]

[a]Data presented as mean ± standard error of the mean.

[b]Cytotoxicity Index = $100 \times \frac{\%C(\text{antibody+complement}) - \%C(\text{complement})}{100\,\% - \%C\ (\text{complement})}$;

% Cytotoxicity (%C) determined by trypan blue exclusion.

[c]Number of Thy 1.2+ cells calculated by multiplying cytotoxicity index times total nucleated spleen cells from Figure 2B.

[d]$P \leq 0.01$ for comparison of infected to normal mice of either strain B or A.

significantly different in the resistant and susceptible hosts. There was, however, a significant difference in the number of splenic Thy 1.2+ cells between normal A and B mice ($P < 0.001$).

In addition to splenomegaly, malaria also causes severe alterations in the thymus and lymph nodes of rodents infected with *P. berghei* (11,12). There is thymic atrophy and a reduction in the number of identifiable T cells in the thymus and lymph nodes of infected animals (11,12). Therefore, we also examined changes in the size and number of Thy 1.2+ cells in these lymphoid organs during the course of *P. chabaudi* infection in B and A mice. The results of the thymus study, shown in Figure 3A and B, demonstrated that 1) there was a significant difference between normal A and B mice in both thymic weight and the number of thymocytes ($P < 0.05$) and 2) the thymus weight and total cell number declined in both resistant B and susceptible A mice. During the first 9-10 days of infection, the significant differences between the strains in these two parameters were maintained. Almost complete atrophy of the thymus was apparent in both strains at approximately day 9-10 of infection, a time at which less than 50% of susceptible A mice were still surviving and the remaining were visibly near death. Atrophy coincided with a significant decrease of 20% ($P < 0.05$) in the percentage of T cells in both strains. Organ weight and thymocyte number returned to normal levels in resistant B mice by 21 days after infection. Lymph node weight as well as cellular composition did not change significantly throughout the course of *P. chabaudi* infection in either resistant B or susceptible A mice (data not shown).

Previous investigations in the rat demonstrated that young animals are more susceptible to *P. berghei* than older, mature animals (12). This difference in susceptibility was found to correlate with depletion of T cells from the spleen and thymus. However, while these investigators concluded there was a depletion of T cells in the spleen

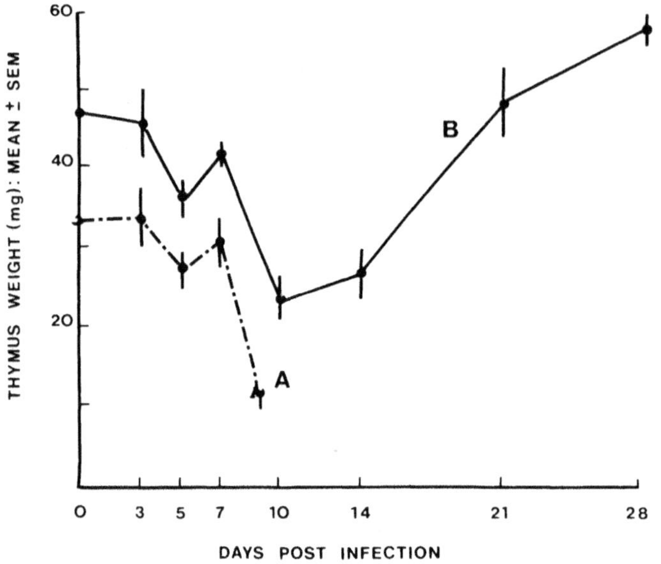

A. Thymus weight (in mg) following IP infection with 1 x 10^6 P. chabaudi P-RBC.

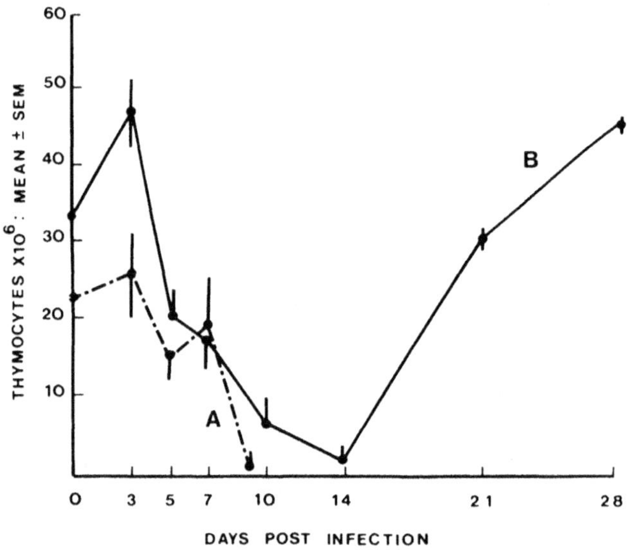

B. Total thymocytes per organ following IP infection with 1 x 10^6 P. chabaudi P-RBC.

Figure 3. Thymic Atrophy During P. chabaudi Infection in Resistant B and Susceptible A Mice.

(by a decrease in the percentage of theta positive cells), they did not take into account that the splenic size and nucleated cell number were concomitantly increasing. Thus, the conclusion of the study was that the loss of T cells from the organs of young rats lead to susceptibility to malaria.

Our results demonstrate that when the increase in splenic cellularity is considered, there is an overall increase in the number of Thy 1.2+ cells in the spleen during P. chabaudi infection. This increase is in spite of a seeming decrease when only the percentage cytotoxicity is considered. More importantly, this increase in Thy 1.2+ cells in the spleen occurs equally in P. chabaudi resistant B and susceptible A mice despite a significant difference in the magnitude of splenomegaly. We have recently demonstrated that marked suppression of antibody formation to the unrelated antigen, sheep erythrocytes, occurred during P. chabaudi infection in both resistant B and susceptible A mice (13).

In a manner similar to the results of previous studies (11,12), we observed severe thymic involution which was apparent in both resistant B and susceptible A mice. During the period of infection with P. chabaudi observed in our study, we found no evidence of changes in the size or cellularity of lymph nodes of infected animals.

In conclusion, our results suggest that a quantitative difference in the number of T cells in the spleen during P. chabaudi infection is not related to the outcome of infection in resistant B and susceptible A hosts. It is possible that a difference in the functional capacity of T cells in the two strains could contribute to the extreme susceptibility of A mice. Future investigations will address this point. The observations of a significant difference between uninfected, normal B and A in the number of Thy 1.2+ spleen cells as well as significant differences in both thymic weight and the number of thymocytes were of interest. At the present time, we do not know the relationship of these observations to the outcome of P. chabaudi infection.

Acknowledgments

This work was supported by the Medical Research Council of Canada. M.M.S. holds an MRC Scholarship. This work was completed by D.R. in partial fulfillment of an M.Sc., McGill University, Montreal, Quebec. We thank Sylvie Pankert for technical assistance and Jean Walker for assistance in preparing the manuscript.

REFERENCES

1. Stevenson, M.M., J.J. Lyanga and E. Skamene. 1982. Murine malaria: genetic control of resistance to Plasmodium chabaudi. Infect. Immun. 38: 80-88.

2. Stevenson, M.M. and E. Skamene. 1985. Murine malaria: resistance of AXB/BXA recombinant inbred mice to Plasmodium chabaudi. Infect. Immun. 47: 452-456.

3. Grun, J.L. and W.P. Weidanz. 1981. Immunity to Plasmodium chabaudi adami in the B-cell-deficient mouse. Nature (London) 290: 143-146.

4. Grun, J.L., C.A. Long and W.P. Weidanz. 1985. Effects of splenectomy on antibody-independent immunity to Plasmodium chabaudi adami malaria. Infect. Immun. 48: 853-858.

5. Roberts, D.W. and W.P. Weidanz. 1978. Splenomegaly, enhanced phagocytosis and anemia are thymus dependent responses to malaria. Infect. Immun. 20: 728-731.

6. Cavacini, L.A., C.A. Long and W.P. Weidanz. 1986. T-cell immunity in murine malaria: adoptive transfer of resistance to Plasmodium chabaudi adami in nude mice with splenic T cells. Infect. Immun. 52: 637-643.

7. Brake, D., W.P. Weidanz and C.A. Long. 1986. Antigen-specific, interleukin 2-propagated T lymphocytes confer resistance to a murine malarial parasite Plasmodium chabaudi adami. J. Immunol. 137: 347-352.

8. Taliaferro, W.H. and H.W. Mulligan. 1937. The histopathology of malaria with special reference to the function and origin of the macrophages in defence. Indian Med. Res. Mem. 29: 1-138.

9. Moran, C., V. DeRivera and J. Turk. 1973. The immunological significance of histological changes in the spleen and liver in mouse malaria. Clin. Exp. Immunol. 13: 467-478.

10. Weiss, L., U. Geduldid and W. Weidanz. 1986. Mechanisms of splenic control of murine malaria: reticular cell activation and the development of a blood-spleen barrier. Am. J. Anat. 176: 251-285.

11. Krettli, A.U. and R. Nussenzweig. 1974. Depletion of T and B lymphocytes during malarial infection. Cell. Immunol. 13: 440-446.

12. Gravely, S.M., J. Hamburger and J.P. Kreier. 1976. T and B cell population changes in young and in adult rats infected with Plasmodium berghei. Infect. Immun. 14: 178-183.

13. Stevenson, M.M. and E. Skamene. 1986. Modulation of Primary Antibody Responses to Sheep Erythrocytes in Plasmodium chabaudi-infected resistant and susceptible mouse strains. Infect. Immun. 54: 600-602.

CUTANEOUS LEISHMANIASIS: RELATIVE ROLE OF T CELL SUBSETS

Richard Titus, Martine Marchand, Genevieve Milon, Gilles Marchal, Thierry Boon and Jacques Louis

Harvard Medical School, 250 Longwood Avenue, Boston, Massachusetts 02115 U.S.A.; International Institute of Cellular and Molecular Pathology, 75 Avenue Hippocrate, B-1200, Brussels, Belgium; Unite d'Immunophysiologie Cellulaire, Institut Pasteur, 75724 Paris, France; and World Health Organization, Immunology Research and Training Center, Institute of Biochemistry, Epalinges CH-1066, Switzerland

INTRODUCTION

Leishmanias are protozoan parasites which are transmitted to their mammalian host by the bite of a sandfly vector (1). Upon entering the host, the flagellated promastigote form of the parasite which is injected by the sandfly is phagocytized by mononuclear phagocytic cells in which it transforms into the aflagellate amastigote form. Following infection of man by *Leishmania*, several different forms of disease can ensue which depend upon the species of *Leishmania* carried by the sandfly. For example, a cutaneous form of leishmaniasis can be caused by *L. major*, *L. mexicana*, or *L. braziliensis*, a mucocutaneous form by *L. braziliensis* and a visceral form by *L. donovani*. In addition, a spectrum of clinical manifestations can be observed in patients suffering from each of these forms of the disease which suggests that the pathologic changes observed in leishmaniasis are due to both the species of the infecting parasite and to the host response to the parasite.

In the murine model for cutaneous leishmaniasis with *L. major*, it has been shown that the severity of disease is determined by the genetic background of the mouse (2,3). For example, in BALB/c mice the disease progresses inexorably leading to death of the animals, while in CBA mice cutaneous lesions resolve with the concomitant development of immunity to reinfection. Thus, the severity of cutaneous leishmaniasis seen in mice of different genetic backgrounds mimics the spectrum of disease seen in man.

Healing of cutaneous lesions in both human and murine leishmaniasis has been shown to be linked to the activities of cells which mediate parasite-specific delayed-type hypersensitivity (DTH) (4,5), although, in some cases, protection can be mediated by cells which do not express this function (6). In the pioneering work of Mitchell and colleagues, it was shown that athymic nu/nu mice (animals which are exquisitely susceptible to *L. major*) could be protected from disease by the adoptive transfer of Lyt-1^{+} splenic T cells from normal syngeneic mice (7). Interestingly, when BALB/c nu/nu mice were adoptively transferred low numbers (10^6-10^7) of syngeneic lymphoid cells, the animals became resistant to cutaneous leishmaniasis. However, transfer of high numbers ($>10^8$) of lymphoid cells resulted in a mouse as susceptible to cutaneous leishmaniasis as its euthymic BALB/c counterpart. The simplest interpretation of these data (although other factors may participate, e.g., affinity of the T cells involved) is that two kinds of parasite-specific T cells exist in the intact BALB/c mouse: one T cell which is potentially host protective and present in large numbers and a second T cell which can be detrimental for the host which is present in fewer numbers than the protective cell, but this latter cell is capable of overriding the effect of the protective cell. Therefore, when low numbers of lymphoid cells are adoptively transferred from BALB/c donors to nu/nu BALB/c recipients, the effect of the detrimental T cell is diluted out so as to be inoperative which allows the protective cell to express itself. In contrast, when high numbers of cells are transferred, enough of the detrimental cells are present so that their activities ultimately prevail over those of the protective cell. The difference between these two T cells may be the epitope of the parasite recognized by the cells and thus a particular parasite antigen may trigger a protective function and another may trigger a detrimental T cell function. This hypothesis has, in fact, recently been advanced by Mitchell and colleagues (8).

Work by Howard, Liew, and colleagues has shown that $Lyt\text{-}1^+2^-$ T cells mediate host resistance to L. major in mice (9); yet, T cells with this same surface phenotype have also been reported to inhibit parasite-specific cell-mediated immune responses (9-11). Interestingly, these latter cells, termed "suppressor cells" by Howard and Liew, do not have the classical surface phenotype of suppressor cells (i.e., $Lyt\text{-}1^-23^+$, $L3T4^-$, $I\text{-}J^+$) but instead bear the phenotype of the helper/inducer lineage (i.e., $Lyt\text{-}1^+23^-$, $L3T4^+$, $I\text{-}J^-$).

Taken together, these observations indicate that parasite-specific T cells play a central role in resistance to murine cutaneous leishmaniasis. In addition, these observations suggest that more than one subset of parasite-specific T cells, which differ either by epitope recognized or function performed, can operate during the course of cutaneous leishmaniasis. It is possible that the absolute number of each of these T cell subsets present during the course of cutaneous leishmaniasis and the interplay between these T cell subsets can explain the different patterns of infection seen in mice of different genetic backgrounds.

In an effort to explore the participation of various T cell subsets in the immune response to cutaneous leishmaniasis, we have taken advantage of two recent advances in murine T cell immunology: 1) the ability to propagate lines and clones of T cells of particular specificity in vitro which has allowed us to determine through adoptive transfer studies the effect of T cell populations with defined function(s) on cutaneous leishmaniasis and 2) the demonstration that there are two major subsets of T cells. One of these subsets of T cells is activated by antigen presented in the context of class II major histocompatibility antigens (e.g., I-A molecules on macrophages) and the other is activated by antigen seen in the context of class I major histocompatibility antigens (H-2 molecules). The former subset of T cells can be thought of as being composed predominantly of T helper cells which have a unique surface marker, termed L3T4, and the latter as being composed predominantly of cytotoxic T cells, or T cells with the unique $Lyt\text{-}2^+$ surface phenotype (12). The existence of these two unique surface markers and the availability of monoclonal antibodies (mAb) specific for the markers has made it possible to a) produce T cells of a given antigen specificity that are of a particular T cell subset, b) monitor the activities of T cells of the two subsets during the course of an immune response in vivo and c) modulate the activities of either of these two T cell subsets in vivo by treating mice with mAb specific for T cell markers (i.e., either specific for L3T4 or Lyt-2). Taking advantage of these technologies, we have:

1) Determined the effect that adoptively transferring T cells with defined functions and surface phenotypes would have on the course of cutaneous leishmaniasis in mice

2) Analyzed the frequency and surface phenotype of parasite-specific T cells responding in genetically-susceptible (BALB/c) and in genetically-resistant (CBA) mice infected with L. major

3) Determined the effect that depleting T cell subsets (both $L3T4^+$ and $Lyt\text{-}2^+$) in vivo would have on cutaneous leishmaniasis

4) Analyzed the nature of the protective effect for cutaneous leishmaniasis seen in mice immunized with chemically-mutagenized non-infective forms of L. major

Effect of L. major-specific T cells on the course of cutaneous leishmaniasis in the mouse

Because of the importance of T cells in resistance to cutaneous leishmaniasis, efforts were made to derive homogeneous populations of L. major-specific T cells, to characterize the cells both phenotypically and functionally and to determine their effect on cutaneous leishmaniasis by adoptive transfer studies. As a source of T cells sensitized to L. major, draining lymph nodes from mice injected subcutaneously at the base of the tail with L. major antigen emulsified in complete Freund's adjuvant were utilized since this route of injection has been shown to induce potent T cell responses (13) and to dramatically increase the frequency of L. major-specific T cells in the sensitized lymph nodes (14). In order to further increase the frequency of L. major-specific T cells in the sensitized lymph node cells, the cells were cultured in vitro in the presence of L. major antigen and the resulting blast cell population was propagated in a culture system containing interleukin-2 (IL-2) (15). Such manipulations have been shown to achieve a final frequency of approximately one L. major-specific T cell in every 25 cells in the IL-2-propagated T cell population (14). These highly enriched L. major-specific T cell populations were found 1) to express almost exclusively an $L3T4^+$, $Lyt\text{-}2^-$, $Thy1.2^+$ surface phenotype, 2) to provide parasite-specific helper activity, 3) to activate L. major-infected macrophages in vitro resulting in destruction of the parasite and 4) to adoptively transfer L. major-specific DTH to naive syngeneic recipients (15).

In order to determine the effect that these L. major-specific T cells would have on the course of cutaneous leishmaniasis in the mouse, adoptive transfer studies were performed. It was anticipated that the T cells would convey protection for cutaneous leishmaniasis in light of the observations above that the cells could activate macrophages in vitro to destroy L. major and could transfer parasite-specific DTH in vivo and this latter function, as mentioned in the Introduction, has been correlated with protection in cutaneous leishmanisis. L. major-specific T cells were derived from BALB/c (genetically-susceptible) and CBA (genetically-resistant) mice. The cells were transferred to syngeneic naive recipients (10^7 cells per mouse injected intravenously) and the animals were challenged 24 hours later with 10^7 L. major promastigotes subcutaneously in the footpad. Surprisingly, rather than protecting the adoptive transfer recipients, the L. major-specific T cells induced an exacerbated course of infection in both susceptible BALB/c mice and in resistant CBA animals as reflected by dramatically increased lesion sizes in mice receiving T cells (Fig. 1).

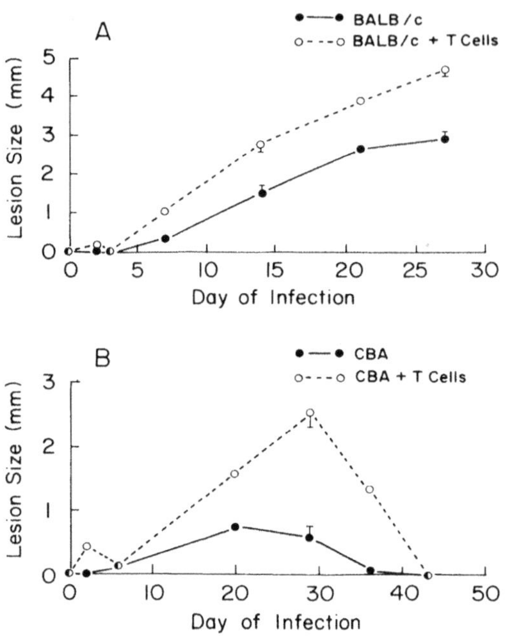

Figure 1. Effect of L3T4$^+$ L. major-specific T cells on the course of cutaneous leishmaniasis in BALB/c and CBA mice

Groups of 5 BALB/c (panel A) or 5 CBA (panel B) mice each received 10^7 syngeneic L3T4$^+$ L. major-specific T cells intravenously (o---o). 24 hours later, these mice and groups of untreated control mice (●——●) were challenged with 10^7 L. major promastigotes subcutaneously in the footpad. Lesion size (mm ± SD) was determined by measuring the infected foot with a vernier caliper and determining the increase in footpad thickness as compared to the uninfected contralateral control footpad.

The exacerbative effect on murine cutaneous leishmaniasis of adoptively transferring L3T4$^+$ L. major-specific T cells could have been the consequence of an accelerated influx of inflammatory cells to the lesion site which enhanced lesion size and/or the consequence of elevated numbers of parasites in the lesions. It thus became important to quantify the number of L. major parasites present in the lesion. In order to enumerate L. major parasites in the lesions of cutaneous leishmaniasis, a sensitive limiting dilution assay for determining the frequency of L. major in mouse tissues was developed (16). Using this assay, it was found that the exacerbative effect of L3T4$^+$ L. major-specific T cells on cutaneous leishmanisis brought about profound increases in parasite numbers in the lesions (between 10 to 1000-fold more parasites in the lesions of mice receiving T cells as compared to control mice not receiving cells) (16, unpublished observations). Thus, the exacerbative effect on cutaneous leishmaniasis of L3T4$^+$ L. major-specific T cells resulted in not only larger lesions but lesions that contained dramatically larger numbers of L. major.

Other studies were performed in which it was shown that the exacerbative effect of L3T4$^+$ L. major-specific T cells on cutaneous leishmaniasis was specific for such cells (15) and that clonally-derived lines of $L3T4^+$ L. major-specific T cells also had an exacerbative effect on the disease (unpublished observations). In addition, $L3T4^+$ L. major-specific T cells were tagged with ^{131}I and injected into syngeneic naive recipients in adoptive transfer studies identical to those described in the legend of Figure 1. The number of L. major-specific T cells which migrated to developing L. major lesions could then be calculated from the levels of radioactivity found in the lesions. Using this approach, it was determined that L. major-specific T cells rapidly entered the developing lesion and that by day 9 of infection 20% of the remaining injected cells had localized in the lesion. This number of cells was more than could be found in any other organ, including the spleen (16.2%). This suggested that the exacerbative effect of adoptively transferring $L3T4^+$ L. major-specific T cells on cutaneous leishmaniasis was associated with the migration of large numbers of the transferred T cells to the exacerbated lesion.

Finally, in order to determine the involvement of host T cells in the exacerbative phenomenon, $L3T4^+$ L. major-specific T cells were adoptively transferred to T cell deficient mice, that is, to adult-thymectomized, lethally-irradiated, bone marrow-reconstituted (AT x BM) mice. It was found (Table 1) that the degree of exacerbation for cutaneous leishmaniasis observed in T cell deficient mice adoptively transferred L. major-specific T cell was equivalent to that seen in normal control animals receiving L. major T cells. This result suggested that host T cells need not participate in the exacerbative effect of $L3T4^+$ L. major-specific T cells on cutaneous leishmaniasis.

In summary, the results thus far indicate that $L3T4^+$ L. major-specific T cells can be detrimental to the host in cutaneous leishmaniasis resulting in accelerated lesion development and enhanced parasite numbers in the lesion. This exacerbative effect of L. major-specific T cells is specific for the cells and is associated with the presence of the cells in the exacerbated lesion. In addition, host T cells need not be involved in the phenomenon indicating that the $L3T4^+$ L. major-specific T cells are not acting via the induction of host T cells (e.g., T suppressor cells). Taken collectively, these observations suggest that $L3T4^+$ L. major-specific T cells can be responsible for lesion progression in cutaneous leishmaniasis. This hypothesis will be tested in the experiments detailed in the next two sections.

Table 1. Adoptive transfer of $L3T4^+$ L. major-specific T cells to AT x BM mice

Day of infection	Lesion size, mm (± SD) — Treatment: None	L. major T cells	AT x BM	AT x BM, L. major T cells
11	0.2 (.05)	1.1 (.06)	0.2 (.03)	1.0 (.05)
21	0.5 (.13)	1.7 (.14)	0.3 (.04)	2.1 (.20)
41	0.7 (.11)	0.9 (.09)	1.4 (.10)	1.4 (.09)
53	0.2 (.05)	0.4 (.13)	1.1 (.11)	0.9 (.08)

Groups of 5 normal CBA or AT x BM CBA mice were injected intravenously with 10^7 syngeneic L. major-specific T cells. 24 hours later, these mice and control mice not receiving cells were challenged with 10^7 L. major promastigotes subcutaneously in the footpad. The resulting lesions were measured as described in the legend of Fig. 1.

Analysis of the frequency and surface phenotype of parasite-specific T cells generated during the course of cutaneous leishmaniasis in BALB/c (genetically-susceptible) and CBA (genetically-resistant) mice. Because it was possible that $L3T4^+$ L. major-specific T cells could cause lesion progression in cutaneous leishmaniasis, the frequency of such cells that evolved during an infection with L. major was determined. It was reasoned that if $L3T4^+$ L. major-specific T cells cause lesion progression, these cells should predominate in BALB/c mice infected with L. major since these animals develop lesions which progress. In contrast, $L3T4^+$ L. major-specific T cells should be less prevalent in infected CBA mice since these animals are resistant to cutaneous leishmaniasis.

The number of L. major-specific T cells present in mice infected with the parasite was assessed by limiting dilution analysis to determine the frequency of cells which mediate L. major-specific DTH (17). At various intervals after infection with L. major, lymph nodes draining the site of infection were removed from BALB/c and CBA mice. A dilution series was made from cell suspensions derived from the lymph nodes and aliquots of each dilution, admixed with a constant number of parasites (3×10^6) as a source of antigen, were injected into the footpad of from 10 to 12 syngeneic normal recipients for each dilution of cells. Fourteen to 16 hrs later, the DTH response was quantified by measuring the increase in footpad thickness as compared to the contralateral control footpad. Frequencies of parasite-specific DTH-mediating T cells were estimated by minimum Chi-squared analysis of the Poisson distribution relationship between the number of lymphoid cells transferred and the percentage of footpads exhibiting no DTH (17). The surface phenotype of the cells transferring L. major-specific DTH reactivity was determined by depleting the lymph node cells of either $L3T4^+$ or $Lyt\text{-}2^+$ T cells prior to transfer into recipient mice. Depletion of $L3T4^+$ or $Lyt\text{-}2^+$ T cells was accomplished by incubating the lymph node cells with mAb specific for either the L3T4 or Lyt-2 marker plus complement (17).

As seen in Figure 2, the number of L. major-specific T cells capable of mediating parasite-specific DTH present in the lymph nodes draining the lesion in BALB/c mice was substantially greater than the number observed in CBA mice. The data given in Figure 2 were obtained at 60 days of infection, however, similar results were obtained at other timepoints (days 16,30,90) (17). In addition, the surface phenotype of T cells capable of mediating L. major-specific DTH in BALB/c and CBA mice infected with the parasite was analyzed. It can be seen (Fig. 2) that the great majority of DTH-mediating cells in the BALB/c was of the $L3T4^+$ phenotype whereas, in contrast, the phenotype of T cells in the CBA mouse was approximately equally divided between the L3T4 and Lyt-2 subsets. These results indicate that susceptibility to cutaneous leishmaniasis in the mouse correlates with the presence of high numbers of $L3T4^+$ L. major-specific T cells during the course of infection with the parasite. As such, the results corroborate those described in the previous section in which $L3T4^+$ L. major-specific T cells were adoptively transferred to mice and suggest that $L3T4^+$ L. major-specific T cells are involved in lesion progression in cutaneous leishmaniasis.

Effect of depleting $L3T4^+$ or $Lyt\text{-}2^+$ T cells in mice on the course of cutaneous leishmaniasis. Since susceptibility to cutaneous leishmaniasis correlated with the presence of large numbers of $L3T4^+$ L. major-specific T cells during the course of the disease (see previous section), the effect that depleting $L3T4^+$ T cells from mice infected with L. major would have on the outcome of the infection was examined. Depletion of $L3T4^+$ T cells in mice was accomplished by injecting the animals with mAb specific for the L3T4 surface marker on mouse T cells (18). Initially, BALB/c mice were injected with the anti-L3T4 mAb since these mice are susceptible to cutaneous leishmaniasis and generate large numbers of $L3T4^+$ L. major-specific T

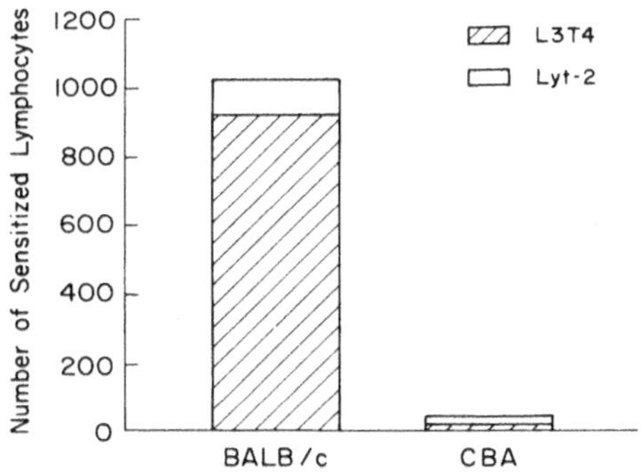

Figure 2. Frequency and surface phenotype of parasite-specific T cells in BALB/c and CBA mice infected with *L. major*

BALB/c and CBA mice were injected with 10^7 *L. major* promastigotes subcutaneously in the shaved rump. At day 60 of infection, the draining inguinal and para-aortic lymph nodes were removed and the number of *L. major*-specific T cells of the L3T4 or Lyt-2 subsets present in the lymph nodes was determined as detailed in the text.

cells during the course of the infection, and, therefore, inhibiting the activities of L3T4$^+$ T cells in these animals might be of therapeutic value.

BALB/c mice were infected with *L. major* and then initiated on a program of intraperitoneal injections of anti-L3T4 mAb. Results of such an experiment are shown in Table 2 and demonstrate that treatment of BALB/c mice with anti-L3T4 mAb had a pronounced therapeutic effect on the course of cutaneous leishmaniasis in the animals which resulted not only in substantially smaller lesions (Table 2) but also in the destruction of parasites in the lesions (18). In addition, the therapeutic effect of anti-L3T4 mAb treatment on cutaneous leishmaniasis in BALB/c mice was found to correlate with a 60-80% depletion of L3T4$^+$ T cells in the lymphoid tissues of the treated animals and was shown not to be due to a negative effect of the mAb either on *L. major* itself or on macrophages (18).

In order to further investigate the therapeutic effect of anti-L3T4 mAb treatment on the course of cutaneous leishmaniasis in BALB/c mice, BALB/c mice that had been treated with anti-L3T4 mAb and had resolved their primary infection with *L. major* were rechallenged with the parasite to determine whether the therapeutic effect of anti-L3T4 mAb treatment led to the development of resistance to a secondary challenge. Results in Fig. 3 demonstrate that prior treatment with anti-L3T4 mAb imparted substantial resistance to a secondary challenge with *L. major* (panel B) and, in fact, even to a tertiary challenge with the parasite (panel C). It should be emphasized that treatment with anti-L3T4 mAb was carried out only through day 56 of the experiment, that is during the time of the primary challenge with *L. major*, and not at the time of secondary challenge (day 134) or tertiary challenge (day 244). Therefore, unless residual anti-L3T4 mAb in the mice from injections of the mAb during day 0 to 56 of the experiment was still present at a level to be biologically active, resistance to the secondary and tertiary challenge with *L. major* must have been due to an effect of the anti-L3T4 mAb during the primary infection only. Thus, treatment with anti-L3T4 mAb had a therapeutic effect not only on a primary infection with *L. major* in susceptible BALB/c mice but also imparted protection to reinfection with the parasite. These results corroborate the findings described in the previous two sections and suggest that L3T4$^+$ *L. major*-specific T cells, or at least an excessive number of such cells, can be detrimental to the course of cutaneous leishmaniasis in the mouse.

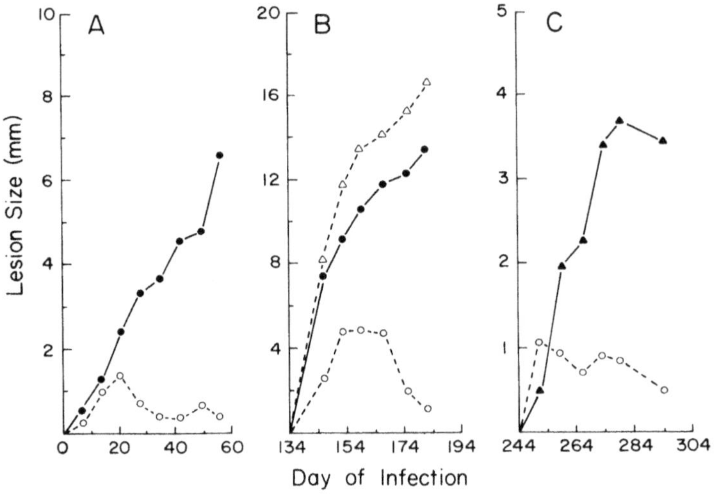

Figure 3. Resistance to rechallenge with L. major in BALB/c mice depleted of L3T4$^+$ T cells

Panel A. On day zero, 10 BALB/c mice were each challenged with 10^7 L. major promastigotes subcutaneously in the right footpad. Three hours later, 5 of the mice (o---o) were begun on treatments with anti-L3T4 mAb as detailed in the legend of Table 2. These animals were not treated with anti-L3T4 mAb beyond day 56 of infection. The other 5 mice were not treated with mAb and served as controls (●——●).

Panel B. At 134 days after the primary infection, the same 2 groups of mice as described in Panel A (o---o and ●——●) were rechallenged in the shaved rump subcutaneously with 10^7 L. major promastigotes. In addition, 5 normal BALB/c mice were similarly challenged and served as controls (Δ---Δ).

Panel C. At 244 days after the primary infection, the mice that had been originally challenged with L. major and treated with anti-L3T4 mAb in Panel A and then rechallenged with L. major in Panel B (o---o) were again rechallenged with 10^7 L. major promastigotes subcutaneously in the left footpad. Five normal BALB/c mice were similarly challenged and served as controls (▲——▲).

The figure depicts lesion development which was followed in the footpad in Panels A and C, as described in the legend of Figure 1 or on the rump (Panel B) by determining the average diameter (mm) of the lesions with a vernier caliper.

Table 2. Therapeutic effect of anti-L3T4 mAb on cutaneous leishmaniasis in BALB/c mice

Day of Infection	Lesion size, mean (± SE) Treatment: None	Treatment: anti-L3T4 mAb
7	0.08 (.06)	0.10 (.02)
14	1.10 (.28)	0.73 (.15)
20	1.62 (.40)	0.77 (.08)
28	2.03 (.23)	0.41 (.23)
35	3.16 (.23)	0.20 (.02)

Two groups of 5 BALB/c mice each were infected with 10^7 L. major promastigotes subcutaneously in the footpad. Three hours later, one of the groups was injected intraperitoneally with 0.5 ml of the culture supernatant of the GK 1.5 (12) anti-L3T4 mAb line. Treatments with mAb GK 1.5 were repeated every day for the first week, 3 times the second week and, thereafter, 2 times/week for the remainder of the experiment. Lesion size was determined as described in the legend of Fig. 1.

It was next reasoned that since $L3T4^+$ L. major-specific T cells can be detrimental to the host infected with the parasite, it was possible that T cells other than those of the $L3T4^+$ subset might be able to mediate protection against infection with L. major. To investigate this possibility, mice were injected with an anti-Lyt-2 mAb (H35-17.2, see reference 19) in an attempt to deplete Lyt-2-bearing T cells from the mice and to determine the effect that this would have on an infection with L. major. For these experiments, CBA mice were utilized since this animal is normally resistant to cutaneous leishmaniasis so that if Lyt-2-bearing cells were involved in resistance to the disease, depletion of these cells in CBA mice would have dramatic effects on the course of cutaneous leishmaniasis. In order to maximize depletion of $Lyt\text{-}2^+$ cells, anti-Lyt-2 mAb was injected before infection with L. major and was injected every day of the experiment which led to a depletion of from 83% to 87% of Lyt-2 bearing cells in various lymphoid tissues of the mice. As can be seen in Table 3, CBA mice depleted of Lyt-2-bearing cells developed lesions which were larger than those seen on control mice; however, the animals were still able to control their infection. Examination of the lesions for numbers of L. major present did not consistently show differences in the number of parasites present in the anti-Lyt-2 mAb treated mice as compared to control animals. Interpretation of these results is difficult since the worsening of lesions in anti-Lyt-2 mAb treated mice could have been either the consequence of depletion of $Lyt\text{-}2^+$ cells which were protective cells or the consequence of enhanced proliferation of $L3T4^+$ L. major-specific T cells to fill the void left by the deleted $Lyt\text{-}2^+$ cells and, from the experiments described above, excessive numbers of $L3T4^+$ L. major-specific T cells always leads to exacerbation of cutaneous leishmaniasis. Nevertheless, it is interesting that CBA mice depleted of $Lyt\text{-}2^+$ T cells by injection of anti-Lyt-2 mAb were still able to control an L. major infection, however, the exact role of $Lyt\text{-}2^+$ T cells in cutaneous leishmaniasis can only be determined by deriving $Lyt\text{-}2^+$ T cells specific for L. major and assessing their effect on cutaneous leishmaniasis in adoptive transfer studies.

Finally, it is interesting that when CBA mice were treated with daily injections of anti-L3T4 mAb in parallel with the anti-Lyt-2 mAb treated mice described in the previous paragraph, the effect on cutaneous leishmaniasis was one of profound exacerbation of the disease (Table 3). These CBA mice treated with anti-L3T4 mAb were found to have as many as 1445-fold more parasites in their lesions compared to control mice. Examination of their lymphoid tissues revealed a depletion of 97 to 100% of $L3T4^+$ T cells and it should also be mentioned that similar severe depletion of $L3T4^+$ T cells in BALB/c mice led to similar substantial exacerbation of cutaneous leishmaniasis (data not shown). These data should be compared to those in Table 2 in which a 60-80% depletion of $L3T4^+$ T cells had a therapeutic effect on cutaneous leishmaniasis in BALB/c mice. Taken together, these observations would suggest that although large numbers of L. major-specific $L3T4^+$ T cells acting during the course of cutaneous leishmaniasis in the mouse can lead to lesion progression (as docomented by many of the experiments presented thus far), severe depletion of such cells also leads to lesion progression which argues that some (or certain) $L3T4^+$ T cells are absolutely necessary for resolution of the disease.

Nature of the protective effect for cutaneous leishmaniasis in mice immunized with chemically-mutagenized non-infective forms of L. major. Mutant forms of L. major were produced in hopes of being able to elicit with these mutant parasites a T cell response different from the exacerbative L. major-specific T cells described above. Non-infective mutant forms of L. major were derived by chemical mutagenesis with N-methyl-N'-nitro-N-nitrosoguanidine (20). Several rounds of mutagenesis were required to obtain three cloned mutants (numbers 75, 79, and 81) which were found to be totally non-infective for normally susceptible BALB/c mice (Table 4). Challenges with as many as 10^7 mutant L. major subcutaneously in the footpad did not produce any noticeable pathologic change in BALB/c or CBA (resistant) mice for over 100 days of observation. Interestingly, although there was no difference in the growth pattern of mutagenized and virulent (wild type) promastigotes in vitro, there were striking differences in the interaction of the mutant parasites with cultured macrophages. Following uptake by macrophages, the mutant parasites were spontaneously destroyed within 24 hr; in contrast, wild type L. major survived and multiplied within macrophages throughout the period of observation. This spontaneous killing of the mutant parasites by normal macrophages was observed with macrophages derived from various sources (bone marrow, resident peritoneal, peritoneal exudate) and from mice with varying susceptibilities to L. major (BALB/c, susceptible; CBA/T6 and C3H/HeJ, resistant; DBA/2 intermediate.)

Table 3. Effect of depleting $Lyt\text{-}2^+$ or $L3T4^+$ T cells in CBA mice on the course of cutaneous leishmaniasis

	Lesion size, mean (± SE)		
		Treatment	
Day of Infection	None	Anti-Lyt-2 mAb	Anti-L3T4 mAb
9	1.3 (.04)	0.9 (.06)	0.6 (.04)
16	1.3 (.03)	1.2 (.08)	1.2 (.04)
22	1.5 (.05)	1.7 (.11)	1.7 (.04)
30	0.4 (.10)	1.8 (.23)	2.7 (.57)
39	0.0 (0.0)	0.4 (.19)	3.3 (.60)

Groups of 5 CBA mice each were injected intraperitoneally with 0.5 ml of the culture supernatant of the anti-Lyt-2 mAb line H35-17.2 or the anti-L3T4 mAb line GK 1.5 on a daily basis from day -6 to day 39. On day 0, these mice and 5 control animals were challenged with L. major and resulting lesions were measured as described in the legend of Fig. 1.

Experiments were conducted to determine whether injection of mice with the mutant parasites would protect the animals from a subsequent challenge with virulent L. major. BALB/c mice (susceptible) were chosen for study since any immunizing effect of the mutants would be more easily detected in mice which are normally susceptible to cutaneous leishmaniasis. It was found that large doses of mutant number 79 (100 to 200 x 10^6) mutant parasites injected intravenously on day -17, -11, and -7) protected the animals from a subsequent challenge on day 0 with 2 x 10^6 virulent L. major subcutaneously (Fig. 4). Lesions on the mutant treated mice reached only a small size and persisted as chronic but contained lesions for over 100 days of observation. In contrast, control BALB/c mice, which were not pretreated with mutant parasites, developed large progressing lesions. It should be mentioned that injection of identical numbers, or fewer numbers (e.g. 2 x 10^7), of virulent L. major intravenously had no protective effect on a subsequent subcutaneous challenge with virulent L. major. In fact, intravenous pretreatment with virulent L. major resulted in death of the mice between days 30 to 40.

It is interesting that the protective effect of immunization with mutant 79 on a subsequent infection with virulent L. major was most pronounced when the mutant was injected intravenously. Protection of a slightly lesser degree ensued when the mutant was injected intraperitonally and no protection was observed (and in some cases exacerbation of a subsequent infection with L. major occurred) when the mutant was injected subcutaneously. These findings are in accordance with observations made by Mitchell (21) and Liew (10,11) and colleagues in which a similar exacerbative effect on cutaneous leishmaniasis was observed if the immunizing procedure was performed subcutaneously.

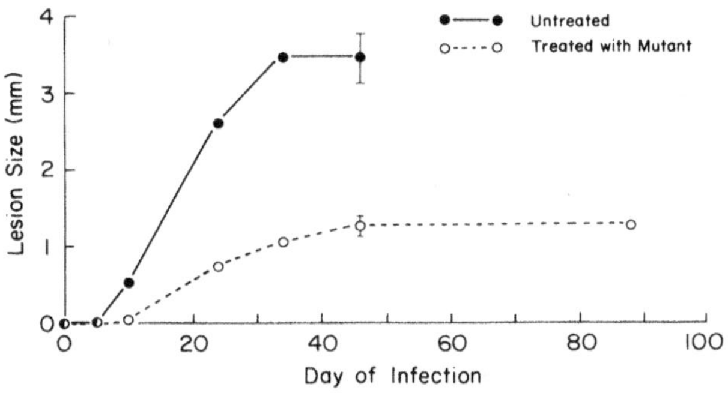

Figure 4. Protection to L. major infection in BALB/c mice incurred by pretreatment with chemically-mutagenized non-infective L. major parasites

Five BALB/c mice were injected intravenously with 100 x 10^6 mutant number 79 on days -17, -11 and -7. On day 0, these mice and 5 normal BALB/c control mice were challenged with 2 x 10^6 virulent L. major subcutaneously in the footpad. Lesion development was followed as detailed in the legend of Figure 1.

Table 4. Lack of infectivity of chemically-mutagenized L. major for BALB/c mice

Day of Infection	Lesion size (mean ± SE) in mice injected with Virulent L. major	Mutant 75	Mutant 79	Mutant 81
18	1.40 (.12)	0 (0)	0 (0)	0 (0)
30	2.22 (.32)	0 (0)	0 (0)	0 (0)
60	3.58 (.59)	0 (0)	0 (0)	0 (0)

Groups of 5 BALB/c mice each were injected subcutaneously in the footpad with 10^7 each of virulent L. major or the mutant forms of the parasite. Lesion development was followed as described in the legend of Fig. 1.

Future work will be aimed at determining the nature of the protective effect on cutaneous leishmaniasis that is engendered by immunization with mutant 79. Initial studies indicate that the protective effect of mutant 79 treatment can be adoptively transferred to naive syngeneic recipients using spleen cells from treated mice. It will be most interesting to characterize the cells involved in this protective effect and to compare their activities with those of the $L3T4^+$ L. major-specific T cell described above that are capable of exacerbating the course of cutaneous leishmaniasis.

CONCLUSIONS AND DISCUSSION

1) There are $L3T4^+$ T cells specific for L. major that can exacerbate cutaneous leishmaniasis caused by L. major. These T cells are capable of activating L. major-infected macrophages to destroy the parasite in vitro and of adoptively transferring parasite-specific DTH in vivo. When susceptible (BALB/c) and resistant (CBA) mice are assessed for the frequency of $L3T4^+$ L. major-specific T cells that are capable of mediating parasite-specific DTH during the course of the disease, it is found that many more of such cells are present in BALB/c mice than in CBA animals. When BALB/c mice are depleted of 60-80% of their L3T4-bearing cells by treatment with anti-L3T4 mAb, the mice are converted from susceptible to resistant to cutaneous leishmaniasis. In contrast, if nearly all the $L3T4^+$ T cells are depleted from these mice, the mice are extremely susceptible to cutaneous leishmaniasis. These observations imply that the presence of large numbers of $L3T4^+$ L. major-specific T cells (the case naturally in BALB/c mice or artificially in mice adoptively transferred $L3T4^+$ L. major-specific T cells) causes progression of cutaneous leishmaniasis. On the other hand, the presence of moderate numbers of $L3T4^+$ L. major-specific T cells (the case naturally in CBA mice or artificially in BALB/c mice partially depleted of $L3T4^+$ T cells) leads to resistance to the disease. However, severe depletion (97 to 100%) of $L3T4^+$ T cells results in extreme susceptibility to cutaneous leishmaniasis in both BALB/c and CBA mice. Thus, some (or certain) $L3T4^+$ T cells are needed for resistance to L. major, but an excessive number of $L3T4^+$ T cells leads to chronic disease.

2) Depletion of $Lyt\text{-}2^+$ T cells from mice by treating the animals with anti-Lyt-2 mAb leads to an enhanced course of cutaneous leishmaniasis. Although this does not prove a role for $Lyt\text{-}2^+$ T cells in cutaneous leishmaniasis, it points to the importance of determining the participation of such cells in the disease by deriving $Lyt\text{-}2^+$ L. major-specific T cells and assessing their effect on the disease using adoptive transfer techniques.

3) By immunizing with non-infective mutant forms of L. major, it is possible to induce a protective response for virulent L. major even in normally susceptible BALB/c mice. Since preliminary results indicate that the protective effect is cell mediated, it will be interesting to compare this cell to the L3T4$^+$ T cell which exacerbates cutaneous leishmaniasis.

When one incorporates the results reported here into those that exist in the literature, a concensus emerges. A number of laboratories, including those of Mitchell, Howard and Liew and colleagues as well as those included in this report, have described procedures which are either beneficial or detrimental for the host in murine cutaneous leishmaniasis. The T cells mediating the opposing effects are difficult to distinguish from each other: they have the same surface phenotype in the work of Howard and Liew (9-11), their effects can be seen only when either low numbers or high numbers of cells are adoptively transferred in the work of Mitchell (7) and one or the other outcome of disease is seen depending on the number of L3T4$^+$ L. major-specific T cells acting during the course of murine cutaneous leishmaniasis as described in the work reported here. It is hoped that by employing the in vitro propagation and cloning techniques for T cells that have been described here, it will become possible to isolate both the protective and exacerbative cell in cutaneous leishmaniasis and to analyze the characteristics of each of these T cells. Since L. major is an obligate intracellular parasite of macrophages, it is likely that the protective and exacerbative T cells will differ in one or more of the following ways: the functions they express, the lymphokines they produce or the manner in which they interact with macrophages. Such information may help explain the pathogenesis of disease in cutaneous leishmaniasis and may have relevance to the mechanism of disease with other intracellular pathogens.

REFERENCES

1. Markell, E.K. and M. Voge. 1971. Medical Parasitology. W.B. Saunders, Philadelphia, p. 129.
2. Behin, R., J. Mauel and B. Sordat. 1979. Exp. Parasitol. 48:81.
3. Handman, E., R. Ceredig and G.F. Mitchell. 1979. Aust. J. Exp. Biol. Med. Sci. 57:9.
4. Convit, J., M.E. Pinardi and A.J. Rondon. 1972. Trans. Roy. Soc. Trop. Med. Hyg. 66:603.
5. Howard, J.G., C. Hale and F.Y. Liew. 1980. J. Exp. Med. 152:594.
6. Liew, F.Y., J.G. Howard and C. Hale. 1984. J. Immunol. 132:456.
7. Mitchell, G.F., R.F. Anders, G.V. Brown, E. Handman, I.C. Roberts-Thomson, C.B. Chapman, K.P. Forsyth, L.P. Kahl and K.M. Cruise. 1982. Immunol. Rev. 61:137.
8. Mitchell, G.F., E. Handman. 1985. Parasitology Today. 1:61.
9. Liew, F.Y., C. Hale and J.G. Howard. 1982. J. Immunol. 128:1917.
10. Liew, F.Y., C. Hale and J.G. Howard. 1985. J. Immunol. 135:2095.
11. Liew, F.Y., A. Singleton, E. Cillairi and J.G. Howard. 1985. J. Immunol. 135:2102.
12. Dialynas, D.P., D.B. Wilde, P. Marrack, A. Pierres, K.A. Wall, W. Havran, G. Otten, M.R. Loken, M. Pierres, J. Kappler and F.W. Fitch. 1983. Immunol. Rev. 74:29.
13. Corradin, G., H.M. Etlinger and J.M. Chiller. 1977. J. Immunol. 119:1048.
14. Louis, J.A., R.H. Zubler, S.G. Coutinho, G. Lima, R. Behin, J. Mauel and H.D. Engers. 1982. Immunol. Rev. 61:215.
15. Titus, R.G., G.C. Lima, H.D. Engers and J.A. Louis. 1984. J. Immunol. 133:1594.
16. Titus, R.G., M. Marchand, T. Boon and J.A. Louis. 1985. Parasite Immunol. 7:545.
17. Milon, G., R.G. Titus, J.-C. Cerottini, G. Marchal and J.A. Louis. 1986. J. Immunol. 136:1467.

18. Titus, R.G., R. Ceredig, J.-C. Cerottini and J.A. Louis. 1985. J. Immunol. 135:2108.
19. Golstein, P., C. Goridis, A.M. Schmitt-Verhulst, B. Hayot, A. Pierres, A. van Agthoven, Y. Kaufmann, Z. Eshhar and M. Pierres. 1982. Immunol. Rev. 68:5.
20. Marchand, M., S. Daoud, R.G. Titus, J. Louis, and T. Boon. 1987. Parasite Immunol., in press.
21. Mitchell, G.F., E. Handman and T.W. Spithill. 1984. Aust. J. Exp. Biol. Med. Sci. 62:145.

WHICH T CELLS ARE RELEVANT TO RESISTANCE AGAINST LISTERIA MONOCYTOGENES INFECTION?

Stefan H. E. Kaufmann

Department of Medical Microbiology and Immunology
University of Ulm
79, Ulm
Federal Republic of Germany

INTRODUCTION

Listeria monocytogenes is an intracellular bacterial pathogen for many mammals including man. Although endemic outbreaks of listeriosis have been reported it appears that the incidence of this disease is greatly underrated. While our knowledge about the epidemiology of listeriosis is still limited, a great deal of information has been gathered about the immune response against this pathogen. This is mostly due to the pioneering work of Mackaness, North and other investigators who have introduced L.monocytogenes to experimental immunology (summarized in 1). In these studies it has been shown that protective immunity depends on the interaction between specific T lymphocytes and mononuclear phagocytes (1-3). With the realization that the peripheral T-cell system consists of at least two well defined populations (summarized in 4) the question arose which of these T cell sets is relevant for the acquisition of resistance and which mechanisms are utilized.

In principle two different T-cell functions could be used: activation or lysis of target cells (1,5). Although exceptions exist, these functions are generally mediated by distinct T-cell subsets (1,4,5): CD4 T-cells ($L3T4^+$ in mice, $T4^+$ in humans) which recognize foreign antigen in association with class II major histocompatibility (MHC) molecules (H-2I in mice, HLA-DR,DP,DQ in humans) preferentially fulfill helper functions. CD8 T cells ($Lyt2^+$ in mice, $T8^+$ in humans) which recognize foreign antigen in association with class I MHC molecules (H-2K,D in mice, HLA-A,B,C in humans) are preferentially programmed for cytolytic functions.

In the original scheme of how T cells contribute to protection it was thought that T cells activate macrophages via the secretion of soluble mediators (1-3). When it was found that lymphokine secretion is the typical feature of CD4 T cells it was conluded that they represent the relevant T-cell population of antibacterial immunity. In support of this notion, it was shown by Zinkernagel et al. (6) that adoptive protection against L.monocytogenes is class II restricted. Therefore, it was somehow surprising that subsequently Kaufmann et al. (7) demonstrated that $Lyt2^+$ T cells were required for adoptive protection. This finding was further substantiated by Cheers and Sandrin (8), showing that adoptive anti-listerial protection was class I restricted. With the availability of monoclonal (mab) antibodies directed against the L3T4 molecule (4) Kaufmann et al.(9) could show that adoptive protection against L.monocytogenes depends on both $L3T4^+$ and $Lyt2^+$ T lymphocytes. These findings could best be accomodated in a scheme in which both class II restricted L3T4$^+$ and class I restricted Lyt2$^+$ T cells contribute to protection. It was assumed that both T cells collaborated with each other and that this collaboration resulted in granuloma formation and macrophage activation.

However, none of these findings could provide direct information about the functional activities of these T-cell sets. Information of this type became available when cloned long term cultured T-cell lines of either subset were established from L.monocytogenes infected mice. In these studies it was found that L3T4$^+$, class II restricted T-cell lines upon antigenic stimulation produce multiple lymphokines and provide help for B cells (10,11). In contrast, Lyt2$^+$ T-cell lines which were either class I restricted or lacked any apparent genetic restriction, were able to lyse macrophages expressing listerial antigens (12,13).

On the basis of these as well as other findings (14-18) it was proposed that within granulomata protection proceeds via three major steps (20): (1) Lysis by cytolytic T cells of infected tissue macrophages unable to destruct intracellular bacteria; (2) subsequent uptake of these bacteria by monocytes with high antibacterial potential; (3) final activation of bacteriocidal capacities in these blood monocytes by helper T lymphocytes. Under less organized conditions tissue destruction and bacterial dissemmination would be the primary outcome and hence pathogenic effects would predominate. It is the purpose of this article to review the findings which led to the hypothesis briefly outlined above and to discuss them in more detail.

RESULTS

The Model: Experimental Listeriosis of Mice

When mice are infected with sublethal doses of L.monocytogenes by the intraveneous route the vast majority of bacteria is found within mononuclear phagocytes of spleen and liver (1-3). Bacteria will grow for several days until the host has developed specific immunity which allows reduction and finally elimination of the infectious agent. Virulence of L.monocytogenes like that of other intracellular bacteria, therefore, is best monitored by determination of bacterial numbers in infected organs. On the left hand panel of Figure 1, a representative listerial growth curve is shown. On the right hand panel of this figure results from an adoptive transfer experiment are illustrated. It can be concluded from this type of experiments that protection can be transferred by lymphocytes from immune mice. Treatment of the cells with anti-Thyl antibodies abrogates adoptive protection and hence this cell type is responsible for acquisition of resistance (21-23).

In Vivo Studies with Serologically Selected T-Lymphocyte Subsets

To further characterize the T cells involved in protection we selected T cells by virtue of their surface phenotype (7). Peritoneal exudate T lymphocytes from L.monocytogenes immune mice were treated with anti-Lytl or anti-Lyt2 antibodies and complement and afterwards selected populations were transferred upon recipients that were subsequently infected with viable L.monocytogenes. As can be seen in Figure 2, protective activity against L.monocytogenes could not be transferred by specific T lymphocytes treated with either anti-Lytl or anti-Lyt2 antibodies plus complement, respectively. Furthermore, a mixture of both selected T-cell populations failed to reconstitute this effect. From these findings it was concluded that T cells of the Lytl$^+$2$^+$ phenotype must be involved in protection.

At this time anti-L3T4 antibodies were not available and it was generally thought that the Lytl molecule represented a unique marker of helper T-cells. Later, it was shown that this molecule is expressed on both helper and cytolytic T

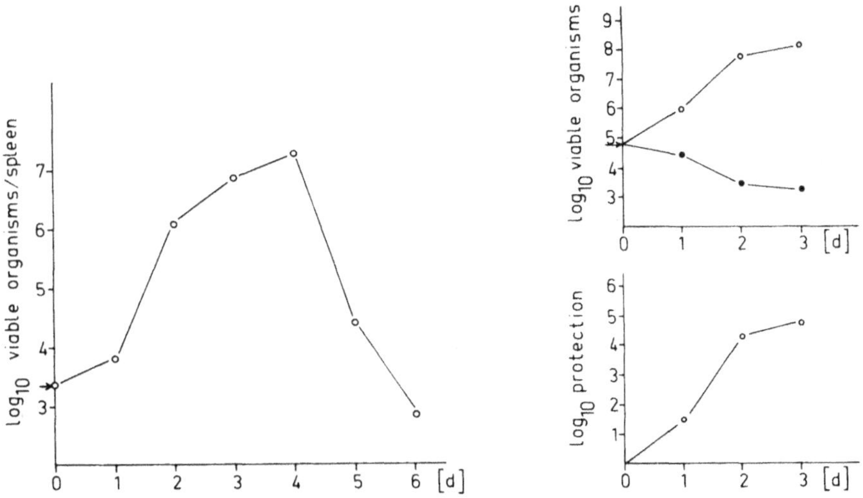

Figure 1. Experimental infection of mice with L.monocytogenes. Left hand panel: Mice were infected with viable L.monocytogenes strain EGD organisms and bacterial numbers in spleens determined at daily intervals. For determination of listerial numbers, spleens were homogenized and appropriate aliquots plated out on trypticase soy plates and incubated at 37°C overnight. Right hand upper panel: Course of infection in adoptively protected mice. Mice received T cells from L.monocytogenes immune donor mice (•) or were sham injected (o). Afterwards, recipient mice were infected with viable L.monocytogenes organisms. Listerial numbers in spleens were determined at daily intervals. Right hand lower panel: Protection in T-cell recipients. The difference between L.monocytogenes organisms in spleens of sham-injected controls and those in spleens of T-cell recipients is termed adoptive protection.

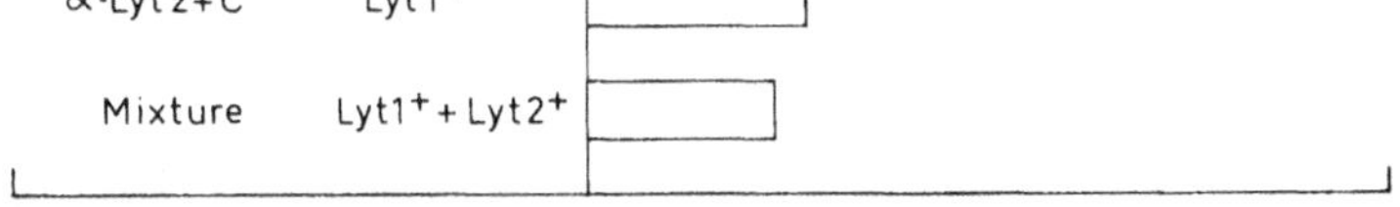

Figure 2. Effect of anti-Lyt antibodies plus complement on adoptive protection by T cells from L.monocytogenes immune mice. Equivalent T-cell numbers were transferred upon recipients which were challenge infected with viable L.monocytogenes organisms. Protection in spleens was determined 2d later. Data adapted from the Journal of Experimental Medicine 150:1033-1038 (1979) by copyright permission of The Rockefeller University Press.

cells and that both cell types differ only quantitatively with helper T cells having a much higher cell surface density of the Lyt1 molecule (24). It therefore became obvious that our finding demonstrated an involvement of $Lyt2^{+}$ T cells but did not provide any information as to the possible role of helper T cells. The role of this T-cell type could only be analyzed following identification of the L3T4 molecule as a unique marker of helper T cells (4). Using anti-L3T4 and anti-Lyt2 mab we could show that successful transfer of protection depends on both $L3T4^{+}$ and $Lyt2^{+}$ T cells (Figure 3). In an attempt to get a deeper insight into the functional role of $L3T4^{+}$ and $Lyt2^{+}$ T cells in the immune response against L.monocytogenes we have generated T-cell lines and clones from infected mice and analyzed their functional capacities (10-12).

Helper Functions of Class II Restricted T-Cell Lines

In our initial strategy we cloned peritoneal exudate T lymphocytes from L.monocytogenes infected (i.v.) C57Bl/6 mice in double layer soft agar (10). Later, lymph node cells from L.monocytogenes infected (s.c.) C57Bl/6 mice were cloned by limiting dilution (25). In both cases, T cells of $Lyt1^{+}2^{-}$ (probably $L3T4^{+}$) phenotype were established. The biological activities of several T-cell lines of this type were assessed in different in-vitro assays (Figure 4). In the presence of listerial antigen and accessory cells these lines showed significant proliferative responses and produced high amounts of interleukins (probably interleukin 2, IL-2). Furthermore, in the presence of accessory cells, listerial antigen and the bystander antigen, sheep erythrocytes, these T cells helped small B cells to mature into immunoglobulin secreting plasma cells. Also, the T cells produced IFN-γ in an antigen-specific way (Figure 5). Based on several criteria the IFN produced belonged to the IFN-γ class. Furthermore, we found that native T cells from L.monocytogenes infected mice which produce IFN-γ after antigen stimulation are $Lyt1^{+}2^{-}$ (probably $L3T4^{+}$); $Lyt1^{-}2^{+}$ T-cells failed to secret this molecule (Figure 6). Thus, these T cells had the functional characteristics of helper/inducer T cells. Proliferation, interleukin secretion, and by-stander help were only demonstrable in the presence of syngeneic accessory cells sharing the H-2I-locus indicating that the T cells were class II restricted (Figure 7).

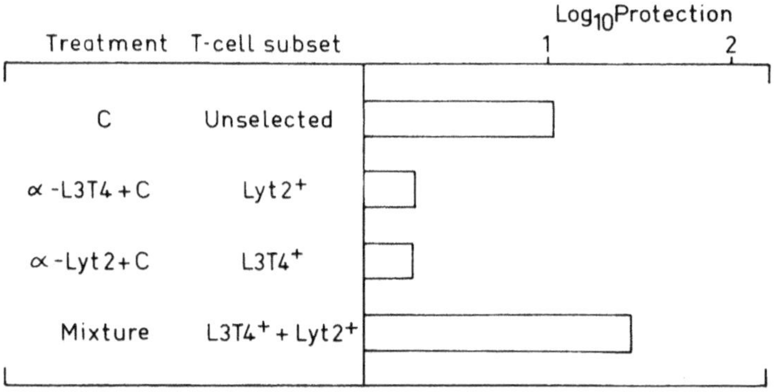

Figure 3. Effect of anti-L3T4 and anti-Lyt 2 mab plus complement on adoptive transfer of protection by T cells from L.monocytogenes immune mice. Equivalent T-cell numbers were transferred upon recipients which were infected with viable L.monocytogenes organisms. Protection in spleens was determined 2 d later. Data reproduced with permission from (9).

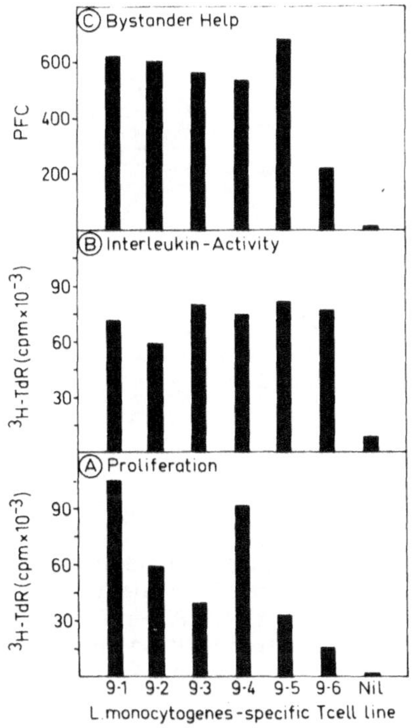

Figure 4. Proliferation (A), interleukin secretion (B), and bystander help (C) of L.monocytogenes reactive T-cell lines. (A) Cloned T cells were cultured with accessory cells and listerial antigen. Proliferative responses were determined by ^{3}H-thymidine incorporation (18h pulse) after 4d. (B) For determination of interleukin activities supernatants of similar cultures were tested on Concanavalin A prestimulated spleen cells. (C) T cells were cultured with small B cells, accessory cells, listerial antigen, and sheep erythrocytes. After 4d, direct sheep-erythrocyte specific plaques were determined. Data adapted from the Journal of Experimental Medicine 155, 1754-1765 (1982) by copyright permission of The Rockefeller University Press (10).

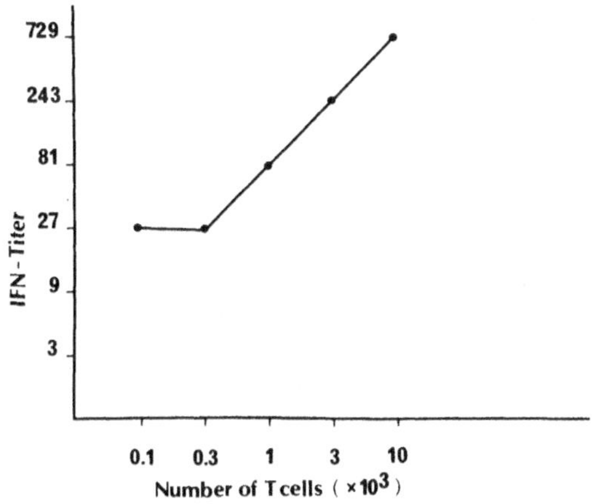

Figure 5. IFN production by a cloned L.monocytogenes-specific T-cell line. Graded numbers of T cells were cultured with accessory cells and listerial antigen. Supernatants were collected and serial dilutions added to L929 cells which were infected with vesicular stomatitis virus. Inhibition of cytopathic effects was determined after 2d. Data reproduced with permission from (11).

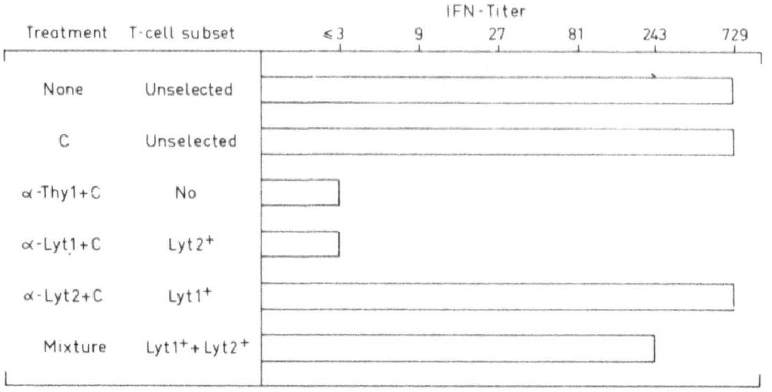

Figure 6. Effect of Lyt antisera plus complement on IFN secretion by T cells from L.monocytogenes immune mice. Equivalent T-cell numbers were cultured with accessory cells and listerial antigen. After 24 h, supernatants were collected and IFN titers determined. Data adapted with permission from (11).

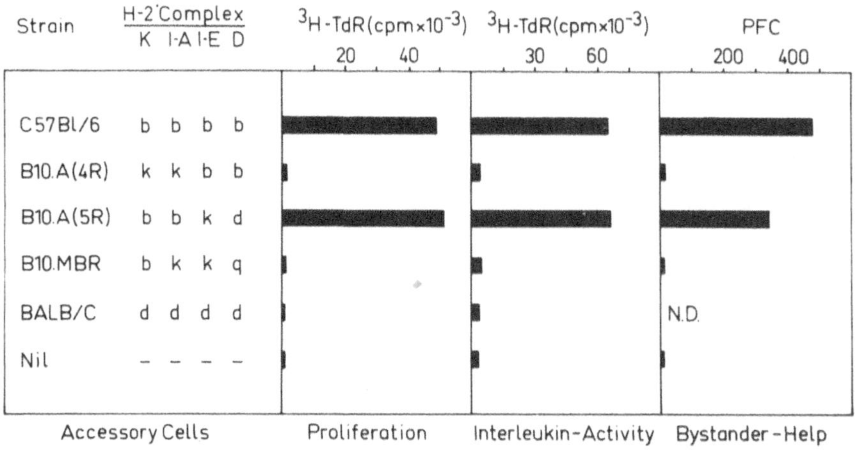

Figure 7. Genetic restriction of a cloned L.monocytogenes specific T-cell line. T cells were cultured with listerial antigen and accessory cells of different haplotype. Proliferative responses, interleukin activities, and bystander help were determined as described in Figure 4. Data adapted from the Journal of Experimental Medicine 155, 1754-1765 (1982) by copyright permission of the Rockefeller University Press (10).

Functions of Lyt2$^+$ T-Cell Lines

Based on the findings (a) that Lyt2$^+$ T cells are involved in adoptive protection of mice against L.monocytogenes and (b) that Lyt2$^+$ T cells typically express cytolytic functions (4) we attempted to identify L.monocytogenes specific Lyt2$^+$ T cells which could lyse macrophages expressing listerial antigens. Because our earlier cloning strategy yielded only L3T4$^+$ T cells we postively selected Lyt2$^+$ T cells from L.monocytogenes infected mice by cytofluorometry (12). Selected Lyt2$^+$ T cells were cultured and cloned in the presence of L.monocytogenes infected stimulator cells and T-cell factors. Using this protocol, L3T4$^-$, Lyt 2$^+$ T-cell clones could be established. Cultures of cloned T cells, infected stimulator cells, and r-IL-2 produced significant IFN-γ activities while cultures containing normal stimulator cells did not (Figure 8). The cytolytic activities of the two T-cell clones 1D7 and 1F1 against peritoneal cells from L.monocytogenes infected mice or L.monocytogenes primed bone marrow macrophages (BMMØ) are shown in Figure 9. With both clones, specific target cell lysis was observed. In contrast, the tumor cells YAC-1 and P815, were not lysed. Furthermore lysis was class I restricted and antigen specific based on the findings that macrophages of mutant H-2K haplotype or expressing the unrelated antigen, Mycobacterium bovis, were not lysed (Figure 9).

Results obtained in a low cell density split culture system indicate that the Lyt2$^+$ L.monocytogenes reactive T-cell population consists of both antigen specific H-2 restricted and antigen specific apparently non-restricted T-cell clones (13). In the meantime we have succeeded to isolate L.monocytogenes specific Lyt2$^+$ T-cell clones which lyse BMMØ of different haplotype but only in the presence of listerial antigen. One of these clones is recognized by the KJ 16.133 mab (26) which reacts with the T-cell receptor of the $V_{\beta 8}$ family. Antigen specific, apparently H-2 nonrestricted cytolysis by this T-cell clone is blocked by the KJ 16.133 mab strongly indicating that the T-cell receptor is involved in this promiscuous cytolytic activity. Studies are in progress to decide whether this T-cell clone recognizes listerial antigen independent from self structures or in association with a monomorphic H-2 epitope shared by macrophages of different haplotypes.

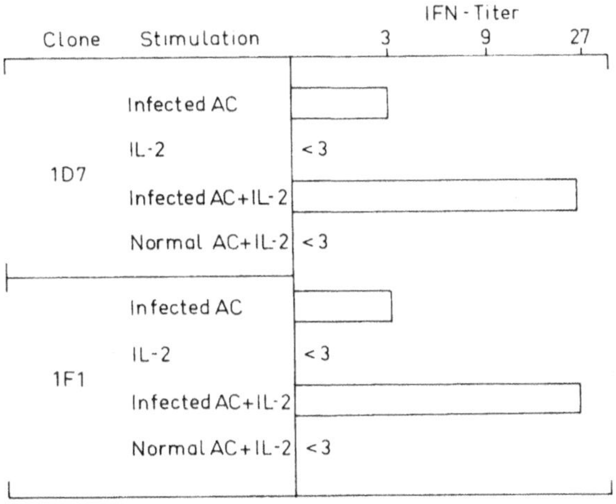

Figure 8. IFN production by cloned L.monocytogenes specific Lyt 2$^+$ T-cell lines. T cells were cultured with accessory cells from L.monocytogenes infected or normal mice in the presence of absence of r-IL-2. Supernatants were collected and IFN-activities determined as described in Figure 5. Data adapted from the Journal of Experimental Medicine 164, 363-368 (1986) by copyright permission of the Rockefeller University Press (11).

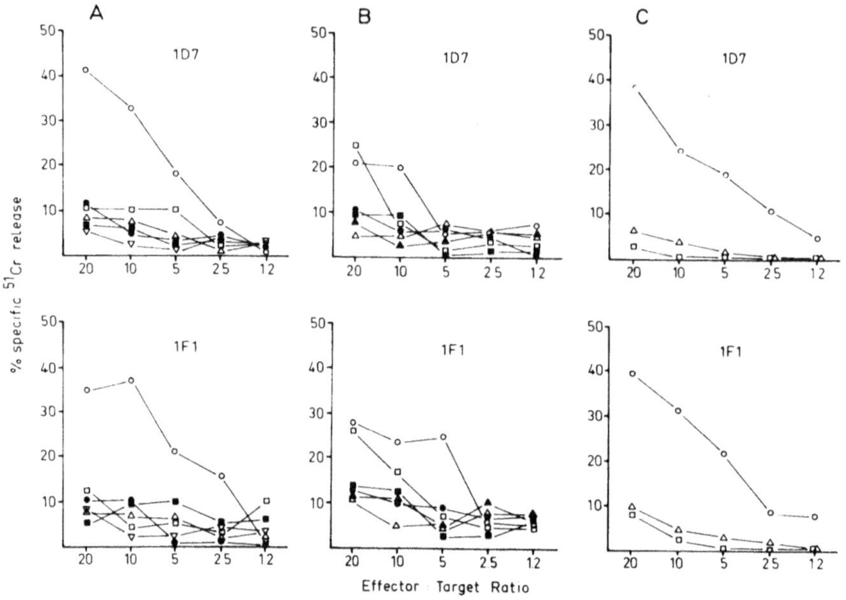

Figure 9. Cytolytic activities of cloned L.monocytogenes specific Lyt2$^+$ T cell lines. Clones 1D7 and 1F1 were tested for their cytolytic activity against different ^{51}Cr labelled target cells. A: (o) peritoneal cells from L.monocytogenes-infected C57Bl/6 mice, (●) peritoneal cells from untreated C57Bl/6 mice, (□) peritoneal cells from L.monocytogenes-infected DBA/2 mice, (■) peritoneal cells from untreated DBA/2 mice, (△) YAC-1, (△) P815. B: (o) peritoneal cells from L.monocytogenes-infected C57Bl/6 mice, (●) peritoneal cells from untreated C57Bl/6 mice, (△) peritoneal cells from L.monocytogenes-infected B6.C-H2bm1 mice, (▲) peritoneal cells from untreated B6.C-H2bm1 mice, (□) peritoneal cells from L.monocytogenes-infected B6.C-H2bm12 mice, (■) peritoneal cells from untreated B6.C-H2bm12 mice. C: (o) L.moncytogenes-infected C57Bl/6 BMMØ, (□) M.bovis infected C57Bl/6 BMMØ, (△) uninfected C57Bl/6 BMMØ. Data reproduced from the Journal of Experimental Medicine 164, 363-368 (1986) by copyright permission from the Rockefeller University Press (11).

Cytolytic Functions of Class II Restricted L3T4$^+$ T-Cell Lines

We wanted to assess whether L3T4$^+$ class II restricted T cells with reactivity for L.monocytogenes possess specific cytolytic activity. For this study a new panel of L3T4$^+$ T-cell clones was established by cloning and recloning under limiting dilution conditions (27). The majority of these clones was capable of lysing P815 tumor cells in the presence of the lectin phytohemagglutinin indicating that they possessed a cytolytic potential. Three L3T4$^+$ T-cell clones derived from spleens, lymph nodes, or peritoneal exudates, respectively, were used for further studies. In contrast to the Lyt 2$^+$ T-cell clones, these cells failed to lyse L.monocytogenes infected BMMØ. Phenotypic analysis, however, revealed that these BMMØ were totally devoid of class II molecules. After stimulation with r-IFN-γ they expressed high amounts of Ia molecules (Figure 10). When IFN-γ stimulated, L.monocytogenes primed BMMØ were used as target cells, specific cytolytic activity by the L3T4$^+$ T-cell clones became demonstrable (Figure 11). Lysis was antigen-specific as indicated by the finding that M.bovis primed BMMØ were not lysed (data not shown). Furthermore, cytolysis was class II restricted since only BMMØ sharing the H-2I-A locus of the MHC were lysed (Figure 12). Taken together, these findings indicate that L3T4$^+$ T-cell clones with reactivitiy to L.monocytogenes are capable of lysing macrophages in an antigen-specific and class II restricted way.

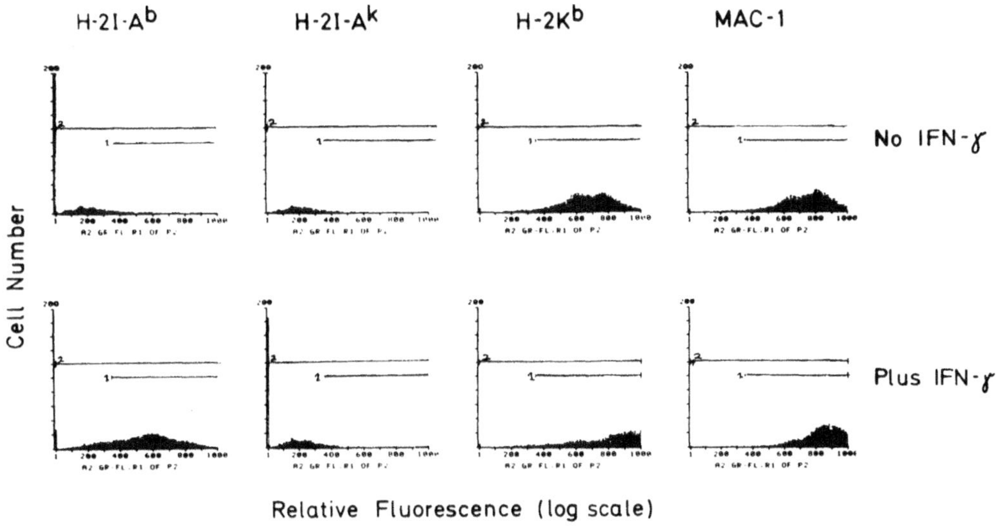

Figure 10. Phenotype of unstimulated and IFN-γ stimulated BMMØ. Unstimulated (no IFN-γ) and stimulated (plus IFN-γ) BMMØ were cultured with anti-H-2I-A^b mab, anti-H-2I-A^k mab, anti-H-2K^b mab, or MAC-1 mab, respectively, and afterwards with fluorescein isothiocyanate labelled goat anti-mouse or anti-rat antiserum. Phenotype analysis was performed on an Ortho Cytofluorograph. Data reproduced with permission from (27).

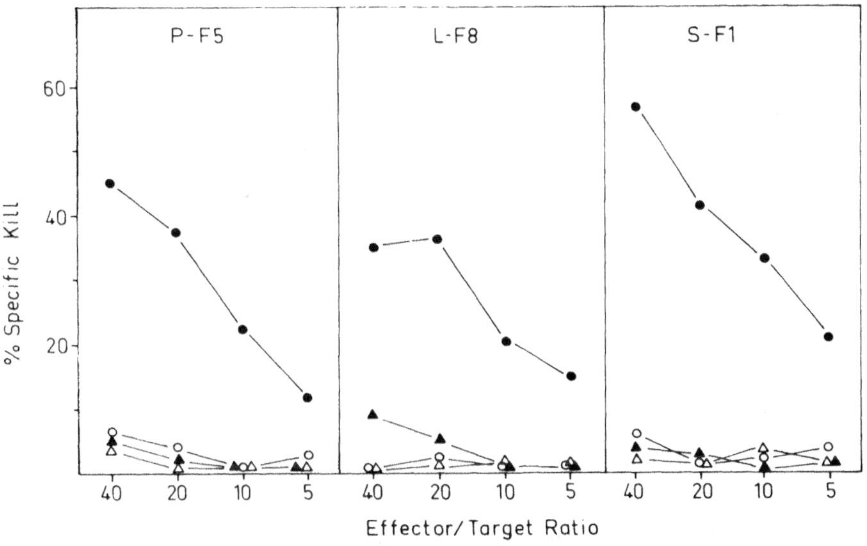

Figure 11. Lysis of IFN-γ stimulated, L.monocytogenes infected BMMØ by L3T4$^+$ T-cell clones. IFN-γ stimulated (o) or unstimulated (Δ) BMMØ, respectively, were infected with viable L.monocytogenes organisms (closed symbols) or remained uninfected (open symbols). ^{51}Cr release was determined after 4h. Data reproduced with permission from (27).

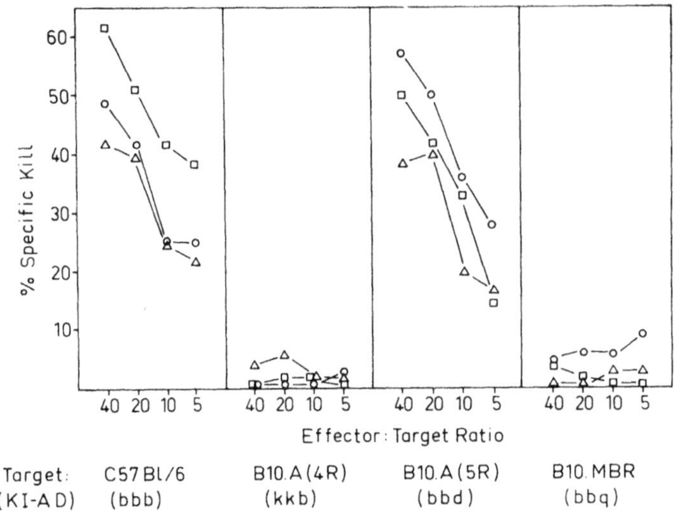

Figure 12. MHC restricted cytolysis by L3T4$^+$ T-cell clones. IFN-γ stimulated BMMØ of different haplotype were primed with L.monocytogenes and afterwards cytolysis was determined. (o) clone P-F5, (Δ) clone L-F8, (□) clone S-F1. Data adapted with permission from (27).

Which Conditions Lead to the Expression of Cytolysis?

It is generally observed in the virus system that the expression of cytolytic activities by Lyt2$^+$ T-cells is markedly facilitated by in-vitro restimulation with antigen. Furthermore, it has been claimed that cytolytic L3T4$^+$ T cells only appear after long term in vitro culture (28). We therefore wanted to assess whether native or short-term cultured T lymphocytes from L.monocytogenes-infected mice of either phenotype were able to lyse BMMØ expressing listerial antigens (27). Splenic T cells from L.monocytogenes infected mice were purified by passage over nylon wool columns and afterwards tested for target cell lysis (Figure 13). This T-cell population which consisted of approximately 60% L3T4$^+$ and 40% Lyt2$^+$ T-cells, failed to express any specific cytolytic activity. Alternatively, spleen cells were restimulated in vitro with accessory cells plus antigen. After 7d of culture this population consisted of 35% L3T4$^+$ and 65% Lyt2$^+$ T cells. Addition of T-cell factors further increased the proportion of Lyt2$^+$ T cells to approximately 95%. Both populations had gained the capacity to lyse IFN-γ stimulated, L.monocytogenes primed BMMØ in an antigen specific way. We then enriched L3T4$^+$ T cells by pretreating the spleen cell population with anti-Lyt2 mab plus complement before restimulation with accessory cells, antigen, and T-cell factors. After restimulation for 7d this population consisted of 95% L3T4$^+$ T cells which had gained the capacity to specifically lyse IFN-γ stimulated, L.monocytogenes primed BMMØ. We conclude from this study that during primary infection with L.monocytogenes, precursor T cells of both phenotypes are triggered and that they express their cytolytic activity rapidly after in-vitro restimulation.

Possible Role of IFN-γ in Antilisterial Resistance

It is generally accepted that IFN-γ is an important mediator of macrophage activation (29). However, although it has been shown that IFN-γ can activate multiple macrophage capacities including leishmanicidal and tumoricidal effects, its role in the activation of anti-listerial macrophage functions is less clear. We therefore analyzed the effects of in vivo application of r-IFN-γ on subsequent L.monocytogenes infection in mice (30). As shown in Figure 14, after systemic

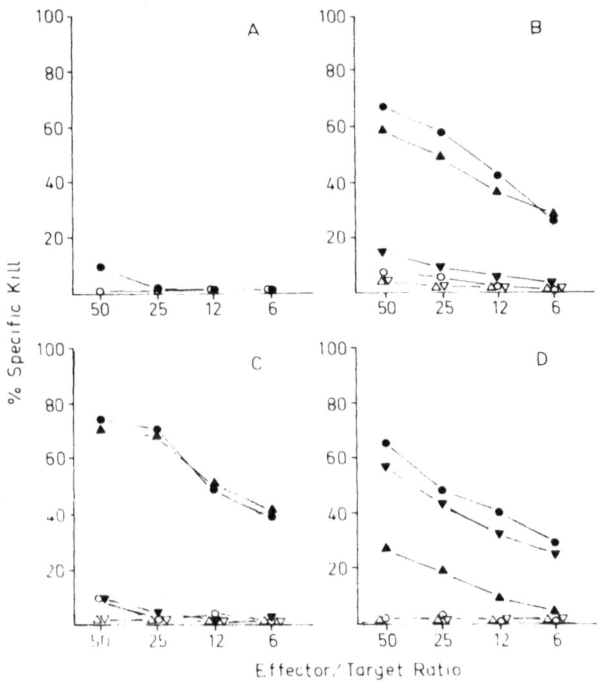

Figure 13. L.monocytogenes-specific lysis by native or short term cultured T cells. The cytolytic activity against IFN-γ stimulated, L.monocytogenes primed (●) or unprimed (o) BMMØ was assessed for the following T-cell populations: (A) native T cells; (B) T cells restimulated with accessory cells plus HKL; (C) T cells restimulated with accessory cells, HKL, plus T-cell factors; (D) selected Lyt2⁻ T cells restimulated with accessory cells, HKL, plus T-cell factors. In some cases, anti-L3T4 mab (△ , ▲), or anti-Lyt 2 mab (△ , ▲) were added to the killer assay. Data reproduced with permission from (27).

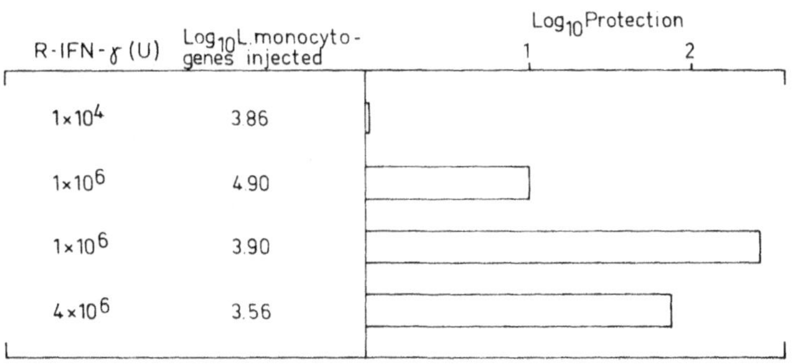

Figure 14. Induction of resistance against L.monocytogenes infection by r-IFN-γ. Mice were treated with different amounts of r-IFN-γ i.v. on d-1. On d0 they received the same amount of r-IFN-γ and viable L.monocytogenes organisms. After another 2d the number of viable L.monocytogenes organisms in spleens was determined. Data reproduced with permission from (30).

application of high r-IFN-γ concentrations listerial growth was significantly reduced. Recently, it was shown that treatment of mice with anti-IFN-γ mab leads to marked exacerbation of listeriosis (31). Taken together these findings suggest that endogeneous IFN-γ is involved in the built up of anti-listerial resistance.

DISCUSSION

Let us briefly summarize the findings reported: (1) Both $L3T4^+$ and $Lyt2^+$ T cells are involved in adoptive protection against L.monocytogenes. (2) Both $L3T4^+$ and $Lyt2^+$ L.monocytogenes specific T-cell lines produce IFN-γ after appropriate stimulation. Native T cells from L.monocytogenes infected mice which produce IFN-γ after antigenic stimulation in vitro are $Lyt2^-$ (probably $L3T4^+$). (3) IFN-γ induces strong anti-listerial effects. The underlying mechanisms, however, remain unknown. (4) Both $L3T4^+$ and $Lyt2^+$ L.monocytogenes specific T-cell lines are capable of lysing L.monocytogenes primed BMMØ. After restimulation in vitro also native T cells from L.monocytogenes infected mice of either phenotype express specific cytolytic activity.

Before integrating these findings into a scheme of acquired antilisterial resistance we need to discuss a few experiments from other laboratories. North (14) has shown that blood monocytes accumulate in the livers of L.monocytogenes infected mice and populate infective foci. Furthermore, evidence was presented in this study that immigrant blood monocytes rather than fixed Kupffer cells in the liver express resistance against L.monocytogenes. Later, Lepay et al. (15) showed that Kupffer cells from normal mice fail to produce reactive oxygen intermediates and to kill intracellular Leishmania donovani or Toxoplasma gondii upon stimulation with lymphokines including IFN-γ. After infection with L.monocytogenes, Kupffer cells remained refractory whereas immigrant mononuclear cells produced high levels of H_2O_2 (16). Finally, not only blood monocytes but also neutrophils are able to kill L.monocytogenes and it appears that the attraction of these cells to rather than their activation at the site of listerial implantation represents the crucial step in resistance (17-19). Recruitment of these inflammatory phagocytes during listeriosis seems to be under the control of specific T cells (18).

With these findings in mind the steps which lead to protection against L.monocytogenes will be discussed in a hypothetical form. Early after systemic infection with L.monocytogenes, the vast majority of organisms is entrapped in mononuclear phagocytes of spleen and liver. Although L.monocytogenes can survive in the phagolysosome of nonactivated macrophages - at least for a certain period of time - some listerial components will be processed and expressed on the phagocyte surface in association with MHC-encoded molecules. Because mononuclear phagocytes can express both class I and class II molecules T cells of Lyt2 and L3T4 phenotype are induced. After second encounter with listerial antigen in association with the adequate restriction element these T-cells will produce multiple lymphokine activities including IL-2 and IFN-γ. Although it is anticipated that these T cells primarily belong to the $L3T4^+$ subset, $Lyt2^+$ T cells in the near vicinity of $L3T4^+$ T cells could produce IFN-γ after costimulation by IL-2 from $L3T4^+$ T cells and listerial antigen plus class I on macrophages. IFN-γ and probably other lymphokines will then activate infected macrophages. Activation of listeriocidal functions, however, can only occur in phagocytes with a high antibacterial potential.

Furthermore, T cells recruit blood monocytes and granulocytes to the site of T cell-macrophage interaction (17-19). Although it appears likely that this step is mediated by lymphokines their nature remains to be identified. Freshly recruited inflammatory phagocytes possess a high antibacterial potential. Hence, stimulation of these cells will induce destruction of intracellular L.monocytogenes. Although certain tissue macrophages may also become listeriocidal upon activation, it appears, that immigrant phagocytes rather than local tissue macrophages are the major effectors of defense. L.monocytogenes organisms residing in Kupffer cells will not be killed because these phagocytes have a low antibacterial potential (15,16). Although Kupffer cells - at least in the beginning - may contribute to protection by facilitating bacillary containment to discrete foci at the same time they represent a habitat that allows bacterial evasion from destructive host defense reactions. Soon after infection the majority of L.monocytogenes are entrapped in Kupffer cells and hence, this event may be of major importance for bacterial survival in the host (1).

Provided that professional phagocytes with high antibacterial potential had been attracted to the site of listerial replication, lysis of infected cells with low antibacterial potential will allow transmission from a surrounding which preferentially supports listerial survival into a more hostile environment. Thus, under well-controlled conditions lysis of infected host cells would be beneficial for the host. A certain degree of tissue destruction due to target cell lysis by T lymphocytes and secretion of harmful molecules by activated phagocytes has to be taken into account as a pathologic side effect.

On the other hand, a primarily detrimental situation must be envisaged when infected host cells are lysed in the absence of phagocytes with high antibacterial potential because this reaction would lead to bacterial dissemination. The situation may worsen when activated macrophages themselves are attacked by cytolytic T lymphocytes and it may be interesting to find out whether lymphokine activation renders macrophages resistant towards lysis by T cells. Obviously, a high degree of regulation is required for a protective outcome of these complex interactions and any dysregulation will favour the occurence of pathogenic effect.

It has been known for a long time that granulomata represent the characteristic tissue response in chronic bacterial infections. Well organized granulomata consisting of epitheloid cells, immigrant blood monocytes as well as CD4 and CD8 T lymphocytes could well represent the microenvironment that fulfills these requirements. Indeed, in established tuberculous granulomata distinct regions of necrosis, cytolysis, and macrophage activation can be identified (32). In these granulomata, release of bacteria through target cell lysis into the center may lead to direct microbial death by hypyoxia. On the other hand, exaggerated target cell lysis may facilitate cavity formation with subsequent bacterial replication and dissemination. Possible cell interactions and mechanisms in T-cell induced granulomata are illustrated in Figure 15.

$L3T4^+$ and $Lyt2^+$ T cells expressing helper and cytolytic functions have also been isolated from M.tuberculosis and M.leprae immune mice (33-36). I therefore assume that similar mechanisms are involved in the host response against tuberculosis and leprosy. M.tuberculosis and M.leprae seem to be more resistant against activated macrophages than L.monocytogenes. Furthermore, replication of M.leprae exclusively depends on an intracellular habitat. Therefore, in mycobacterial infections, cytolytic T cells could gain particular importance.

ACKNOWLEDGEMENTS

I thank R. Schneider, R. Brugger, and G. Eichhorn for their excellent secretarial assitance.

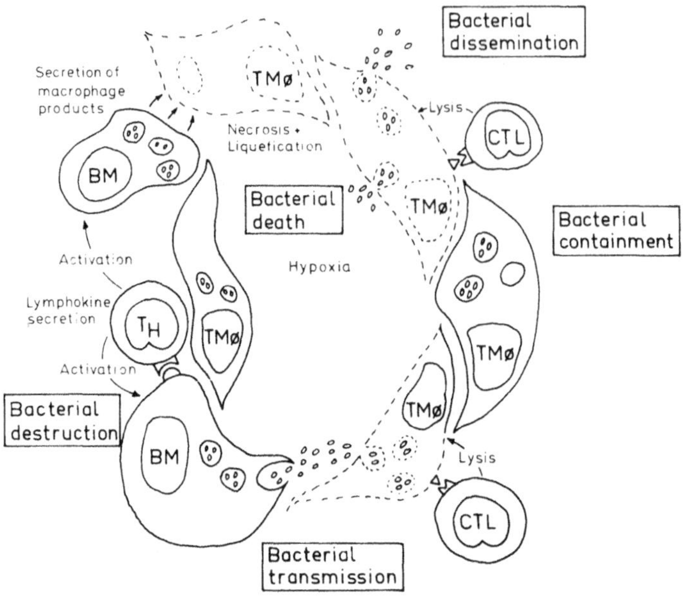

Figure 15. Possible cell interactions and mechanisms in a T-cell induced granuloma.

REFERENCES

1. Hahn, H. and S.H.E. Kaufmann. 1981. Role of cell mediated immunity in bacterial infections. Rev. Infect. Dis. 3: 1221-1250.
2. Mackaness, G.B. 1962. Cellular resistance to infection. J. Exp. Med. 116: 381-406.
3. Mackaness, G.B. 1969. The influence of immunologically committed lymphoid cells on macrophage activity in vivo. J. Exp. Med. 129: 973-992.
4. Fitch, R.W. 1986. T-cell clones and T-cell receptors. Microbiol. Rev. 50, 50-69.
5. Zinkernagel, R.M. and P.C. Doherty. 1979. MHC restricted cytotoxic T cells: Studies on the biological role of polymorphic major transplantation antigens determining T-cell restriction-specificity, function and responsiveness. Adv. Immunol. 27, 51-177.
6. Zinkernagel, R.M., A. Althage, B. Adler, R.V. Blanden, W.F. Davidson, U. Kees, M.B.C. Dunlop, and D.C. Shreffler. 1977. H-2 restriction of cell-mediated immunity to an intracellular bacterium. Effector T cells are specific for Listeria antigen in association with H-2I region-coded self markers. J. Exp. Med. 145: 1353-1367.
7. Kaufmann, S.H.E., M.M. Simon, and H. Hahn. 1979. Specific Lyt123 T cells are involved in protection against Listeria monocytogenes and in delayed-type hypersensitivity to listerial antigens. J. Exp. Med. 150: 1033-1038.
8. Cheers, C. and M.S. Sandrin. 1983. Restriction in adoptive transfer of restance to Listeria monocytogenes. II. Use of congenic and mutant mice show transfer to be H-2K restricted. Cell. Immunol. 7: 199-205.
9. Kaufmann, S.H.E., E. Hug, U. Väth and I. Müller. 1985. Effective antibacterial protection against Listeria monocytogenes and delayed-type hypersensitivity to listerial antigens depend on cooperation between specific $L3T4^+$ and $Lyt2^+$ T cells. Infect. Immun. 48: 263-266.
10. Kaufmann, S.H.E., and H. Hahn. 1982. Biological functions of T cell lines with specificity for the intracellular bacterium Listeria monocytogenes in vitro and in vivo. J. Exp. Med., 155: 1754-1765.

11. Kaufmann, S.H.E., H. Hahn, R. Berger, and H. Kirchner. 1983. Interferon-γ production by Listeria monocytogenes-specific T cells active in antibacterial immunity. Eur. J. Immunol. 13: 265-268.
12. Kaufmann, S.H.E., E. Hug, and G. De Libero. 1986. Listeria monocytogenes reactive T lymphocyte clones with cytolytic activity against infected target cells. J. Exp. Med. 164: 363-368.
13. De Libero, G., and S.H.E. Kaufmann. 1986. Antigen-specific Lyt2$^+$ cytolytic T lymphocytes from mice infected with the intracellular bacterium Listeria monocytogenes. J. Immunol. 137: 2688-2694.
14. North, R.J. 1970. The relative importance of blood monocytes and fixed macrophages to the expression of cell-mediated immunity to infection. J. Exp. Med. 132: 521-534.
15. Lepay, D.A., C.F. Nathan, H.W. Murray, R.M. Steinman, and Z.A. Cohn. 1985. Murine Kupffer Cells: Mononuclear phagocytes deficient in the generation of reactive oxygen intermediates. J. Exp. Med. 161: 1079-1096.
16. Lepay, D.A., R.M. Steinman, C.F. Nathan, H.W. Murray, and Z.A. Cohn. 1985. Liver macrophages in murine listeriosis: Cell-mediated immunity is correlated with an influx of macrophages capable of generating reactive oxygen intermediates. J. Exp. Med. 161: 1503-1512.
17. Campbell, P.A. 1986. Are inflammatory phagocytes responsible for resistance to facultative intracellular bacteria? Immunology Today 7: 70-72.
18. Czuprynski, C.J., P.M. Henson, and P.A. Campbell. 1985. Enhanced accumulation of inflammatory neutrophils and macrophages mediated by transfer of T cells from mice immunized with Listeria monocytogenes. J. Immunol. 134: 3449-3454.
19. Czuprynski, C.J., P.M. Henson, and P.A. Campbell. 1984. Killing of Listeria monocytogenes by inflammatory neutrophils and mononuclear phagocytes from immune and nonimmune mice. J. Leuk. Biol. 35: 193-208.
20. Kaufmann, S.H.E. 1987. Possible role of helper and cytolytic T lymphocytes in antibacterial defense: Conclusions from experimental listeriosis in mice. Rev. Inf. Dis., in press.
21. North, R.J. 1973. Importance of thymus-derived lymphocytes in cell-mediated immunity to infection. Cell Immunol. 7: 166-76.
22. Lane, F.C., and E.R. Unanue. 1972. Requirement of thymus (T) lymphocytes for resistance to listeriosis. J. Exp. Med. 153: 1104-1112.
23. Blanden, R.V., and R.E. Langman. 1972. Cell-mediated immunity to bacterial infection in the mouse. Thymus derived cells as effectors of acquired resistance to Listeria monocytogenes. Scand. J. Immunol. 1: 379-391.
24. Ledbetter, J.A., R.O. Rouse, H.S. Nicklem, and L.A. Herzenberg. 1980. T cell subsets defined by expression of Lyt-1,2,3 and Thy-1 antigens. Two parameter immunofluorescence and cytotoxicity analysis with monoclonal antibodies modified current view. J. Exp. Med. 152: 280-295.
25. Kaufmann, S.H.E. 1984. Acquired resistance to facultative intracellular bacteria: Relationship between persistence, crossreactivity on the T cell level and capacity to stimulate cellular immunity of different Listeria strains. Infect. Immun. 45: 234-241.
26. Roehm, N., L. Herron, J. Cambier, D. Di Guisto, K. Haskins, J. Kappler, and P. Marrack. 1984. The major histocompatibility complex-restricted antigen receptor on T cells: distribution on thymus and peripheral T cells. Cell 38: 577-
584.
27. Kaufmann, S.H.E., E. Hug, U. Väth, and G. De Libero. 1987. Specific lysis of Listeria monocytogenes infected macrophages by class II-restricted L3T4$^+$ T cells. Eur. J. Immunol.
28. Fleischer, B. 1984. Acquisition of specific cytotoxic activity by human T4$^+$ T lymphocytes in culture. Nature 308: 365-367.
29. Nathan, C.F., H.W. Murray, M.W. Wiebe, and B.Y. Rubin. 1983. Identification of interferon as the lymphokine that activates human macrophage oxidative metabolism and antimicrobial activity. J. Exp. Med. 158: 670-689.
30. Kiderlen, A.F., S.H.E. Kaufmann, and M.-L. Lohmann-Matthes. 1984. Protection of mice against the intracellular bacterium Listeria monocytogenes by recombinant immune interferon. Eur. J. Immunol. 14: 964-967.

31. Buchmaier, N.A. and R.D. Schreiber. 1985. Requirement of endogeneous interferon-γ production for resolution of Listeria monocytogenes infection. Proc. Natl. Acad. Sci. USA 82: 7404-7408.
32. Schmidt, F. 1958. Immunbiologie. In "Handbuch der Tuberkulose", J. Hein, H. Kleinschmidt, E. Uehlinger, eds, Thieme, Stuttgart.
33. Kaufmann, S.H.E. 1984. Biological activities of a murine T cell clone with reactivity to Mycobacterium leprae. Cell. Immunol. 83: 215-220.
34. Chiplunkar, S., G. De Libero, and S.H.E. Kaufmann. 1986. Mycobacterium leprae-specific Lyt2$^+$ T lymphocytes with cytolytic activity. Infect. Immun. 54: 793-797.
35. Kaufmann, S.H.E. and I. Flesch. 1986. Function and antigen recognition pattern of L3T4$^+$ T-cell clones from Mycobacterium tuberculosis immune mice. Infect. Immun. 54: 291-296.
36. Kaufmann, S.H.E. and G. De Libero. 1987. Cytolytic T cells in Mycobacterium tuberculosis infections. In: "Tuberculosis: Interactions with the Immune System", H. Friedman and M. Bendinelli, eds, Plenum, New York.

USE OF RECOMBINANT VACCINIA VIRUSES TO EXAMINE CYTOTOXIC T LYMPHOCYTE RECOGNITION OF INDIVIDUAL VIRAL PROTEINS

Jonathan Yewdell[1], Jack Bennink[1], Geoffrey Smith[2,3], and Bernard Moss[3]

[1] Wistar Institute, Philadelphia, Pa.
[2] University of Cambridge, Cambridge, England
[3] Laboratory for Viral Diseases, National Institute of Allergy and Infectious Diseases, National Institutes of Health, Bethesda, Md.

INTRODUCTION

Cytotoxic T lymphocytes (CTL) are believed to play an important role in immunity to tumors and viruses.[1] CTL recognize foreign antigens in conjunction with class I major histocompatibility complex (MHC) molecules, and act by either directly lysing cells bearing the foreign antigen, or by releasing molecules with anti-viral and/or anti-tumor activities.[2-4] Understanding of CTL has been hindered by difficulties in identifying which foreign antigens are recognized on the target cell surface. We have addressed this problem using recombinant vaccinia viruses containing individual cloned genes from two well characterized viruses which have been extensively used in previous studies of CTL specificity and function, influenza virus (a myxovirus), and vesicular stomatitis virus (a rhabdovirus).

STRUCTURE AND ASSEMBLY OF MYXO- AND RHABDOVIRUSES

Myxo- and rhabdoviruses are RNA viruses which obtain their envelope by budding through the host cell plasma membrane. In this process, virions acquire a dense layer of surface spikes consisting of one [rhabdovirus glycoprotein (G)] or two [myxovirus hemagglutinin (HA) and neuraminidase (NA)] integral membrane viral glycoproteins which are present in large quantities on infected cell surfaces. Inside the envelope, matrix or membrane protein (termed M1 for myxoviruses, M for rhabdoviruses) is believed to form a shell which encases the ribonucleoprotein complex. For myxoviruses, this consists of 8 RNA segments along with nucleoprotein (NP) and small quantities of three viral polymerases (PA, PB1, PB2); for rhabdoviruses, this consists of the nucleocapsid protein (N) and two polymerases (NS and L). During the course of a myxovirus infection, three other proteins are produced which appear to be completely excluded from virions (NS1, NS2, and M2).

Myxo- and rhabdoviruses demonstrate a major difference in their replication cycles: a critical portion of myxoviruses transcription occurs in the nucleus, whereas rhabdoviruses require no nuclear functions. This difference is reflected in the cellular localization of viral proteins involved in transcription. Myxovirus NP, NS1, and polymerases are all transported into the nucleus following translation, while rhabdovirus N, NS, and L are located exclusively in the cytoplasm.

CTL RECOGNITION OF INDIVIDUAL INFLUENZA A VIRUS ANTIGENS

Human type A influenza viruses are grouped into three subtypes, designated H1N1, H2N2, and H3N2. H1, H2, and H3 and N1 and N2 each designate non-cross-reactive serotypes of the HA and NA molecules, respectively. Initial studies found that anti-influenza CTL could be divided into two major categories, those specific for the immunizing strain and other strains within the subtype ("strain specific"), and those able to lyse cells infected with any human influenza A virus ("cross-reactive").[5-7] The existence of cross-reactive CTL was surprising since it was thought that only the serologically non-cross-reactive glycoproteins were expressed on infected cell surfaces. It was proposed that either CTL recognized the glycoproteins in a manner different from antibodies, or that one or a number of the highly conserved internal proteins were expressed on infected cell surfaces.

Unambiguous identification of the viral antigens recognized by CTL became possible only through the application of genetic engineering techniques to produce histocompatible cells which express genetically isolated viral components. Two types of vectors have been used for expression of cloned viral genes:

1. DNA constructs containing an influenza virus gene in conjunction with transcriptional promoters and a gene (commonly thymidine kinase or neomycin resistance) conferring a growth advantage to cells when cultured under selective conditions. These constructs are introduced into cells by direct transfection and results in the constitutive biosynthesis of the influenza virus gene product.[8,9]

2. Recombinant vaccinia viruses (Vac) containing influenza virus genes under the control of Vac promoters. Infection of cells with Vac recombinants results in the expression of influenza virus gene products during the course of a lytic Vac infectious cycle.[10,11]

Although cells expressing transfected genes have been successfully used to study CTL specificity, using the currently available vectors it has proven difficult to maintain uniform levels of expression of influenza virus genes in transfected murine cells. This problem is averted using Vac recombinants, which also offer great experimental flexibility due to their broad host range and ability to induce anti-influenza CTL responses in vivo and in vitro.[12] These advantages have led to the widespread adoption of Vac recombinants for studies of CTL specificity.

Using Vac recombinants, we have examined CTL recognition of 8 of the 10 influenza virus gene products. Results obtained using the recombinants to examine the specificity of anti-influenza CTL derived from BALB/c (H-2^d) mice are described below by gene product (references are given where these results have been described in published accounts). CTL activity was measured in ^{51}Cr release assays using influenza or recombinant Vac-infected P815 cells [a DBA/2 (H-2^d) mastocytoma cell line]. To produce CTL populations, splenocytes from mice immunized with live influenza virus or Vac recombinants were co-incubated for 6 days with autologous splenocytes infected with influenza A virus.

HA[12,13]

Recognition of cells infected with Vac recombinants containing cloned H1 or H2 HA genes (termed H1-Vac and H2-Vac) by anti-influenza CTL populations was predominantly strain specific. CTL populations induced by priming and/or in vitro stimulation with H1-Vac or H2-Vac also demonstrated predominantly strain specific recognition. A moderate amount of cross-reactive recognition was detected between H1 and H2 HAs, but did not extend to the H3 HA. This pattern of recognition is consistent with the amino acid homologies of the HAs (H1 and H2 are among the most closely related of the 13 known HA serotypes, while H1 and H3, and H2 and H3 are among the most distantly related HAs.) Unlabelled target inhibition studies confirmed that the HA is, at most, only a minor target antigen for cross-reactive CTL.

NP[14]

NP was found to be a major target antigen for cross-reactive CTL. NP-Vac infected cells were consistently lysed by all cross-reactive CTL populations tested. Unlabelled target inhibition experiments and limiting dilution analysis of CTL precursor frequency confirmed that a substantial portion of secondarily in vitro stimulated BALB/c CTL recognize NP. Inoculation of mice with NP-Vac primed splenocytes for vigorous secondary CTL responses following in vitro stimulation with influenza viruses from all three human subtypes. NP-Vac also primed mice for an accelerated pulmonary CTL response following aerosol infection with influenza virus.

NS1[15]

NS1-Vac infected cells were consistently lysed by cross-reactive CTL, but generally at lower levels than NP-Vac infected cells. The comparative frequencies of BALB/c NP and NS1 specific CTL precursors, as determined by limiting dilution analysis, were consistent with this finding. These findings provide the first evidence that non-structural viral proteins synthesized during a lytic infection can be recognized by CTL.

Polymerases[15]

PB2-Vac infected cells were consistently lysed by cross-reactive BALB/c CTL, and inoculation with PB2-Vac primed mice for secondary in vitro cross-reactive responses. Levels of lysis were generally similar to those observed on NS1-Vac infected cells; again, this was consistent with precursor frequencies. Pa-Vac infected cells were usually lysed by cross-reactive CTL populations. Levels of lysis were always lower than those observed for PB2-Vac infected cells. PB1-Vac infected cells were only occasionally lysed by cross-reactive (or strain-specific) CTL populations, and then, only at low levels.

M1

In a large number of experiments, M1-Vac infected cells were not specifically recognized by anti-influenza CTL populations. This was not due to low levels of expression of M1, since M1-Vac infected cells expressed antigenically active M1 at levels comparable to influenza A virus infected cells. Nor is this attributable to the resistance of these cells to lysis by CTL, since they were lysed by anti-Vac CTL with identical efficiency as cells infected with other Vac recombinants. Inoculation of mice with M1-Vac also failed to prime their splenocytes for secondary in vitro responses.

M2

M2-Vac infected cells were not recognized by most CTL populations tested. Occasionally, using high effector to target ratios, lysis at levels marginally above control values were observed. Whether this represents specific recognition by a very minor CTL population can only be determined using CTL clones. The failure to observe greater levels of CTL recognition is not due to the lack of surface expression of this integral membrane protein, since in the presence of complement, M2-Vac infected cells were efficiently lysed by an antiserum which demonstrates the same cross-reactive recognition of influenza A virus infected cells as CTL. This antiserum was produced by immunization of goats with purified M1, and its cross-reactive recognition of influenza A virus infected cells provided evidence for the expression of M1 on infected cell surfaces.[16] These findings could not be confirmed using monoclonal antibodies specific for M1.[17,18] This cell surface reactivity, and probably the reactivity of other anti-M1 antisera used in other studies,[19-21] is apparently entirely due to its cross-reaction with M2, since we found that it does not lyse cells infected with M1-Vac or with any of the other Vac recombinants. The basis for this cross-reaction is easily explained, since M1 and M2 share the same 9 amino terminal residues, and M2 has been shown to be oriented in the plasma membrane such that at least 18 of its amino terminal residues are exposed at the cell surface.[22]

CTL RECOGNITION OF INDIVIDUAL VSV ANTIGENS

As with anti-influenza CTL, anti-VSV CTL can be divided into cross-reactive and serotype specific categories.[23] Based on the initial findings in this system, it was thought that both of these CTL populations predominantly, if not solely, recognize G.[24,25] CTL recognition of individual VSV components was examined using recombinant Vac viruses containing G genes derived from Indiana and New Jersey serotypes, and the N gene derived from VSV Indiana. The recombinant Vac viruses were used to both elicit anti-VSV CTL and to sensitize target cells for lysis by CTL induced by VSV.

Both N and G were found to be recognized by VSV specific CTL. Recognition of G-Vac infected cells was largely limited to CTL induced by priming and stimulating with the homologous serotype. In contrast, N-Vac infected cells were efficiently lysed by CTL induced with any combination of serotypes in priming and stimulation.[26]

CTL RECOGNITION OF INDIVIDUAL VIRAL ANTIGENS OCCURS IN CONJUNCTION WITH ONLY A LIMITED NUMBER OF THE AVAILABLE CLASS I RESTRICTION ELEMENTS

As described above, BALB/c CTL demonstrated marked differences in responsiveness to individual influenza virus proteins. To examine the strain dependence of this phenomenon, cross-reactive CTL derived from C57BL/6 ($H-2^b$) and CBA ($H-2^k$) mice were tested for their ability to lyse Vac-recombinant infected MC57G ($H-2^b$) and L ($H-2^k$) cells respectively.[15] In contrast to BALB/c CTL, C57BL/6 CTL only consistently recognized NP and NS1. CBA CTL yielded still another pattern of recognition, in only recognizing NP, NS1, and PB1. We failed to detect recognition of either M1 or M2 in any of these experiments.

The differential responsiveness to PB1 and PB2 by BALB/c and CBA/J CTL was further examined using cross-reactive CTL populations derived from BALB/c and BALB/K ($H-2^k$), and B10.D2 ($H-2^d$) and B10.BR ($H-2^k$) congenic strains. Responsiveness to PB1 was found to co-segregate with $H-2^k$, while PB2 responsiveness co-segregated with $H-2^d$. By using target cells derived from C3H X DBA/2 ($H-2^{kxd}$) F1 mice, we eliminated the possibility that these results were due to differential expression of PB1 and PB2 in L cells versus P815 cells, since an identical pattern of recognition of PB1 and PB2 was observed. These data indicate that responsiveness to PB1 and PB2 is controlled by the MHC.

The effect of the MHC on CTL recognition of individual antigens was further studied by testing the ability of cross-reactive CTL derived from A/J (K^kD^d) and C3H.OH (K^dD^k) to lyse Vac recombinant infected P815 and L cells. With a single exception (recognition of PB1 by $H-2^k$ CTL), recognition of individual viral antigens could be mapped to the K or D end of the MHC. These data suggest that CTL recognition of many viral antigens occurs only in association with a limited number of the available MHC class I restriction elements.

CONCLUSIONS

Based on our studies, we can make the following general conclusions regarding CTL recognition of viral antigens.

1. Both external and internal viral proteins can serve as target antigens for CTL. Recognition can include non-structural proteins, as well as proteins present in mature virions. CTL recognition of VSV N indicates that nuclear residence is not an absolute requirement for CTL recognition. The process by which these proteins traverse the plasma membrane and are presented for recognition by CTL is an open question. Whatever the mechanism, CTL recognition of internal viral proteins suggests that internal cellular antigens could play a prominent role in CTL responses to minor histocompatibility antigens and tumor antigens.

2. CTL recognition of internal viral proteins is independent of their relative abundance. Despite the fact that the polymerases are produced in very low amounts during an influenza virus infection, they can be recognized with equal efficiency to NP or NS1, which are produced in 100 to 1000 fold higher amounts. It appears that even lower amounts of internal proteins can be detected in transfected cells,[27,28] which suggests that CTL surveillance of cellular proteins may not often be limited by low levels of expression.

3. Cross-reactive CTL recognition of related proteins generally reflects their degree of amino acid homology. Cross-reactive CTL recognition of influenza or VSV proteins is largely limited to the highly conserved internal proteins. This is not to say that recognition of internal proteins is always cross-reactive; it is now clear that at least two of the internal proteins (PB2[29] and NP[30]) can be recognized in a highly strain specific manner. Indeed, it has been found that under some conditions, most strain specific CTL recognize internal viral proteins.[31] Conversely, a minority of cross-reactive clones are specific for the highly variable glycoproteins.

4. Most, but maybe not all, viral components can serve as CTL recognition structures. It has not been possible to demonstrate recognition of M1 or M2 by CTL derived from BALB/c or CBA mice. If this can be shown to be related to some physical property of these proteins, this would provide valuable insight into the processing of viral antigens into CTL target antigens. It is possible, however, that these antigens can only be recognized in conjunction with a very limited number of class I MHC alleles, and it will be necessary to examine their recognition using CTL restricted to other MHC haplotypes. This idea is favored by the recognition of M1 by human CTL.[32]

5. The prevalence of CTL specific for any given component depends on a number of factors. One major factor is

MHC haplotype, since non-responder class I MHC alleles have been identified for each viral component. Other factors also appear to influence responses to individual proteins, since even in high responder inbred mouse strains, CTL recognition of NP has been found to vary widely between individuals.[33] Whether this is due to specific suppression of anti-NP responses, or to fundamental differences in individual CTL repertoires, remains to be determined.

6. T lymphocyte recognition of internal viral antigens is still consistent with their high degree of conservation. Influenza virus has the ability to mutate rapidly in response to host immunity. This property accounts for the high degree of antigenic variation observed in glycoproteins derived from different virus isolates. Despite this, internal viral proteins exhibit a degree of antigenic variation consistent with random genetic drift (and/or occasional host cell selection for functional variants). As CTL responses are directed against the internal components, this must mean that CTL exert little, if any, evolutionary selection for mutants with antigenically altered internal proteins. As their is no apparent difference between T lymphocyte recognition of internal and external protein, this indicates that antigenic variation in the viral glycoproteins is due solely to antibody mediated selection.

The lack of CTL mediated variant selection is easy to understand. First, the fact that CTL responses are directed against a number of viral proteins (and, in some cases, possibly a number of determinants on a single protein), means that there would be little selective advantage conferred by the failure of a single CTL clonotype to recognize cells expressing a protein with an altered determinant. As the frequency of mutant viruses with multiple alterations is exceedingly low (approximately 10^{-5n}, where n = the number of mutations),[34] variant selection would have to occur in a host producing a monoclonal, or at most, biclonal T lymphocyte response. The existence of individuals with such restricted responses among either human or experimental animal populations has yet to be described.

Second, even in the case of an oligoclonal response, the frequency of cells expressing a given protein solely with a variant phenotype would decrease exponentially with the multiplicity of infection (in this case the frequency of these cells would be approximately 10^{-5n}, where n = the number of infectious virions per cell). This would mean that only cells infected with two infectious particles at most, could act as the source of potential variants. Although the multiplicity of infection in vivo is unknown, it could well be higher than this.

7. Implications for vaccine design. Our findings have two major implications for the design of vaccines meant to elicit maximal CTL immunity. First, these vaccines should include internal viral antigens. From the present work it is clear that many of these proteins can be recognized by CTL, and that their generally high degree of conservation between virus serotypes will insure the broadest induction of immunity. Second, to avoid potential difficul-

ties of MHC linked non-responsiveness to individual viral components, vaccines should be composed of a number of viral proteins.

It must be stressed that the utility of such anti-viral "CTL vaccines" remains to be determined. Although CTL appear to play an important role in eradicating established influenza, vaccinia, and LCM virus infections,[5-39] the anti-viral activity of CTL in other viral infections must be determined for each individual virus. Furthermore, as suggested by Zinkernagel et al.,[40] vaccination for CTL memory may be a pointless exercise since CTL memory could be short-lived, and in any event, primary and secondary in vivo CTL responses differ little in their kinetics and magnitude. However, while such vaccines may not prove to be useful in cases where vigorous CTL responses arise during the immune response, they may be important in circumstances where CTL responses are low or absent such as chronic virus infections and tumors.

ACKNOWLEDGMENTS

We wish to thank P. Palese (Mt. Sinai School of Medicine, New York, N.Y.), J. Rose (Salk Institute, La Jolla, Ca.), R. Lamb (Northwestern University, Evanston, Ill.), and M. Gething (University of Texas, Dallas, Tex.) for providing cloned viral genes used to construct Vac recombinant viruses. This work was supported by grants AI 22114, AI 14162, and AI 20338 from the National Institutes of Health, Bethesda, Md.

REFERENCES

1. R. M. Zinkernagel and P. D. Doherty, MHC-restricted cytotoxic T cells: studies on the biological role of polymorphic major transplantation antigens determining T-cell restriction-specificity function and responsiveness. Adv. Immunol. 27:51 (1979).
2. F. A. Ennis, Some newly recognized aspects of resistance against and recovery from influenza. Arch. Virol. 73:207 (1982).
3. A. G. Morris, Y.-L. Lin, and B. A. Askonas, Immune interferon release when a cloned cytotoxic T-cell line meets its correct influenza-infected target cell. Nature (London) 295:150 (1982).
4. J. R. Klein, D. H. Raulet, M. S. Pasternack, and M. J. Bevan, Cytotoxic T lymphocytes produce immune interferon in response to antigen or mitogen. J. Exp. Med. 155:1198 (1982).
5. R. B. Effros, P. C. Doherty, W. Gerhard, and J. R. Bennink, Generation of both cross-reactive and virus-specific T-cell populations after immunization with serologically distinct influenza A virus. J. Exp. Med. 145:557 (1977).
6. K. L. Yap and G. L. Ada, Cytotoxic T cells specific for influenza virus-infected target cells. Immunology 32:151 (1977).

7. H. J. Zweerink, S. A. Courtneidge, J. J. Skehel, M. J. Crumpton, and B. A. Askonas, Cytotoxic T cells kill influenza virus infected cells but do not distinguish between serologically distinct type A viruses. Nature (London) 267:354 (1977).
8. T. J. Braciale, V. L. Braciale, T. J. Henkel, J. Sambrook, and M. J. Gething, Cytotoxic T lymphocyte recognition of the influenza hemagglutinin gene product expressed by DNA-mediated gene transfer. J. Exp. Med. 159:341 (1984).
9. A. R. M. Townsend, A. J. McMichael, N. P. Carter, J. A. Haddleston, and G. G. Brownlee, Cytotoxic T cell recognition of the influenza nucleoprotein, hemagglutinin expressed in transfected mouse L cells. Cell 39:13 (1984).
10. G. L. Smith, B. R. Murphy, and B. Moss, Construction and characterization of an infectious vaccinia virus recombinant that expresses the influenza hemagglutinin gene and induces resistance to influenza virus infection in hamsters. Proc. Natl. Acad. Sci. USA 80:7155 (1983).
11. M. Mackett, G. L. Smith, and B. Moss, General method for production and selection of infectious vaccinia virus recombinants expressing foreign genes. J. Virol. 49:857 (1984).
12. J. R. Bennink, J. W. Yewdell, G. L. Smith, C. Moller, and B. Moss, Recombinant vaccinia virus primes and stimulates influenza haemagglutinin-specific cytotoxic T cells. Nature (London) 311:578 (1984).
13. J. R. Bennink, J. W. Yewdell, G. L. Smith, and B. Moss, Recognition of cloned influenza virus hemagglutinin gene products by cytotoxic T lymphocytes. J. Virol. 57:786 (1986).
14. J. W. Yewdell, J. R. Bennink, G. L. Smith, and B. Moss, Influenza A virus nucleoprotein is a major target antigen for cross-reactive anti-influenza A virus cytotoxic T lymphocytes. Proc. Natl. Acad. Sci. USA 82:1785 (1985).
15. J. R. Bennink, J. W. Yewdell, G. L. Smith, and B. Moss, Anti-influenza cytotoxic T lymphocytes recognize the three viral polymerases and a nonstructural protein: responsiveness to individual viral antigens is MHC controlled. J. Virol., in press (1987).
16. W. E. Biddison, P. C. Doherty, and R. G. Webster, Antibody to influenza virus matrix protein detects a common antigen on the surface of cells infected with type A influenza virus. J. Exp. Med. 146:690 (1977).
17. C. J. Hackett, B. A. Askonas, R. J. Webster, and K. van Wyke, Quantitation of influenza virus antigens on infected target cells and their recognition by cross-reactive cytotoxic T cells. J. Exp. Med. 151:1014 (1980).
18. J. W. Yewdell, E. Frank, and W. Gerhard, Expression of influenza A virus internal antigens on the surface of infected P815 cells. J. Immunol. 126:1814 (1981).
19. T. J. Braciale, Immunologic recognition of influenza virus-infected cells. II. Expression of influenza A matrix protein on the infected cell surface and its role in recognition by cross-reactive cytotoxic T cells. J. Exp. Med. 146:673 (1977).

20. G. L. Ada and K. L. Yap, Matrix protein expressed at the surface of cells infected with influenza viruses. Immunochemistry 14:643 (1977).
21. C. S. Reiss and J. L. Schulman, Influenza type A M protein: expression on infected cells is responsible for cross-reactive recognition by cytotoxic thymus derived lymphocytes. Infec. Immun. 29:719 (1980).
22. R. A. Lamb, S. L. Zebedee, and C. D. Richardson, Influenza virus M2 protein is an integral membrane protein expressed on the infected-cell surface. Cell 40:627 (1985).
23. K. L. Rosenthal and R. M. Zinkernagel, Cross-reactive cytotoxic T cells to serologically distinct vesicular stomatitis viruses. J. Immunol. 124:2301 (1980).
24. A. H. Hale, D. N. Witte, D. Baltimore, and H. N. Eisen, Vesicular stomatitis virus glycoprotein is necessary for H-2-restricted lysis of infected cells by cytotoxic T lymphocytes. Proc. Natl. Acad. Sci. USA 75:970 (1978).
25. R. M. Zinkernagel, A. Althage, and J. Holland, Target antigens for H-2-restricted vesicular stomatitis virus-specific cytotoxic T cells. J. Immunol. 121:744 (1978).
26. J. W. Yewdell, J. R. Bennink, M. Mackett, L. LeFrancois, D. S. Lyles, and B. Moss, Recognition of cloned vesicular stomatitis virus internal and external gene products by cytotoxic T lymphocytes. J. Exp. Med. 163:1529 (1986).
27. A. R. M. Townsend, F. M. Gotch, and J. Davey, Cytotoxic T cells recognize fragments of the influenza nucleoprotein. Cell 42:457 (1985).
28. L. Puddington, M. J. Bevan, J. K. Rose, and L. Lefrancois, N protein is the predominant antigen recognized by vesicular stomatitis virus-specific cytotoxic T cells. J. Virol., in press (1986).
29. J. R. Bennink, J. W. Yewdell, and W. Gerhard, A viral polymerase involved in recognition of influenza virus-infected cells by a cytotoxic T-cell clone. Nature (London) 296:75 (1982).
30. A. R. M. Townsend, J. J. Skehel, P. M. Taylor, and P. A. Palese, Recognition of influenza A virus nucleoprotein by an H-2 restricted cytotoxic T cell clone. Virology 133:456 (1984).
31. U. Kees and P. J. Krammer, Most influenza A virus-specific memory cytotoxic T lymphocytes react with antigenic epitopes associated with internal virus determinants. J. Exp. Med. 159:365 (1984).
32. F. Gotch, A. McMichael, G. Smith, and B. Moss, Identification of the viral molecules recognized by influenza specific human cytotoxic T lymphocytes. J. Exp. Med., in press (1987).
33. P. Pala and B. A. Askonas, Low responder MHC alleles for Tc recognition of influenza nucleoprotein. Immunogenetics 23:379 (1986).
34. J. W. Yewdell, R. G. Webster, and W. U. Gerhard, Antigenic variation in three distinct determinants of an influenza type A haemagglutinin molecule. Nature (London) 279:246 (1979).
35. K. L. Yap, G. L. Ada, and I. F. C. McKenzie, Transfer of specific cytotoxic T lymphocytes protects mice inoc-

ulated with influenza virus. Nature (London) 273:238 (1978).
36. Y. L. Yin and B. A. Askonas, Biological properties of an influenza A virus-specific killer T cell clone. J. Exp. Med. 154:225 (1981).
37. J. R. Bennink, J. W. Yewdell, A. Feldman, W. Gerhard, and P. C. Doherty, The role of virus-specific CTL in vivo, in: "T Cell Clones," H. von Boehmer and W. Haas, eds., Elsevier, New York (1984).
38. A. E. Lukacher, V. L. Braciale, and T. J. Braciale, In vivo effector function of influenza virus-specific cytotoxic T lymphocyte clones is highly specific. J. Exp. Med. 160:814 (1984).
39. M. B. A. Oldstone, P. Blount, P. J. Southern, and P. W. Lampert, Cytoimmunotherapy for persistent virus infection reveals a unique clearance pattern from the central nervous system. Nature (London) 321:239 (1986).
40. R. M. Zinkernagel, H. Hengartner, and L. Stitz, On the role of viruses in the evolution of immune responses. Brit. Med. Bull. 41:92 (1985).

ROLE OF NATURAL KILLER CELLS IN THE EARLY CLEARANCE OF *RICKETTSIA TYPHI* IN MICE

F. M. Rollwagen

Infectious Disease Department, Naval Medical Research Institute, Bethesda, MD

INTRODUCTION

Clearance of the intracellular bacterium, *Rickettsia typhi*, has been a field of much recent inquiry. Cells which transfer immunity arise late during the course of infection, bear the Thy-1 antigen (1) and are H-2 restricted. Further, H-2 restricted cytotoxic T-cells functional *in vitro* also arise at approximately the same time (2), and are believed to belong to the same lineage as those which transfer immunity (3). Examination of the kinetics of the immune response, however, reveals that the onset of the cellular response, as well as that of IgG antibodies, occurs as much as one week after the organisms have been cleared. How, then, is the early clearance of infection brought about?

It has been shown that tissue culture cells pretreated with interferon-gamma (IFN) can effectively eliminate subsequent infections with *R. prowazekii* (4). IFN has been shown to increase natural killer (NK) activity (5), but not to alter the action of natural cytotoxic (NC) cells (6). In addition, since IFN can be increased following rickettsia infection (7) it was of interest to attempt to differentiate the effects of IFN, NC, and NK activity on the early clearance of *R. typhi in vivo*.

In the experiments described in this report, mice were treated with anti-asialo GM-1 (anti-ASG) a rabbit antibody which eliminates NK activity *in vivo* (8) and *in vitro* (9), but has no effect on the activity of NC cells (10). The subsequent effect on the growth of *R. typhi* was assessed, as well as the state of NK and NC activity. In addition, the ability of spleen cells to lyse NK or NC targets infected with *R. typhi* was examined.

MATERIALS AND METHODS

Mice

BALB/cByJ female mice were obtained from The Jackson Laboratory, Bar Harbor, ME, and used at 6-8 weeks of age.

Rickettsia

Rickettsia typhi, strain Wilmington was propagated in chicken yolk sacs and were purified by density gradient centrifugation as previously described (11). *In vivo* titration of rickettsial burden was carried out as previously described (1). All organisms and *in vivo* mouse titrations were performed courtesy of Dr. G. Dasch, Rickettsial Diseases Division.

Cytotoxicity Assays

The ^{51}Cr release method of estimation of NK activity was carried out by standard means. The ^{3}H-proline method for NC activity was carried out according to the method of Bean et al (12). The only modifications of these two methods was that the target cells were infected with *R. typhi* at a MOI of 3 on day 2 before the cytotoxicity assay, and were subsequently held at 34°C in the presence of 1% fetal calf serum in order to optimize growth of rickettsiae. This procedure did not affect the uptake of isotope in either of the two assay systems (data not shown).

RESULTS

Mice were injected intravenously with anti-ASG about six hours before being infected with $2x10^4$ pfu of *R. typhi*, intraperitoneally. Analysis by fluorescence activated cell sorter revealed that all cells staining with anti-ASG were eliminated from the spleens of treated mice (data not shown). It can be seen in Figure 1A that this procedure completely eliminated spleen cells with NK activity directed toward the NK target, YAC-1 (compare NL with Ab); reactivity toward the NC targets, METH E-4 and METH A were unchanged (Fig. 1B). As has been shown previously (13), NK activity was increased in mice infected with *R. typhi*; this increase in NK activity could not override the elimination of NK activity effected by administration of anti-ASG seen in Fig. 1A (compare INF with INF+Ab). Again, NC activity remained unchanged by these *in vivo* manipulations (Fig. 1B).

The data of Table 1 show that mice which had been injected with anti-ASG and then infected with *R. typhi* had increased growth of organisms in their livers over mice given *R. typhi* alone. These differences could be observed on day 3 and were most apparent on day 5 post infection. By day 7 post infection, the normal animals had begun to clear their infections, so differences were less apparent.

Since rickettsiae are intracellular bacteria, a possible role for NK cells in the early clearance of organisms could lie in the preferential lysis of infected cells over noninfected cells. In order to answer this question, target cells susceptible to either NK or NC cells were infected with *R. typhi* on day 0 and the infection allowed to proceed to day 2, when the NK and NC tests were performed. It can be seen in Table 2 that infected YAC-1 cells, which are NK targets, were lysed to a greater extent in the 4-hour ^{51}Cr release assay than uninfected YAC-1 cells. The same observation can be made using the NC target, METH-E4. Another NC target, METH A, however, was not more susceptible to lysis when infected with *R. typhi* than when uninfected.

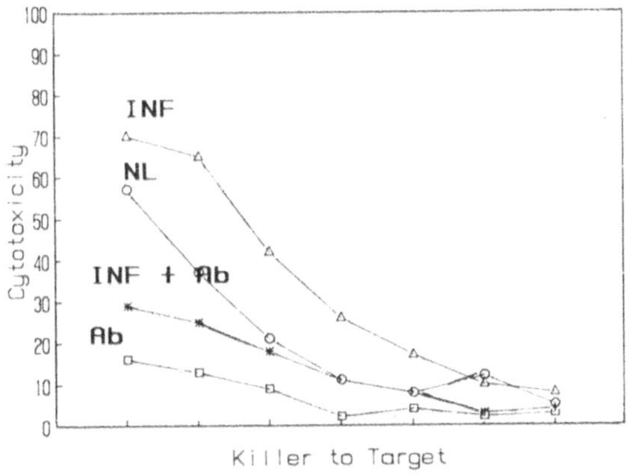

Figure 1, Panel A. ^{51}Cr release assay against Yac-1 target cells by spleen cells taken from mice injected three days previously with anti-asialo GM1 (Ab), Ab and R. typhi (INF+Ab), or with R. typhi alone (INF). INF = infected

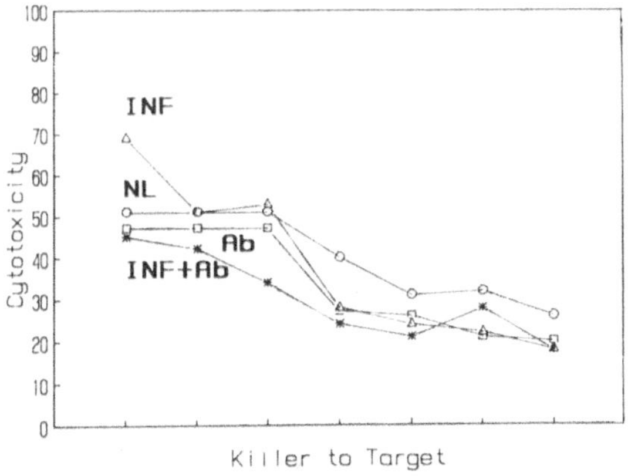

Figure 1, Panel B. ^{3}H-proline cytotoxicity assay against METH E-4 by the same spleen cell populations as described in Panel A.

Table 1. Rickettsial Organisms per Liver

Treatment Group	Log pfu/Liver Day of Assay		
	3	5	7
Uninfected	<1	<1	<1
Infected	5.75	4.0	2.75
Uninfected & α ASGMI	<1	<1	<1
Infected & α ASGMI	6.78	6.0	2.75

Livers from mice treated as described in the footnote to Figure 1 were homogenized and titrated in an *in vivo* assay as described in Ref. 1.

Table 2

Target	*R. typhi* infection	% Cytotoxicity E:T[a]		
		100	50	25
YAC[b]	+	78	68	51
	-	40	28	18
Meth E4[c]	+	62	61	34
	-	60	41	14
Meth A[c]	+	46	30	31
	-	40	32	31
L929[d]	+	9	0	0
	-	0	0	0

a = Spleen cells taken from mice on day 3, post infection with 2 x 10^4 pfu *R. typhi*.
b = 4-hour ^{51}Cr release assay
c = 18-hour ^{3}H-proline cytotoxicity assay
d = L929 is not susceptible to NK or NC mediated killing

DISCUSSION

The roles of NK and NC cells in the clearance of infectious organisms has remained unclear. Examination of clearance of infection in mice treated with anti-ASG reveals that in many cases, *in vivo* compromise of NK activity allows an increase in growth of certain viruses (14). In addition, NK cells have been implicated in the clearance of viral (15,16) and protozoal (17,18) species. These results are often shown to be related to increased susceptibility of NK targets after they have been infected *in vitro* with the organism under study (10,16,19). These observations are by no means universal, however. It has been shown that *in vivo* treatment with anti-ASG has little or no effect on the course of infection with lymphocytic choriomeningitis virus (14). The data presented in this report suggest that *in vivo* elimination of NK activity allows an increase in the numbers of *R. typhi* organisms recovered from the livers of infected mice. That unrestrained growth of the organism was not observed, however, suggests that additional mechanisms may operate to eliminate the organism *in vivo*. NC activity was unchanged by *in vivo* treatment with anti-ASG, suggesting that this activity may act to control the growth of this intracellular bacterium.

It has been shown that pretreatment of adherent cell lines with gamma-interferon (IFN) induces the intracellular destruction of organisms when such cell lines are infected with *R. prowazekii* (4). These data suggest that *in vivo* elevation of IFN subsequent to infection causes infected cells to eliminate intracellular organisms. In addition, the *in vivo* treatment of mice with antibody to IFN allows virtual unrestricted growth of *R. tsutsugamushi* (20). The data presented in this report suggest a simple model for the role of IFN and NK in the clearance of infection with *R. typhi*. Since under some conditions, cloned NK cell lines manufacture IFN (21), the increase in NK activity following infection with rickettsiae may increase the amounts of circulating IFN thereby inducing increased intracellular lysis of organisms. Interruption of the feedback loop between IFN and NK allows the unrestricted growth of organisms. IFN, in addition, acting on infected endothelial cells can induce increased expression of Ia antigens and, presumably, of rickettsial antigens on the cell surface.

ACKNOWLEDGMENTS

The author wishes to thank Dr. G. Dasch for supplying the rickettsiae and for running the mouse *in vivo* titrations. Thanks also to Ms. D. Hicks for typing the manuscript. Special thanks to Ms. Nancy Pacheco for excellent and untiring technical help, especially on the weekends.

This research was supported by the Naval Medical Research and Development Command Project No. 3M161102BS10.AC.423. The opinions and assertions contained herein are the private ones of the author and are not be construed as official or reflecting the views of the Navy Department or the Naval Service at large. The experiments reported herein were conducted according to the principles set forth in the "Guide for the Care and Use of Laboratory Animals", Institute of Laboratory Animals Resources, National Research Council, DHEW, Pub. No. (NIH) 78-23.

REFERENCES

1. Crist, A.E., Jr., C.L. Wisseman, Jr., and J.R. Murphy. 1984. Characteristics of *Rickettsia mooseri* infection of normal and immune mice. Infect. Immun. 43:38.
2. Rollwagen, F.M., G.A. Dasch, and T.R. Jerrells. 1986. Mechanisms of immunity to rickettsial infection: Characterization of a cytotoxic effector cell. J. Immunol. 136:1418.
3. Dasch, G., and F.M. Rollwagen. Characterization of cells which transfer immunity to rickettsial infection. Manuscript in preparation.
4. Turco, J., and Winkler, H.H. 1983. Inhibition of the growth of *Rickettsia prowazekii* in cultured fibroblasts by lymphokines. J. Exp. Med. 157:974.
5. Djeu, J.Y., J.A. Heinbaugh, H.T. Holden, and R.B. Herberman. 1979. Augmentation of mouse natural killer cell activity by interferon and interferon inducers. J. Immunol. 122:175.

6. Stutman, O., E. Feo Figarella, C.J. Paige, and E.C. Lattime. 1980. Natural cytotoxic (NC) cells against solid tumors in mice: general characteristics and comparison to natural killer (NK) cells. In: Natural Cell-Mediated Immunity against Tumors. Ed. by R.B. Herberman, Academic Press, N.Y., p. 187.
7. Palmer, B.A., F.M. Hetrick, and T.R. Jerrells. 1984. Gamma interferon production in response to homologous and heterologous strain antigens in mice chronically infected with Rickettsia tsutsugamushi. Infect. Immun. 46:237.
8. Kasai, M., T. Yoneda, S. Habu, Y. Maruyama, K. Okumura, and T. Tokunaga. 1981. In vivo effect of anti-asialo GM1 antibody on natural killer activity. Nature 291:334.
9. Kasai, M., M. Iwamori, Y. Nagai, K. Okumura, and T. Tada. 1980. A glycolipid on the surface of mouse natural killer cells. Eur. J. Immunol. 10:175.
10. Tang, J., D.C. DeLong, P. Marder, L.D. Butler, and E.W. Ades. 1985. Identification of functional subpopulations of murine natural killer cells based on their cell surface asialo GM1 phenotype. Cell. Immunol. 96:386.
11. Weiss, E., J.C. Coolbaugh, and J.C. Williams. 1975. Separation of viable Rickettsia typhi from yolk sac and L cell host components by Renografin density gradient centrifugation. Appl. Microbiol. 30:456.
12. Bean, M.A., Y. Kodera, and H. Shiku. 1976. Tritiated-proline microcytotoxicity assay for the study of cellular and humoral immune reaction directed against target cells grown in monolayer cultures. In: In vitro Methods in Cell Mediated and Tumor Immunity. B.R. Bloom and J.R. David, eds. Academic Press, New York, p. 471.
13. Jerrells, T.R. 1986. Mechanisms of immunity to Rickettsia species and Coxiella burnetii. In: Biology of Rickettsial Diseases. Walker, D.H., Ed. CRC Press, Boca Raton, FL, in press.
14. Colmenares, C., and C. Lopez. 1986. Enhanced lysis of Herpes simplex virus type 1-infected mouse cell lines by NC and NK effectors. J. Immunol. 136:3473.
15. Kurane, I., D. Hebblewaite, W.E. Brandt, and F.A. Ennis. 1984. Lysis of dengue virus-infected cells by natural cell-mediated cytotoxicity and antibody-dependent cell-mediated cytotoxicity. J. Virol. 52:223.
16. Munoz, A., L. Carrasco, and M. Fresno. 1983. Enhancement of susceptibility of HSV-1-infected cells to natural killer lysis by interferon. J. Immunol. 131:783.
17. Skamene, E., M.M. Stevenson, and S. Lemieux. 1983. Murine malaria: dissociation of natural killer (NK) cell activity and resistance to Plasmodium chabaudi. Parasite Immunol. 5:557.
18. Kirkpatrick, C.E., J.P. Farrell, J.F. Warner, and G. Dennert. 1985. Participation of natural killer cells in the recovery of mice from visceral leishmaniasis. Cell. Immunol. 92:163.
20. Li, H., T.R. Jerrells, and D.H. Walker. 1986. Evidence for the role of gamma-interferon as a crucial host defense against Rickettsia conorii in vivo. Am. Soc. for Rickettsiology, Williamsburg, Va.
21. Handa, K., R. Suzuki, H. Matsui, Y. Shimizu, and K. Kumagai. 1983. Natural killer (NK) cells as a responder to interleukin-2 (IL-2). II. IL 2-induced interferon-γ production. J. Immunol. 130:988.

LOSS OF TUMORIGENICITY FOLLOWING *IN VITRO* MULV INFECTION IS ASSOCIATED WITH INDUCTION OF PERITONEAL NATURAL KILLER CELL ACTIVITY[1]

Karin Thiel, Eugene V. Genovesi[2], J. Dirk Iglehart, Dani P. Bolognesi, and Kent J. Weinhold[3]

Department of Surgery
Duke University Medical Center
Durham, North Carolina 27710

ABSTRACT

Infection by an attenuated replication-competent murine retrovirus (Friend leukemia virus-FLV[4]),but not other non-transforming retroviruses, stimulated rejection of transplantable thymomas (RL-cell line) and subsequent tumor immunity in syngeneic mouse recipients. FLV-infected RL-cells (RL-FLV) were unaltered in their *in vitro* growth, and grew progressively to kill sublethally irradiated animals and nude mice. Primary RL-FLV rejection was due to induction of increased natural killer (NK)-cell activity limited to peritoneal sites of tumor inoculation with a minor cytolytic macrophage population. Syngeneic mutant beige (NK-deficient) mice similarly rejected RL-FLV cells with increased peritoneal NK-cell activity and acquired immunity to the parental RL-tumor. While RL-FLV stimulated far greater peritoneal NK activity than did other tested retrovirus-infected RL-cells, the inherent susceptibility of these cells to lysis by normal NK cells was not altered by virus. RL-FLV induced NK effectors showed an indiscriminant lysis pattern that was independent of target cell type and retrovirus expression. Reconstitution studies revealed a necessary T-lymphocyte component for NK-cell stimulation by RL-FLV in mice, which may be lymphokine-mediated, but not

---

[1]This work was supported by PHS, NCI grant 5P01-CA25863-05.

[2]Present address: USDA Plum Island Animal Disease Center, P.O. Box 848, Greenport, Long Island, NY 11944

[3]To whom requests for reprints should be addressed at P.O. Box 2926, Duke University Medical Center, Durham, NC 27710

[4]Abbreviations used in this paper:
AM, activated macrophage; anti-ASGM-1, anti-asialo GM-1 antiserum; BALB-I, endogenous ecotropic virus of BALB/c mice; CTL, cytolytic thymus-derived lymphocytes; FLV, Friend leukemia virus; LCMV, lymphocytic choriomeningitis virus; MoLV, Moloney leukemia virus; MSV, murine sarcoma virus; MuLV, murine leukemia virus; NK, natural killer cell; PC, peritoneal cells; RadLV, radiation leukemia virus; RIA, radioimmunoassay.

interferon dependent.

INTRODUCTION

Murine leukemia viruses (MuLV) have long been utilized as experimental tools in a number of varied fields of research. Their utility in tumor immunology is due in large part to the well-characterized antigens present on virions and expressed on virus-infected cells. As such, these antigens can act as potent immunogens, stimulating a variety of host components - most notably virus-specific cytotoxic thymus-derived lymphocytes (CTL) (1,2) and accessory macrophages (3). Additionally, virus antigens have been shown to greatly enhance the immunogenicity of pre-existing tumor-associated antigens (4,5).

The present study was begun in order to evaluate any quantitative or qualitative differences in the immune response generated against a virus-negative tumor cell line infected with a variety of different non-transforming MuLV. Quite unexpectedly, one particular virus isolate converted a highly lethal tumor into a cell line which failed to grow in conventional syngeneic recipients. Our studies subsequently focussed on the mechanism whereby large tumor cells were rapidly rejected. Our findings, detailed herein, show that activated NK cells were responsible for this potent tumor cell rejection.

MATERIALS AND METHODS

Mice - Female C57BL/6J and C57BL/6J-bg (beige) mice were purchased from the Jackson Laboratories, Bar Harbor, Maine and were used at 8-14 weeks of age.

Cells - BL/RL_{12}-NP, hereafter referred to as RL-12, is a transformed suspension cell line derived by Liebermann *et al.* (6) from a radiation-induced thymic lymphoma of a C57BL/Ka mouse. YAC-1 cells were a gift from Dr. Hillel Koren. Ha MSV-NP cells were obtained from Dr. Edward Scolnick. Mink lung cells were a gift of Dr. Miles Cloyd. The AKR thymocyte cell line was derived in our laboratory from the thymus of an overtly leukemic AKR mouse. The remaining cell lines were obtained from various stock culture collections and are routinely maintained in our laboratory. All cell lines were grown *in vitro* in either McCoy's 5a or RPMI 1640 medium containing 10% fetal calf serum (FCS), 100U/ml penicillin, 100 ug/ml streptomycin, and 2mM glutamine.

Viruses - Ecotropic MuLV used for *in vitro* infection of RL-12 cells was obtained from clarified culture supernatants of the following virus-producing cell lines: Friend leukemia virus (FLV) produced by Friend Eveline suspension cells (7), Moloney leukemia virus (MoLV) propagated in 3T3-FL cells, the B-tropic virus of Balb/c mice (BALB-I) propagated in B6-3T3 cells, and radiation leukemia virus (RadLV) produced by VL_3 cells. Viruses were obtained from 72-hr cultures of the appropriate cell lines. Virus was pelleted from cell-free supernatants, resuspended in medium without FCS, aliquoted and frozen at -70°C. The amount of infectious virus in each preparation was determined by S^+L^- infectivity assays (8) and expressed as PFU/ml.

In Vitro Infection of RL-12 Cells - Infection of RL-12 cells was attempted with various MuLV (see above) according to the following protocol. Log phase cells were grown overnight in medium containing 1 ug/ml of Polybrene (Sigma Chemical Co., St. Louis, Mo.), after which time 10^6 cells were pelleted by low speed centrifugation. Cell pellets were gently resuspended in 0.5 ml of medium containing 10^6- 10^7 PFU of the various MuLV isolates. The cultures were incubated for 30 min in a 37°C waterbath. Following incubation, 10 ml of medium was added and the cells were cultured in T-25 flasks at 37°C. When cell densities reached approximately 10^6/ml, the cells were washed and seeded in new flasks at $5x10^4$ cells/ml. After 5 such passages the cells were examined for viral antigen expression by competition RIA and immunofluorescence.

Sera - The preparation and reactivity of a rabbit anti-p30 serum has been previously described (9). Goat anti-AKA virus gp71 serum, obtained from the NCI Biological Carcinogenesis Branch Repository, was passaged over an affinity column containing Rauscher leukemia virus polypeptides linked to cyanogen bromide-activated Sepharose 4B. In this procedure, type-specific anti-AKR antibodies were contained in the column effluent, whereas MuLV group-specific antibodies bound to the column and were subsequently eluted with 3M guanidine. The purely group-specific activity of these antibodies was confirmed and they were subsequently utilized for cytofluorometry. Anti-NK 1.1 serum and anti-Qa5 monoclonal antibody were generous gifts from Dr. Gloria Koo and Dr. Mary Kirch, respectively. Anti-Thy 1.2, anti-Lyt 1.2, and low-toxicity rabbit complement were purchased from Accurate Chemical and Scientific Corp., Westbury N.Y. Rabbit anti-asialo GM1 (anti-ASGM-1) serum was purchased from Wako Chemicals, Dallas, Texas.

Preparation of Effector Cells - Normal and tumor inoculated mice were killed by cervical dislocation. Spleen cell suspensions were prepared by gentle disaggregation between the frosted ends of sterile glass slides. Debris was removed by passage through a sterile nylon mesh screen. Peritoneal cells (PC) were collected by vigorous lavage with 5 ml of phosphate-buffered saline (PBS) per animal. Cells were separated into plastic adherent and non-adherent fractions using the technique described by Schon-Hegrad and Holt (10). Nylon wool separations were performed according to the method of Julius *et al*. (11).

Serologic Assays - Radioiodination of purified antigens and details of the competition RIA have been previously described (12). For cytofluorographic analysis of gp71 expression, $2x10^6$ cells of the various RL lines were resuspended in cold PBS containing 2% FCS and 0.1% sodium azide. Cells were incubated on ice for 45 min in the presence of a 1:50 final dilution of group-specific goat anti-AKR gp71 serum (see above). Cells were washed twice and incubated an additional 45 min on ice in the presence of fluorescein-conjugated rabbit anti-goat IgG (Cappel Laboratories, Cochranville, Pa.). Finally, cells were washed twice and resuspended to 10^6 cells/ml. Analysis of fluorescent intensity vs. cell number was performed with a Coulter EPICS IV cytofluorograph.

Cell Depletions - Single cell suspensions of peritoneal and splenic effector cells from normal and tumor-inoculated mice were exposed to specific antibody and complement using a single step cell depletion technique. Briefly, 10^7 viable cells were resuspended in 1 ml of cytotoxicity medium (Accurate Chemical and Scientific Corp., Westbury, N.Y.) and dilutions of specific antibodies were added. Low-toxicity rabbit complement was then added to yield a final dilution of 1:15, and the mixtures were incubated with occasional shaking in a 37°C water bath for 1 hr. Cells were washed twice and resuspended to original volumes prior to assessment of their cytolytic activities.

Cell-mediated Cytolytic Assays - Both 4 and 18 hr ^{51}Cr release assays were utilized to assess the cytolytic activity of peritoneal and splenic effectors. Four million tumor cell targets were resuspended in 1 ml of supplemented McCoy's 5a medium and incubated at 37°C for 90-120 min with

TABLE I

Virus Expression in RL-12 Cell Lines Infected In Vitro

Cell Lines	MuLV p30 (ng/mg)[a]	Infectious Virus[b]
RL-12	50	0
RL-FLV	1600	35 ± 9
RL-BALB-I	2000	16 ± 5
RL-MoLV	7400	44 ± 8
RL-RadLV	1300	N.D.[c]

[a]MuLV p30 expression was assayed by competition RIA with cell extracts and a monospecific goat anti-p30 antiserum.

[b]Infectious virus was determined in an S^+L^- assay using 24 hr culture supernatants of cells seeded at a density of 5×10^5 cells/ml. Values represent infectious virus per ml of cell-free supernatant.

[c]Not done.

120 uCi of $Na_2{}^{51}CrO_4$ (sp. act. 250-500 mCi/mg, Amersham Corp., Chicago, IL).[2] After incubation, the labeled cells were washed four times and resuspended to 10^5 cells/ml in supplemented McCoy's 5a medium. A modification of the procedure described by Thorn *et al.* (13) was used for the cytolytic assays. Briefly, 0.1 ml of effector cells (10^7/ml for 100:1 E:T) was added in triplicate into wells of a flat-bottomed 96-well plate (Costar, Cambridge, Mass.) followed by the addition of 0.1 ml (10^4 cells) of targets. Plates were incubated for 4 or 18 hr at 37°C in a 5% CO_2 humidified atmosphere. After incubation, 0.1 ml of the supernatant was removed from each well and the release of ^{51}Cr determined. Spontaneous release ranged from 4-10% in 4 hr assays and from 14-26% in 18 hr assays. Maximum release from Triton X-100 treated cells ranged from 88-98%. The percent specific ^{51}Cr release was determined by the formula:

$$\frac{\text{cpm released in test samples} - \text{cpm of spont. rel.}}{\text{cpm of max. rel.} - \text{cpm of spont. rel.}} \times 100$$

Cold target competition assays were performed as above except that effectors were added in 0.05 ml followed by addition of unlabeled cells in 0.05 ml. Labeled target cells were added immediately thereafter.

RESULTS

In Vitro Infection of Tumor Cells with MuLV Isolates

As a first step in determining the feasibility of utilizing MuLV antigens as targets for immunotherapy, we selected a virus-negative lymphoma cell line and attempted *in vitro* infection of these cells with a variety of non-transforming MuLV isolates. RL-12 (14) cells were exposed to FLV, BALB-I virus, MoLV, and RadLV as described in the Methods section. After a 2-week culture period to allow for stabilization, cell lines were established and tested for virus expression. As shown in Table I, the parental RL-12 cell line was devoid of detectable ecotropic

MuLV and contained very low amounts of MuLV p30 antigen. Following virus infection, all cell lines exhibited greatly increased amounts of MuLV p30 antigen. Of the infected cell lines tested, all produced low, but detectable levels of infectious virus. Periodic assessment of antigen expression and virus production revealed only minor fluctuations. We concluded, therefore, that *in vitro* infection of RL-12 cells with various ecotropic MuLV isolates resulted in the establishment of stable virus-expressing sublines. Cytofluorographic analysis of cell surface gp71 expression revealed uniformly high levels of antigen among the infected sublines compared to the parental RL-12 cells (not shown).

To examine the effects of virus infection on subsequent tumorigenicity, we determined the LD_{50} for each cell line in syngeneic B6 recipient mice. As shown in Table II, parental RL-12 cells displayed moderate tumorigenicity with an LD_{50} of approximately 10^4 cells. This level remained unchanged for RL-BALB-I cells, while the LD_{50} values for RL-MoLV and RL-RadLV were slightly increased. Quite unexpectedly, however, RL-FLV cells failed to produce tumors at any level tested. As footnoted, attempts to determine tumorigenic doses using up to $2x10^8$ cells have been uniformly negative. Thus, the RL-FLV cell line, although expressing quantities of viral antigens similar to the other infected sublines, failed to induce tumors *in vivo*. When RL-FLV cells were inoculated into sublethally irradiated (450 rads) recipients, 10^6 cells were uniformly lethal, indicating a possible radiation-sensitive component in RL-FLV cell rejection.

Host Anti-RL-FLV Immune Reactivity

Because of the dramatic alteration of tumorigenicity seen with RL-FLV cells, as well as the influences of sublethal irradiation, we focused our attention on possible host rejection mechanisms for this tumor line. For these and all subsequent studies, B6 mice were inoculated i.p. with 10^7 RL-FLV cells. To assess anti-tumor immune responses, mice were killed at various times after tumor cell inoculation and their peritoneal, spleen, and lymph node cells were tested in 18 hr ^{51}Cr-release assays against RL-FLV targets. Likewise, sera were collected and assayed for anti-gp71 antibodies by RIA. The data in Figure 1 shows the cytolytic activity of peritoneal cells (PC) as well as the anti-gp71 antibody response.

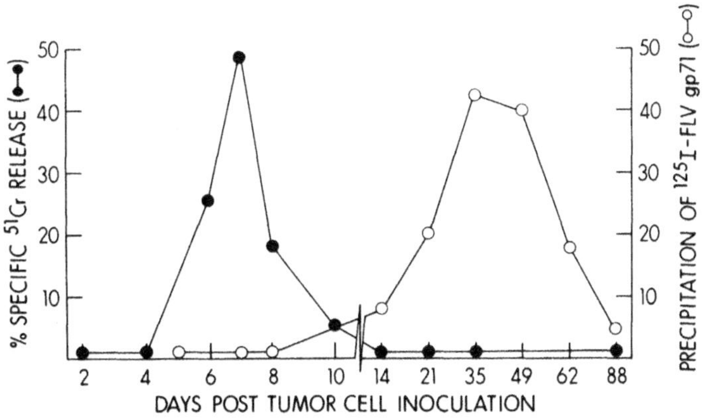

Figure 1. Serum anti-gp71 antibody (open circles) and peritoneal cell 18-h cytolytic activity (closed circles) (E:T=200:1) following i.p. inoculation of RL-FLV cells in B6 mice.

TABLE II

LD_{50} of RL-12 Cell Lines in Syngeneic B6 Mice

	Tumor Associated deaths/Number of Mice Tested (%)				
Cell Inoculum (i.p.)	RL-12	RL-FLV	RL-BALB-I	RL-MoLV	RL-RadLV
$1x10^7$	10/10 (100)	0/10 (0)	10/10 (100)	10/10 (100)	10/10 (100)
$1x10^6$	10/10 (100)	0/10 (0)	10/10 (100)	6/10 (60)	10/10 (100)
$1x10^5$	8/10 (80)	0/10 (0)	9/10 (90)	0/10 (0)	5/10 (50)
$1x10^4$	4/10 (40)	0/10 (0)	5/10 (50)	0/10 (0)	0/10 (0)
LD_{50}[a]	$10^{4.3}$	$>10^{7}$[b]	10^4	$10^{5.8}$	10^5

[a]LD_{50} determined by the method of Reed and Muensch

[b]Inocula from 10^7 - $2x10^8$ cells i.p. have also failed to produce tumors

Anti-RL-FLV lysis by PC is first apparent by 5-6 days post-tumor cell inoculation, peaking on day 7 and declining rapidly thereafter. Neither spleen nor lymph node cells exhibited detectable cytolytic activity during the time interval tested. Antibody to gp71 appeared by day 14 and reached maximum titers by 5 weeks. Intraperitoneal tumor cell burden declined to undetectable levels by day 12 (not shown).

To test the possibility that anti-RL-FLV PC recognized FLV-specific antigens as cell surface targets, we examined the lytic specificity of these cells against the parental and the various virus-infected RL cell lines. Normal B6 PC were included for comparison. As shown in Table III, none of the RL lines were susceptibile to lysis by normal PC. Day 7 anti-RL-FLV PC, on the other hand, lysed all of the RL cell lines indiscriminately. We attempted to examine the relevance of these findings to in vivo rejection by challenging RL-FLV inoculated mice on day 7 with the other RL cell lines. Tumor cells failed to grow out in any of the groups (data not shown), thus confirming the lack of apparent FLV specificity and emphasizing the importance of the PC response in tumor cell rejection.

Characterization of B6 Anti-RL-FLV Effector PC

We next attempted to characterize our day 7 cytolytic effector cells with respect to expression of phenotypic markers. For this, we selected a panel of specific antibodies which would allow us to categorize these cells as cytolytic T cells (CTL), activated macrophages (AM), natural killer cells (NK), or natural cytotoxic cells (NC). The data contained in Table IV represent results obtained from cytolytic depletions using the designated antibodies plus complement. Treatment with any of these antibodies alone failed to produce any depletion of cytolytic activity beyond that seen with complement alone. In order to confirm the specificity of these reagents, we also used them to deplete a known NK response (ie B6 spleen vs YACO) as well as a known allogeneic CTL response (ie L5178Y-immune B6 PC vs L5178Y). Using YAC cells as a standard NK target, we also examined their susceptibility to lysis by B6 anti-RL-FLV PC.

The specificity of reagents used in this analysis was confirmed by the expected depletions of CTL and NK cell lytic activities. CTL expressed Thy 1.2 and to a lesser extent Lyt 1,2, whereas NK cells present in normal B6 spleens were $Qa5^+$, NK 1.1^+, ASGM-1^+ and showed partial depletion with Thy 1.2 and Lyt 1.2. Both CTL and NK cells were contained in the plastic non-adherent populations. The depletion patterns of either anti-YAC or anti-RL-FLV lytic activities in day 7 B6 anti-RL-FLV PC were nearly identical and were compatible with an NK cell phenotype. The sole exception was the effect of anti-Thy 1.2 on anti-YAC vs anti-RL-FLV activity. Whereas this antibody plus complement treatment reproducibly had little effect upon anti-YAC activity, it actually enhanced the lytic activity against RL-FLV cells, possibly by lysing RL-FLV contained in the PC population. Subsequent cold target competition studies revealed that RL-12, RL-FLV, and YAC cells competed for anti-RL-FLV lytic activity with YAC cells showing the greatest level of competition. These findings have several important implications. First, although RL-FLV cells were seemingly potent 'inducers' of this NK activity, they were extremely poor lytic targets. This could explain our inability to detect significant lysis of RL-FLV by PC in short term assays, thus dictating the need for 18-20 hr cytolysis assays. More importantly, despite the poor susceptibility of RL-FLV to 4h in vitro lysis, these cells failed to grow out in vivo at any cell inoculum. We will elaborate further on this apparent paradox in the 'Discussion' section.

TABLE III

Lysis of RL cell Lines by B6 Anti-RL-FLV PC

Effector Cells[b]	E:T Ratio	% Specific Lysis of Target Cells[a]				
		RL-12	RL-FLV	RL-BALB I	RL-MoLV	RL-RadLV
Normal PC	200:1	2.6	2.1	2.8	2.0	1.7
	100:1	1.4	0.6	0.9	1.1	0.1
	50:1	-0.5	-0.3	-1.1	-0.6	-1.2
Day 7 anti-RL-FLV PC	200:1	48.4	53.4	40.4	34.4	64.2
	100:1	13.4	51.7	14.7	28.8	34.3
	50:1	12.1	41.1	11.1	27.2	19.6

[a]Specific lysis was measured in an 18 hr ^{51}Cr release at the indicated E:T ratios.

[b]Effector cells were obtained from pools of normal and tumor inoculated animals.

TABLE IV

Characterization of B6 Anti-RL-FLV Cytolytic Effector PC

	B6 anti-L5178Y PC (CTL)[a]	Normal B6 SPC (NK)[b]	B6 anti-RL-FLV PC[c]	
Treatment	L5178Y Targets	YAC Targets	YAC Targets	RL-FLV Targets
None	81.7	27.6	72.9	41.9
C' alone	79.5	21.4	65.3	31.8
Anti-Thy 1.2 + C'	5.9 (92.6)[d]	18.2 (15.0)	57.5 (12.0)	55.9
Anti-Qa5 + C'	81.0	3.5 (83.7)	6.7 (89.8)	2.7 (91.6)
Anti-NK 1.1 + C'	80.6	5.0 (76.7)	20.3 (69.0)	9.5 (70.2)
Anti-Lyt 1.2 + C'	70.1 (11.9)	14.6 (31.8)	48.1 (26.4)	21.0 (34.0)
Anti-ASGM-1 + C'	78.3	1.2 (94.3)	3.8 (94.2)	1.5 (96.3)
Adherent[e]	0.2	2.4	11.4	13.2
Non-adherent	90.4	33.8	91.6	65.4

[a]L5178Y immune PC were tested at an E:T of 100:1 in 6 hr ^{51}Cr release assays.

[b]Normal B6 spleen cells were tested at an E:T of 100:1 in 6 hr ^{51}Cr release assays.

[c]Day 7 B6 anti-RL-FLV PC were tested at an E:T of 100:1 in 4 hr assays against YAC targets and 18-hr assays against RL-FLV targets.

[d]Values in parentheses represent percent reduction in lytic activity compared to complement alone. Pretreatment cell numbers were not restored after antibody plus complement treatment.

[e]Following plastic adherence, both adherent and non-adherent populations were assayed at 100:1 E:T ratios.

Examination of NK Induction

In attempting to further substantiate a role for NK cells in the rejection of RL-FLV, we inoculated RL-FLV cells into B6 beige mice - a mutant strain previously described as partially deficient in lytic NK activity (23). The NK lesion in beige mice is not an absolute deficiency of NK cells, but rather the presence of cells which bind but cannot lyse NK targets (24). As in conventional B6 mice, RL-FLV cells failed to grow out at any level of cell inoculation (data not shown). If RL-FLV cells were potent 'inducers' of NK lytic activity in conventional mice, we reasoned that perhaps these tumor cells somehow conferred lytic activity on beige NK cells. To test this, we inoculated B6 beige mice with 10^7 RL-FLV and examined anti-YAC and anti-RL-FLV lytic activities of peritoneal and spleen cells 7 days later. The data in Table V clearly demonstrate that RL-FLV inoculation of B6 beige mice induced both anti-YAC as well as anti-RL-FLV lytic activity. This effect is most apparent with PC, although an increase in anti-YAC activity also occurs in the spleen. Subsequent studies revealed that RL-FLV inoculated conventional mice had substantially higher NK activity than mice inoculated with the other RL cell lines (not shown).

As noted in the first section of the results, rejection of RL-FLV cells in B6 mice involves a radiation-sensitive host function. This, coupled with the finding that RL-FLV cells routinely produced tumors in either BALB/c or NIH nude mice (K. Weinhold, unpublished observation) suggested a possible T cell involvement in the NK 'induction cascade'. We approached this question experimentally by sublethally irradiating B6 mice and attempting to reconstitute their ability to reject RL-FLV cells with selected cell populations from normal mice. Groups of mice were irradiated, received spleen cell populations 24 hrs later, and were immediately inoculated i.p. with 2×10^6 RL-FLV cells.

TABLE V

Induction of NK Activity in RL-FLV Inoculated Beige Mice

	% Specific Lysis[a]			
	YAC Targets		RL-FLV Targets	
Effector Cells	200:1	50:1	200:1	50:1
N-B6 Beige PEC	3.1	0.2	-0.5	-2.2
B6 Beige anti-RL-FLV PC	58.1	48.0	20.2	1.0
N-B6 Beige SPC	5.2	1.6	-2.1	-3.3
B6 Beige anti-RL-FLV SPC	18.2	7.1	-3.7	-3.4

[a]Lysis was measured in 4-hr assays using YAC targets and 18-hr assays using RL-FLV targets.

As shown in Table VI, normal spleen cells fully reconstituted the ability of mice to reject RL-FLV tumor cells. The predominant cell type responsible for this effect resided in the nylon wool non-adherent fraction of

TABLE VI

Reconstitution of Sublethally Irradiated RL-FLV Inoculated Mice

Cell Population Transferred[a]	Survivors at 40DPI[b]
Normal B6-SPC	10/10
Nylon wool adherent B6-SPC	1/10
Nylon wool non-adherent B6 SPC	9/10
Thy 1.2 depleted B6-SPC[c]	0/10
Qa-5 depleted B6-SPC[c]	2/10
ASGM-1 depleted B6-SPC[c]	9/10

[a]Mice in each group received $3x10^7$ viable i.v. 24-hrs after a 450 rad dose of whole body gamma irradiation.

[b]Number mice alive and showing no visible signs of ascites at 40 days post inoculation (DPI) of $2x10^6$ RL-FLV cells.

[c]Spleen cell populations were treated with the respective antibodies plus C and 3×10^7 viable cells were injected i.v.

B6 spleen cells. Depletion of Thy 1.2 bearing cells completely abolished reconstitution and Qa5-depleted cells had only a slight restorative activity. Relative to Qa5 depletion, it should be noted that although Qa5 is an excellent marker for splenic NK cells, approximately 30% of splenic T cells also express this antigen (25). In this respect anti-asialo GM-1 (ASGM-1) antiserum is, perhaps, more specific for splenic NK cells than anti-Qa5 serum. Spleens depleted of ASGM-1 bearing NK cells fully retained their ability to reconstitute irradiated mice for the rejection of RL-FLV cells. While this experiment does not conclusively identify the radiation-sensitive cell as being either a T-cell or resident NK cell, it does strongly suggest a T-cell component in the cascade leading to the rejection of RL-FLV.

DISCUSSION

The data presented here demonstrate that infection of a virus-negative tumor with FLV can completely abolish its tumorigenicity. The failure of this virally-infected cell line to grow in syngeneic animals was not due to a physiologic alteration of its growth potential, but rather was a reflection of the ability of such cells to induce a potent host rejection response mediated by peritoneal NK cells.

It has been known for several years that activation of NK cells accompanies host infection by a wide variety of viruses (reviewed in 26). Both interferon (27) and viral glycopeptides (28) can directly activate NK cells. These agents by themselves cannot, however, elicit the levels of activity achieved following _in vivo_ virus infection. Regarding this latter point, it should be emphasized that our current model of NK induction with RL-FLV cells does not involve infectious spread of FLV from tumor to host cells. The FLV utilized for *in vitro* infection of RL cells is predominantly N-tropic and, although capable of infecting B6 tumor cells, will infect and replicate poorly in normal B6 tissues (29). We have extensively analyzed various tissues of RL-FLV inoculated mice and have not found any evidence of virus infection (unpublished observations). A number of established mammalian cell lines which are normally resistant to lysis by NK cells become highly susceptible when acutely or persistently infected with a variety of viruses (reviewed in 30). Evidence that this is not the case with RL-FLV cells is amply demonstrated by the lack of anti-YAC cold target competition activities with both the RL-12 and RL-FLV cell lines. This observation likewise casts doubt on the contention that viral antigens may serve as cytolytic target antigens for NK cells (31).

Clearly the major change in RL cells brought about by *in vitro* infection with FLV is at the level of NK induction *in vivo*. We have used the general term 'induction' to describe the increased lytic potential of anti-RL-FLV PC primarily because we do not know whether this is due to an increase in the relative proportion of NK cells in the peritoneum (*ie*. elicitation or rapid proliferation) or to an increase in the rate of lysis (*ie*. local activation) by resident NK populations. It is likely that both effects are participating to some degree; absolute numbers of peritoneal cells are increased over those seen in normal animals and whether there is an additional activation phase will be determined using single cell cytotoxic assays. Certainly, the absence of target cell specificities with RL-FLV-induced NK cells would be more consistent with an activated NK population (32).

The induction of NK activity by RL-FLV cells was entirely restricted to peritoneal cell populations, with little or no enhancement of 'spontaneous NK' activities in the spleen. This localized induction was observed in both conventional B6 and B6 beige mice and was somewhat unexpected since most models of NK activation following either virus infection (26) or interferon induction (27) involves a primary splenic effect with lesser activities seen in peritoneal cells. A possible explanation for this discrepancy may be that, unlike viruses and soluble agents, RL-FLV cells remain in the peritoneum and are not found in the spleen or distal organs at any time following injection (unpublished observations).

Although we presently have no evidence as to the nature of the induction cascade, these effects may be mediated, at least in part, by the production of interferon. Both interferon and poly I:C have been shown to augment NK activity *in vivo* (33). Likewise, Welsh and Kiessling have shown that LCMV-infected beige mice exhibit greatly increased cytolytic NK activities, presumably mediated via interferon 34). Again, in order to be consistent with the restricted activities seen in both conventional and beige mice in the present model, the induction of interferon would have to occur locally within the confines of the peritoneal cavity. In this regard, we are presently attempting to examine interferon levels in peritoneal fluid following inoculation with RL-FLV cells. Interferon production, or NK induction in general, might also require a T cell component, perhaps involving IL-2 (35), which would be consistent with our findings that RL-FLV cells grew progressively in nude and sublethally irradiated mice and that reconstitution with whole, but not Thy 1.2 depleted spleen cells restored the rejection response.

Phenotypically, the anti-RL-FLV-generated NK cell population closely resembled resident NK cells found in normal B6 spleens. Kiessling *et al*. have reported that NK cells, following activation by LCMV, exhibited changes in cell surface properties - most notably increased sensitivity to anti-Thy 1.2 + C treatment (36). Our failure to document this in the present system may be related to differences in the mode and degree of activation, as well as differences in the serologic reagents and conditions used for depletions. Clearly, resident NK cells as a group represent a phenotypically heterogenous population possibly derived from multiple cell types (37), and it is likely that activation of NK cells could result in a similar form of phenotypic and functional heterogeneity.

The apparent paradox that RL-FLV cells were potent inducers of, but poor targets for NK cells may be biologically relevant to the *in vivo* behavior of these cells. Specifically, RL-FLV cells grew progressively in B6 recipients for 4-5 days until high levels of NK activity were established, following which tumor cell rejection occured over the next 5 days. One could speculate that if RL-FLV cells were better NK targets, they would not be present in animals for an equivalent time interval and the levels of NK activity seen would be dramatically reduced. Their status as poor NK targets thus insures an extended presence in the peritoneal cavity, thereby augmenting the level of NK activity induced.

The major strength of the present system lies not only in the NK induction capacities of RL-FLV cells, but also in the ability of such augmented effector cells to mediate the rejection of large tumor cell inocula. Future studies will focus on the precise mechanism of augmentation, as well as any immunotherapeutic applications which may become evident.

REFERENCES

1. Gorczynski, R.M. (1974). Evidence for *in vivo* protection against murine sarcoma virus induced tumors by T lynphocytes from immune animals. *J. Immunol.* 112:533.
2. Shellam, G.R., R.A. Knight, N.A. Mitchinson, R.N. Gorczynski and A. Maoz. 1976. The specificity of effector T cells activated by tumours induced by murine oncornaviruses. *Transplant. Rev.* 29:249.
3. Gomard, E., J. Wybier-Franqui, and J.P. Levy. 1981. Accessory cells in the *in vitro* generation of type C virus specific T killer lymphocytes. I. Role of macrophages in primary anti-FMR reaction. *J. Immunol.* 126:891.
4. Al-Ghazzouli, I.K., R.M. Donahue, K. Huang, B. Sass, R.L. Peters and G.J. Kelloff. 1976. Immunity to virus-free syngeneic tumor cell transplantation in the BALB/c mouse after immunization with homologous tumor cells infected with type C virus. *J. Immunol.* 117:2239.
5. Boone, C.W., N. Takeichi, F.C. Austin, E. Gotohda, T. Oikawa and R. Gillette. 1979. Virus augmentation: increased immunogenicity of tumor-associated transplantation antigens in tumor cell extracts after infection with surface budding viruses. *In*: GANN Monograph on Cancer Research, #23, p. 7.
6. Liberman, M., A. DeCleve, P. Ricciardi-Castagnoli, J. Boniver, O.J. Finn, and H.S. Kaplan. 1979. Establishment, characterization, and virus expression of cell lines derived from radiation- and virus-induced lymphomas of C57Bl/Ka mice. *Int. J. Cancer* 24:168.

7. Seifert, E., M. Claviez, H. Frank, G. Hunsmann, H. Schwarz, and W. Schafer. 1975. Properties of mouse leukemia viruses. XII. Production of substantial amounts of Friend Leukemia virus by a suspension tissue culture line (Eveline suspension cells). Z. Naturforsch 30:698.
8. Bassin, R.H., N. Tuttle, and P.J. Fischinger. 1971. Rapid cell culture assay technique for murine leukemia viruses. Nature 229:564.
9. Green, R.W., D.P. Bolognesi, and W. Schafer. 1973. Polypeptides of mammalian oncornaviruses. I. Isolation and serological analysis of polypeptides from murine and feline C-type viruses. Virology 56:565.
10. Schon-Hegard, M.A. and P.G. Holt. 1981. Improved method for the isolation of purified mouse peritoneal macrophages. J. Immunol Methods 43:169.
11. Julius, M.H., E. Simpson, and L.A. Herzenberg. 1973. A rapid method for the isolation of functional thymus-derived murine lymphocytes. Eur J. Immunol. 3:645.
12. Bolognesi, D.P., J.J. Collins, J.P. Leis, V. Moennig, W. Schafer and P.H. Atkinson. 1975. Role of carbohydrate in determining the immunochemical properties of the major glycoprotein (gp71) of Friend murine leukemia virus. J. Virol. 16:1453.
13. Thorn, R.M., J.C. Palmer, and L.A. Manson. 1974. A simplified ^{51}Cr-release assay for killer cells. J. Immunol. Methods 3:301.
14. Fischinger, P.J., H.-J. Thiel, M. Lieberman, H.S. Kaplan, N.M. Dunlop, and W.G. Robey. 1982. Presence of a novel recombinant murine leukemia virus-like glycoprotein on the surface of virus-negative C57BL lymphoma cells. Cancer Res. 42:4650.
15. Weinhold, K.J., L.T. Goldstein, and E.F. Wheelock. 1979. The tumor dormant state: Quantitation of L5178Y cells and host immune responses during the establishment and course of dormancy in syngeneic DBA/2 mice. J. Exp. Med. 149:732.
16. Corer, P.A. and D.B. Amos. 1956. Passive immunity in mice against C57BL leukosis EL4 by means of iso-immune serum. Cancer Res. 16:338.
17. Patuleia, M.C. and C. Friend. 1967. Tissue culture studies on murine virus-induced leukemia cells: Isolation of single cells in agar-liquid medium. Cancer Res. 27:726.
18. Law, L.W., T.B. Dunn, P.J. Boyle, and J.H. Miller. 1949. Observations on the effects of a folic-acid antagonist on transplantable lymphoid leukemias in mice. J. Natl. Cancer Inst. 10:179.
19. McCoy, J.L., A. Fefer, and J.P. Glynn. 1967. Comparative studies on the induction of transplantation resistance in BALB/c and C57BL/6 mice in three murine leukemia systems. Cancer Res. 27:1743.
20. Klein, E., and G. Klein. 1964. Antigenic properties of lymphoma induced by the Moloney agent. J. Natl. Cancer Inst. 32:547.
21. Iglehart, J.D., E.C. Ward, K. Thiel, G. Huper, S.S. Geier, and D.P. Bolognesi. 1981. In vivo antigenic modification of tumor cells. I. Introduction of murine leukemia virus antigens on non-virus-producing murine sarcomas. J. Natl. Cancer Inst. 67:107.
22. Henderson, I.C., M.M. Lieber, and G.J. Todaro. 1974. Mink cell line MulLu (CCL 64). Focus formation and the generation of 'nonproducer' transformed cell lines with murine and feline sarcoma viruses. Virology 60:282.
23. Roder, J.C. 1979. The beige mutation in the mouse. I. A stem cell predetermined impairment in natural killer cell function. J. Immunol. 123:2168.
24. Roder, J.C., M.-L. Lohmann-Mathes, W. Domzig, and H. Wigzell. 1979. The beige mutation in the mouse. II. Selectivity of the natural killer (NK) cell defect. J. Immunol. 123:2174.
25. Hammerling, G.J., Un Hammerling, and L. Flaherty. 1979. Qat-4 and Qat-5, new murine T-cell antigens governed by the Tla region and identified by monoclonal antibodies. J. Exp. Med. 150:108.

26. Welsh, R.M. 1981. Natural cell-mediated immunity during viral infections. Curr. Top. Microbiol. Immunol. 92:83.
27. Welsh, R.M. 1978. Cytotoxic cells induced during lymphocytic choriomeningitis virus infection of mice. I. Characterization of natural killer cell induction. J. Exp. Med. 148:163.
28. Casali, P., J.G.P. Simmons, M.J. Buchmeier, and M.A. Oldstone, 1981. In vitro generation of human cytotoxic lymphocytes by virus. Viral glycoproteins induce nonspecific cell-mediated cytotoxicity without release of interferon. J. Exp. Med. 154:840.
29. Iglehart, J.D., E.C. Ward, G. Huper, K. Thiel, and D.P. Bolognesi. 1981. In vivo antigenic modification of tumor cells. II. Distribution of virus in sarcoma-bearing mice. J. Natl. Cancer Inst. 67:117.
30. Rager-Zisman, B., and B.R. Bloom. 1982. Natural killer cells in resistance to virus-infected cells. In: Springer Semin. Immunopathol. 4:397, Springer-Verlag.
31. Lane, M.A. 1980. Murine retrovirus-specific natural killer cell activity. In: Natural cell-mediated immunity against tumors. Edited by R.B. Herberman. Academic Press, New York. Pp. 921-938.
32. Welsh, R.M., R.M. Zinkernagel and L.A. Hallenbeck. 1979. Cytotoxic cells induced during lymphocytic choriomeningitis virus infection of mice. II. 'Specificities' of the natural killer cells. J. Immunol. 122:475.
33. Djeu, J.Y., J.A. Heinbaugh, J.T. Holden, and R.B. Herberman. 1979. Augmentation of mouse natural killer cell activity by interferon and interferon inducers. J. Immunol. 122:175.
34. Welsh, R.M. and R.W. Kiessling. 1980. Natural killer cell response to lymphocytic choriomeningitis virus in beige mice. Scand. J. Immunol. 11:363.
35. Henney, C.S., K. Kuribayashi, D.E. Kern and S. Gillis. 1981. Interleukin-2 augments natural killer cell activity. Nature 291:235.
36. Kiessling, R., E. Eriksson, L.A. Hallenbeck, and R.M. Welsh. 1980. A comparative analysis of the cell surface properties of activated vs endogenous mouse natural killer cells. J. Immunol. 125:1551.
37. Minato, N., L. Reid, and B.R. Bloom. 1981. On the heterogeneity of murine natural killer cells. J. Exp. Med. 154:750.

ACKNOWLEDGEMENTS

The authors wish to thank Drs. Koo andKirch for their generous gifts of anti-NK 1.1 and anti-Qa-5 reagents respectively. We wish to acknowledge G. Huper and G. Johnson for their excellent technical assistance and R. Weisner for typing the manuscript.

VALIDATION OF A ROLE FOR ENDOGENOUSLY PRODUCED IFNγ IN RESOLUTION OF LISTERIA MONOCYTOGENES INFECTION IN MICE

Robert D. Schreiber

Department of Pathology
Washington Univ. School of Medicine
St. Louis, Missouri

INTRODUCTION

It is now well recognized that activated macrophages can express enhanced levels of cytocidal activity toward a variety of microbial targets and neoplastic cells (1-6). Three to five years ago, work from several laboratories indicated that IFNγ was one of the major classes of lymphokines capable of activating macrophages under well-defined *in vitro* conditions (7-14). Recently, there has been an explosive growth of experiments directed at defining IFNγ's mechanism of action at the molecular level. These investigations have led to the identification and characterization of a specific IFNγ receptor on the macrophage plasma membrane (15-17), have provided insights into the mechanism of transmembrane signal transduction, (18-20), and have elucidated the ultimate fate of receptor bound ligand (16,21).

In contrast to the extensive number of *in vitro* studies conducted with IFNγ, it has been difficult to perform the *in vivo* experiments needed to validate IFNγ's physiologic role. In part this difficulty was due to the lack of specific molecular reagents needed to undertake such an analysis. Recently, a few laboratories have circumvented this obstacle by generating neutralizing monoclonal antibodies against murine IFNγ (10,22-24). My laboratory produced a unique set of high affinity, hamster monoclonal anti-murine IFNγ which, depending on their epitope specificity, could either inhibit or enhance IFNγ's functional activity when tested *in vitro* (10). The purpose of this report is to summarize the studies we have conducted during the past two years which used these antibodies to elucidate the *in vivo* role of endogenously produced IFNγ (25). Specifically, data will be presented that will support the concept that IFNγ plays an obligatory role in promoting resistance to *Listeria monocytogenes* infection in mice.

RESULTS

Correlation of IFNγ Production and Resolution of Listeria Monocytogenes Infection in Mice.

In an attempt to validate IFNγ's *in vivo* role we used the model of *Listeria monocytogenes* infection in mice. This model was specifically chosen for two reasons: (1) historically, it was the experimental system used by Mackaness which first introduced the concept of the activated macrophage (1,26,27) and (2) results of subsequent studies performed in other laboratories indicated that resolution of Listeria infection occurred roughly concomitant with lymphokine production and macrophage activation (28-30). We therefore set as our first goal the use of modern improved assays to quantitate the levels of IFNγ production and macrophage activation during the course of an unperturbed sublethal Listeria infection in mice.

Mice were infected with a sublethal dose of Listeria (3×10^4 colony forming units (CFU)) and then, after various periods of time, groups of animals were sacrificed to obtain blood (to detect IFNγ in the circulation) or T cells (to measure cellular capacity to produce IFNγ). Cells were cultured in medium alone to quantitate constitutive production of the lymphokine or in the presence of antigen or the T cell mitogen Concanavalin A (Con A) to measure inducible production. IFNγ was quantitated with an IFNγ-specific enzyme linked immunosorbant assay which utilized the monoclonal antibodies that we raised against purified, murine recombinant IFNγ (10,25).

IFNγ was not detected in the circulation at any time during the Listeria infection. However, this observation is not entirely surprising since little free IFNγ would be expected in the presence of the many somatic and hematopoeitic cells which carry high affinity IFNγ receptors on their surface (14,16). We therefore took the alternative approach of studying cellular production of IFNγ <u>in vitro</u>. As seen in Figure 1, cells from normal, uninfected mice (day 0) showed neither constitutive nor antigen-induced IFNγ production in culture but did secrete the lymphokine when stimulated with mitogen (25). Con A stimulated normal peritoneal cells produced 80 IRU IFNγ/ml while stimulated normal spleen cells produced 65 units/ml. In contrast, cells derived from infected mice showed an accentuated mitogen-induced production of IFNγ. When stimulated with Con A, spleen cells from 6 day infected mice produced almost 40 times more IFNγ than the uninfected controls. Peritoneal cells also showed augmented IFNγ production. However, in the latter case the response was biphasic. The first phase occurred 2-4 days after infection while the second phase developed after 8-10 days of infection. Thus, these observations indicated that cells from Listeria-infected mice displayed an enhanced capacity to produce IFNγ.

We next measured the kinetics of bacterial clearance from the spleen and peritoneal cavity. Viable bacteria from these two anatomical sites increased during the first four days of infection to over 10^5 CFU/mouse. Thereafter, bacteria were rapidly killed and eliminated such that by day 6, no viable bacteria were detected in the peritoneal cavity and by day 8, the infection was totally resolved. When this data was compared with the kinetics of IFNγ production, a correlation was observed between enhanced IFNγ production and bacterial clearance (Fig. 2).

Finally, we studied the elaboration of activated macrophages in infected mice. Activated macrophages were identified by their ability to express nonspecific tumoricidal activity in an <u>in vitro</u> assay system (15,25). This assay was specifically chosen because past experience had shown that it was a quantitative indicator of the activation state of peritoneal macrophage populations. To perform this analysis macrophages from control or infected animals were plated into wells of tissue culture plates and incubated with cytoplasmically labeled P815 mastocytoma tumor cells in the presence or absence of a second or triggering signal (25). After 18 hours, culture supernatants

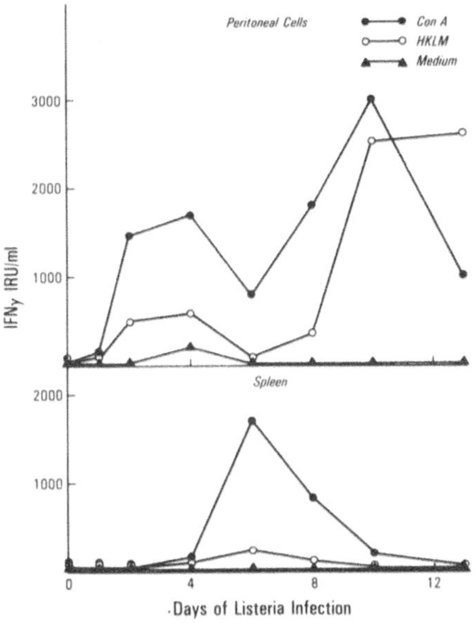

Fig. 1. Production of IFNγ by cultured spleen and peritoneal cells from Listeria-infected mice. (25)

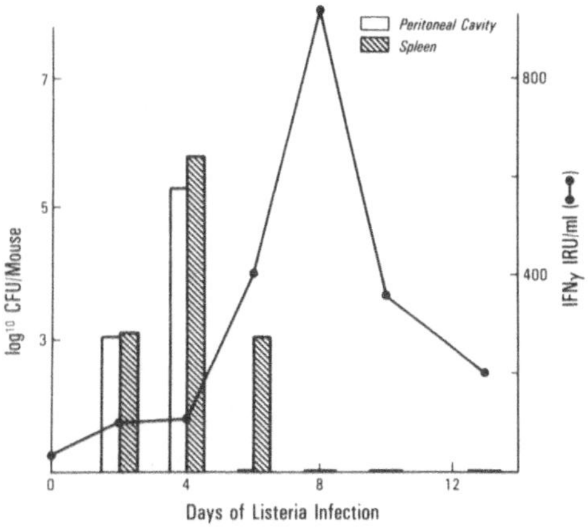

Fig. 2. Correlation between IFNγ production and clearance of Listeria from spleen and peritoneal cavity. (25)

were harvested, counted and the percentage of specific isotope release quantitated according to the following formula:

$$\% \text{ Specific Release} = \frac{\text{Experimental Release-Control Release}}{\text{Total (SDS) Release-Control Release}}$$

Fully activated macrophages were defined as those cells capable of directly lysing the tumor cells in the absence of an exogenous second signal. Partially activated or primed cells were defined as those which had been exposed to IFNγ in vivo but required the addition of a second signal in order to trigger the tumoricidal response in vitro. Nonactivated macrophages did not express tumoricidal activity either in the presence or absence of a triggering signal.

Using a variety of different triggering signals such as heat killed Listeria monocytogenes, Poly I-C or Lipopolysaccharide (LPS), partially activated macrophages were detected in the peritoneal cavity as early as two days after infection and maximal accumulation of fully activated cells occured on day 4 (Fig 3). Thus, taken together the results of these analyses indicated that there was an apparent three way correlation between IFNγ production, macrophage activation and resolution of the bacterial infection.

Immunochemical neutralization of endogenous IFNγ abrogates induction of activated macrophages in infected mice and prevents resolution of the infection.

Based on the correlative data presented above, we investigated whether the IFNγ that was produced in vivo during the infection was directly responsible for the generation of activated macrophages and ultimately to the eventual resolution of the infection. To answer this question we examined whether the course of a normal sublethal infection could be altered if we blocked the functional activity of endogenously

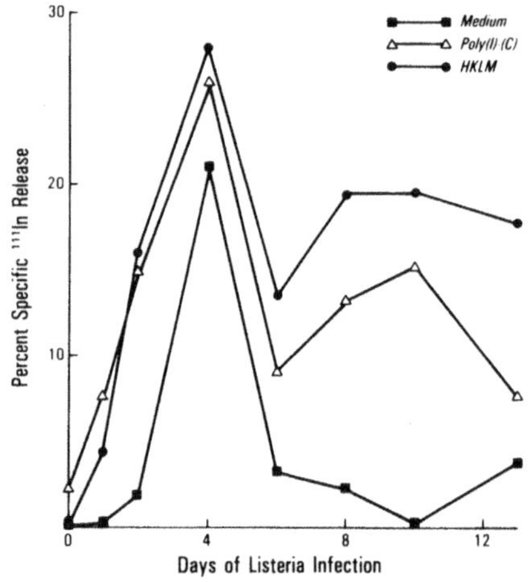

Fig. 3. Generation in vivo of activated macrophages during Listeria infection. (25)

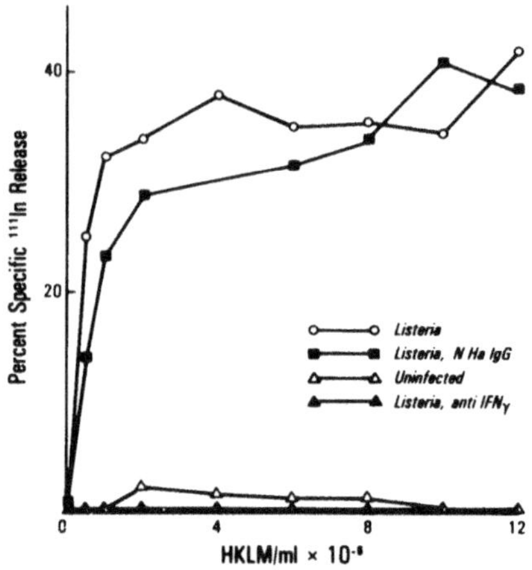

Fig. 4. Monoclonal anti-IFNγ inhibits generation of activated macrophages during Listeria infection. (25)

produced IFNγ (25). This was accomplished by treating mice with a neutralizing monoclonal antibody that we raised to murine IFNγ (10).

The characteristics of this antibody, known as H22, are summarized in Table 1. To eliminate any interference caused by endotoxin that may have been present in the antibody preparations, we performed these experiments both in normal mice and in LPS unresponsive C3H/HeJ mice. On day 0, mice were injected with a sublethal dose of Listeria. Twenty-four hours later, groups of animals were either left untreated or were given a single intraperitoneal injection of 125μg of either the H22 monoclonal anti-IFNγ or normal hamster IgG. At various times thereafter, groups of mice were sacrificed to access the activation state of peritoneal macrophages and the bacterial loads in the peritoneal cavity and spleen.

As would be expected peritoneal macrophages from uninfected mice were not activated and did not display significant levels of antitumor activity while cells derived from infected, untreated mice were activated and lysed 30-40% of labelled P815 target cells (Fig. 4). Injection of normal hamster IgG into infected mice did not diminish elicitation of activated macrophages thereby documenting that normal immunoglobulin did not nonspecifically inhibit expression of macrophage antitumor activity. In contrast, tumoricidal activity was completely suppressed in peritoneal macrophages derived from infected mice that had been treated with a single dose of monoclonal anti-IFNγ. Thus, immunologic neutralization of endogenously produced IFNγ during Listeria infection, abrogated the in vivo elaboration of activated macrophages.

In parallel experiments, the anti-IFNγ monoclonal also blocked the in vivo induction of Ia bearing macrophages in a dose-dependent fashion. Whereas peritoneal macrophages obtained from infected mice treated with either normal hamster IgG or a second, nonneutralizing hamster monoclonal anti-IFNγ were approximately 80% positive for Ia

TABLE 1

Characteristics of Hamster Monoclonal Anti-murine IFNγ (H22)

Immunogen: Purified, recombinant murine IFNγ
Immunized Animal: Armenian hamster
Fusion: Hamster splenocytes x murine myeloma (P3X63.Ag8.653)

Antigenic Specificity:

A. High avidity reaction with natural and recombinant murine IFNγ.
B. No crossreaction with murine IFNα or IFNß or human IFNγ.

Functional Inhibitory Activity

A. Inhibits binding of IFNγ to cellular IFNγ receptors.
B. Inhibits IFNγ dependent induction of tumoricidal activity.
C. Inhibits IFNγ dependent induction of antimicrobial activity.
D. Inhibits IFNγ dependent induction of Ia antigens.
E. Inhibits IFNγ dependent modulation of macrophage surface receptors.
F. Inhibits IFNγ dependent antiviral activity in fibroblasts.

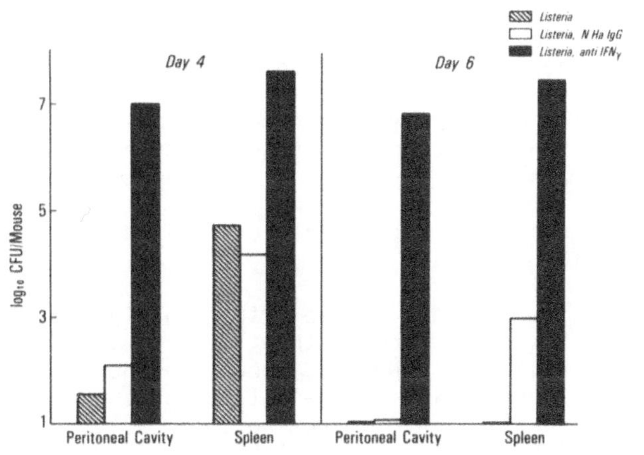

Fig. 5. Inhibition of Listeria clearance from spleen and peritoneal cavity by monoclonal anti-IFNγ. (25)

antigen expression, cells from H22 treated mice displayed Ia levels that were actually below the background levels expressed in uninfected, untreated mice. Injection of as little as 10-30 μg of H22 was sufficient to produce this inhibition.

In the final experiment, we determined whether in vivo administration of the anti-IFNγ monoclonal effected the overall outcome of the Listeria infection. As seen in Figure 5, Listeria-infected animals that were subsequently left untreated or injected with normal hamster IgG were perfectly capable of resolving the infection. Cells from the two control groups effectively eliminated the bacteria such that by day 4 peritoneal cells of untreated infected mice contained only 60 CFU per animal and those from normal hamster IgG treated mice only 100 CFU. By day 6, no viable bacteria were detected in peritoneal cells of either group of infected control mice. In contrast, the peritoneal cavity of infected mice treated with the anti-IFNγ monoclonal carried 10^7 CFU of bacteria on day 4 and $8x10^6$ CFU on day 6. Thus immunochemical blocking of IFNγ in vivo abrogated the in vivo clearance of Listeria. Similar results were also obtained for spleen colony counts. Spleens of anti-IFNγ-treated infected mice contained ~1000 fold more bacteria on Day 4 and 50,000 fold more Listeria on Day 6 than control mice. The blockage of bacterial clearance directly correlated with the death of the animals. Whereas all the untreated and normal hamster IgG treated infected animals recovered from the sublethal bacterial challenge, the majority of the anti-IFNγ-treated, infected mice died during the course of the experiment.

CONCLUSIONS

The results presented herein are some of the first to document that endogenously produced IFNγ plays a relevant role in vivo in promoting host resistance to Listeria infection. The data that supports this concept is as follows:

1. The production of IFNγ during Listeria infection correlates with the in vivo activation of macrophages and the clearance of bacteria from the spleen and peritoneal cavity.

2. IFNγ produced during Listeria infection is accessory for the in vivo activation of macrophage cytocidal activity and increased expression of macrophage MHC Class II antigens.

3. IFNγ is required for the clearance of Listeria and resolution of the infection.

At the present time, we are not able to identify the distinct step(s) in the anti-Listeria response that is (are) influenced by IFNγ. Whereas the ability of IFNγ to directly enhance cytocidal activity of host macrophages may be one site of action, we cannot rule out more indirect effects of the lymphokine such as its ability to promote generation of other cytokines which activate macrophages or other effector cells to kill the bacteria or, as has been suggested by Campbell and colleagues, to cause an increased accumulation of effector cells at the sites of bacterial sequestration (31,32). Nevertheless, the demonstration that endogenously produced IFNγ plays an obligatory role in promoting host defense to Listeria represents the first step in establishing the physiologic role of this lymphokine in vivo.

REFERENCES

1. Mackaness, G.B. 1970. The monocyte in cellular immunity. Sem. Hematol. 7:172.
2. Nogueira, N. and Z.A. Cohn. 1978. Trypanosoma cruzi: in vitro induction of macrophage microbicidal activity. J. Exp. Med. 148:284.
3. Nacy, C.A., M.S. Meltzer, E.J. Leonard, and D.J. Wyler. 1980. Intracellular replication and lymphokine-induced destruction of Leishmania tropica in C3H/HeN macrophages. J. Immunol. 127:2380.
4. Evans, P. and R. Alexander. 1970. Cooperation of immune lymphoid cells with macrophages in tumor immunity. Nature 228:620.
5. Meltzer, M.S. 1981. Tumor cytotoxicity by lymphokine-activated macrophages: Development of macrophage tumoricidal activity requires a sequence of reactions. Lymphokines 3:319.
6. Fidler, I.J. and A. Raz. 1981. The induction of tumoricidal capacities in mouse and rat macrophages by lymphokines. Lymphokines 3:345.
7. Roberts, W.K. and A. Vasil. 1982. Evidence for the identity of murine gamma interferon and macrophage activating factor. J. Interferon Res. 2:519.
8. Schreiber, R.D., J.L. Pace, S.W. Russell, A. Altman, and D.H. Katz. 1983. Macrophage-activating factor produced by a T cell hybridoma: physiochemical and biosynthetic resemblance to γ-interferon. J. Immunol. 131:826.
9. Svedersky, L.P., C.V. Benton, W.H. Berger, E. Rinderknecht, R.N. Harkins, and M.A. Palladino. 1984. Biological and antigenic similarities of murine interferon-γ and macrophage activating factor. J. Exp. Med. 159:812.
10. Schreiber, R.D., L.J. Hicks, A. Celada, N.A. Buchmeier, and P.W. Gray. 1985. Monoclonal antibodies to murine γ-interferon which differentially modulate macrophage activation and anti-viral activity. J. Immunol. 134:1609.
11. Le, J. and J. Vilcek. 1984. Lymphokine mediated activation of human monocytes: neutralization by monoclonal antibody to interferon-γ. Cell Immunol. 85:278.
12. Nathan, C.F., H.W. Murray, M.E. Weibe, and B.Y. Rubin. 1983. Identification of interferon-γ as the lymphokine that activates human macrophage oxidative metabolism and antimicrobial activity. J. Exp. Med. 158:670.
13. Nacy, C.A., A.H. Fortier, M.S. Meltzer, N.A. Buchmeier, and R.D. Schreiber. 1985. Macrophage activation to kill Leishmania major: Activation of macrophages for intracellular destruction of amastigotes can be induced by both recombinant interferon-γ and non-interferon lymphokines. J. Immunol. 135:3505.
14. Schreiber, R.D. and A. Celada. 1985. Molecular characterization of gamma interferon is a macrophage activating factor. Lymphokines 11:87.
15. Celada, A., P.W. Gray, E. Rinderknecht, and R.D. Schreiber. 1984. Evidence for a gamma-interferon receptor that regulates macrophage tumoricidal activity. J. Exp. Med. 160:55.
16. Celada, A., R. Allen, I. Esparza, P.W. Gray, and R.D. Schreiber. 1985. Demonstration and partial characterization of the interferon-gamma receptor on human mononuclear phagocytes. J. Clin. Invest. 76:2196.

17. Finbloom, D.S., D.L. Hoover, and L.M. Wahl. 1985. The characteristics of binding of human recombinant interferon-γ to its receptor on human monocytes and human monocyte-like cell lines. J. Immunol. 135:300.
18. Hamilton, T.A., D.L. Becton, S.D. Somers, P.W. Gray, and D.O. Adams. 1985. IFN-γ modulates protein kinase C activity in murine peritoneal macrophages. J. Biol. Chem. 260:1378.
19. Somers, S.D., J.E. Weiel, T.A. Hamilton, and D.O. Adams. 1986. Phorbol esters and calcium ionophore can prime murine peritoneal macrophages for tumor cell destruction. J. Immunol. 136:4199.
20. Celada A. and R.D. Schreiber. 1986. Role of protein kinase C and intracellular calcium mobilization in the induction of macrophage tumoricidal activity by interferon-γ. J. Immunol. 137:2373.
21. Celada A. and R.D. Schreiber. 1986. Internalization and degradation of receptor bound interferon-γ by murine macrophages: Demonstration of receptor recycling. Submitted.
22. Spitalny G.L. and E.H. Havell. 1984. Monoclonal antibody to murine gamma interferon inhibits lymphokine-induced antiviral and macrophage tumoricidal activities. J. Exp. Med. 159:1560.
23. Prat, M., G. Gribaudo, P.M. Comoglio, G. Cavallo, and S. Landolfo. 1984. Monoclonal antibodies against murine γ interferon. Immunol. 81:4515.
24. Russell, J.K., M.P. Hayes, J.M. Carter, B.A. Torres, B.M. Dunn, S.W. Russell and H.M. Johnson. 1986. Epitope and functional specificity of monoclonal antibodies to mouse interferon-γ: the synthetic peptide approach. J. Immunol. 136:3324.
25. Buchmeier N.A. and R.D. Schreiber. 1985. Requirement of endogenous interferon-γ production for resolution of Listeria monocytogenes infection. Proc. Natl. Acad. Sci. (USA) 82:7404.
26. Mackaness, G.B. 1964. The immunological basis of acquired cellular resistance. J. Exp. Med. 120:105.
27. Mackaness, G.B. 1969. The influence of immunologically committed lymphoid cells on macrophage activity in vivo. J. Exp. Med. 129:973.
28. Jones T. and G. Youmans. 1973. The in vitro inhibition of growth of intracellular Listeria monocytogenes by lymphocyte products. Cell. Immunol. 9:353.
29. Farr, A., W. Wechter, J-M. Kiely, and E. Unanue. 1979. Induction of cytocidal macrophages after in vitro interactions between Listeria-immune T cells and macrophages - role of H-2. J. Immunol. 122:2405.
30. Havell, E.A., G.L. Spitalny, and P.J. Patel. 1982. Enhanced production of murine interferon-γ by T cells generated in response to bacterial infection. J. Exp. Med. 156:112.
31. Campbell, P.A. 1986. Are inflammatory phagocytes responsible for resistance to facultative intracellular bacteria. Immunol. Today 7:70.
32. Campbell, P.A. 1987. What T cells tell macrophages to do during resistance to Listeriosis. In: "Host Defenses and Immunomodulation to Intracellular Pathogens." Eisenstein, Hana, Ward and Bullock, eds. Plenum Publishing Corp., New York, NY.

IN VIVO AND *IN VITRO* ROLE OF GAMMA INTERFERON IN IMMUNE CLEARANCE OF *Rickettsia species*

Thomas R. Jerrells, Han Li, and David H. Walker

Department of Pathology
Route F-09
University of Texas Medical Branch
Galveston, Texas 77550

INTRODUCTION

Members of the genus *Rickettsia* are obligate intracellular bacteria, and due to the intracellular location of their growth, they present a unique challenge to the immune system. Since antibody cannot gain entrance to viable cells, it has been argued that antibody does not play a major role in the effector phase of immunity to these organisms.

A number of studies have suggested that the cellular immune response is of primary importance in clearance of rickettsiae from infected animals.[1-4] Care should be taken in interpreting this generalization since it was shown that the antibody response to *R. tsutsugamushi* is completely dependent on the presence of antigen-reactive T-cells.[4]

The most distinguishing characteristic of T-cells that are of the helper/inducer type is their production of lymphokines after stimulation with specific antigen. It has been suggested that T-helper cells can be placed functionally in two groups based on the lymphokines that the cells produce.[5] One type of T-helper cell produces factors that act on B-cells to induce their responsiveness, proliferation, and ultimately antibody production. In contrast the other group seems to produce T-cell helper factors such as interleukin 2 and effector substances such as gamma interferon (IFN-γ).

In earlier studies from this laboratory a strong association between the production of IFN-γ following *in vivo* administration of antigen or stimulation of immunocompetent cells *in vitro* with antigen and protective immunity was noted.[6,7] These findings, with minor differences, also were noted in a primate model of scrub typhus[8] and suggest that IFN-γ production during the immune response to this organism is a general finding and not restricted to the murine model. The role of IFN-γ in immunity is complex but it has been shown to be the molecule responsible for the induction of class II major histocompatibility antigens on macrophages and other antigen-presenting cells; thus, it is critical for the induction of immune responses.[9,10]

IFN-γ also is a major effector molecule involved in macrophage activation to kill tumors, bacteria, and rickettsiae,[11] and it induces antirickettsial activity in "nonimmunological" cells such as fibroblasts and endothelial cells.[12,13] Unrestrained rickettsial growth in experimental animals has been shown to be associated with defects in IFN-γ activity but not necessarily production.[14]

The majority of the described studies that have defined the role of IFN-γ in antirickettsial immunity have been performed *in vitro*. Although the evidence for IFN-γ activity in rickettsial immunity is compelling, the relative *in vivo* importance of IFN-γ still is not known. With the development of monoclonal antibodies that neutralize the antirickettsial activity of IFN-γ,[15] it is possible to approach the problem of IFN-γ activity *in vivo*. The present study was designed to assess the importance of IFN-γ in resistance to rickettsial infection by depleting IFN-γ *in vivo* using repeated injection of monoclonal antibody specific for murine IFN-γ.

MATERIALS AND METHODS

Female Swiss-Webster mice were used at 6 to 8 weeks of age. Animals were administered monoclonal antibodies to IFN-γ or to Vero cells as ascites prepared in athymic (nu/nu) mice. The ascites containing anti-IFN-γ contained 4.2×10^6 neutralizing units of antibody per milliliter. Animals were injected with 0.1 ml of the appropriate material on days 0, 1, 3, 5, and 7, relative to the time of rickettsial infection. Treated and untreated mice were infected with 12 $TCID_{50}$ of *R. conorii*, strain 7 (Malish). This dose of rickettsiae routinely produces a lethal infection in susceptible C3H/HeJ mice. Animals were observed for signs of the infection including lethargy, ruffled fur, anorexia, and death.

In other experiments animals were bled at various times after infection to assay for IFN and anti-IFN activity in sera and randomly chosen animals were sacrificed to determine the number of rickettsiae in various organs. Interferon and anti-IFN levels in sera were determined using cytopathic effect in L929 cells produced by vesicular stomatitis virus as previously described[6] as the end point. Rickettsiae numbers were estimated in kidney, liver, and spleen sections using a direct immunofluorescence assay.[16]

In separate studies BALB/c mice were treated with anti-IFN-γ using an identical protocol as described and infected with the Gilliam strain of *R. tsutsugamushi*; macrophage influx was evaluated for Ia antigen expression using an immunofluorescent assay as previously described.[17]

In another study BALB/c mice were depleted of T-helper cells (L3T4) by injection of antibody produced by the GK.15 hybridoma. On three consecutive days 250 μg of antibody was given intraperitoneally, and two weeks after the last injection animals were infected subcutaneously with a sublethal dose of Karp strain, *R. tsutsugamushi*.

RESULTS

Administration of antibody-containing ascites to either Swiss-Webster or BALB/c mice without further treatment had no noticeable effect on the animals (data not shown). Treatment of animals with monoclonal anti-IFN-γ, however, had a marked effect on the outcome of infection with *R. conorii*. As can be seen from the data in Table 1 Swiss-Webster mice are normally resistant to infection with *R. conorii*, strain 7 (Malish); however, administration of monoclonal anti-IFN-γ resulted in 100% of the treated animals showing signs of infection and in the three experiments performed a total of 47% of the infected animals died. Administration of a control monoclonal antibody with Vero cell reactivity had no effect on the outcome of

Table 1. Effect of Anti-Murine IFN Gamma on Resistance to Rickettsial Challenge

Treatment[a]	% Morbidity[b]	% Mortality
None	0	0
Anti-Vero Cell Antibody	0	0
Anti-IFN-γ Antibody	100 (40/40)	47 (17/36)

[a]Antibodies or diluent (0.1 ml) given on days 0, 1, 3, 5, and 7 intraperitoneally. Infected with 12 $TCID_{50}$ of R. conorii, strain 7 (Malish) on day 0 intraperitoneally.
[b]Data represent mean of three experiments.

the infection. Since the infecting rickettsiae were grown in Vero cell cultures this is an appropriate control monoclonal antibody.

Table 2. Serum IFN Levels in Treated Mice at Various Times Following Infection with R. conorii, Strain 7 (Malish)

Treatment[a]	Day After Infection	IFN Titer[b]	Anti-IFN Activity[c]
Anti-Vero Cell Antibody	2	10	-
	4	<10	-
	6	160	-
	8	40	-
	10	160	-
	12	10	-
	14	<10	-
Anti-IFN-γ Antibody	2	40 (40)[d]	+ (16)[e]
	4	<10	+ (32)
	6	10 (5)[d]	+ (16)
	8	<10	+ (16)
	10	<10	+ (8)
	12	<10	-
	14	<10	-

[a]See footnote to Table 1.
[b]Determined by inhibition of cytopathic effects of vesicular stomatitis virus on L929 cells.
[c]Determined by neutralization of 10μ IFN as described by Spitalney and Havell.[15]
[d]IFN titer after treatment at pH 2.0.
[e]Anti-IFN-γ titer.

To determine if IFN-γ is produced by animals resistant to *R. conorii* sera obtained during the infection were evaluated for antiviral activity. It was found (Table 2) that relatively high levels of IFN were produced during this infection by untreated mice and interestingly this response was lacking in anti-IFN-treated animals. A relatively low IFN response was noted early in the infection in IFN-γ depleted animals and this IFN was resistant to pH 2 indicating it was not of the gamma type. Sera obtained from anti-IFN-treated animals also contained anti-IFN activity indicating sufficient antibody was given to these animals.

As it was possible that factors other than rickettsiae were producing morbidity and mortality in the anti-IFN-treated mice we estimated rickettsial numbers in tissue sections using the direct immunofluorescence method. These studies showed that the administration of anti-IFN resulted in markedly higher numbers of rickettsiae in the liver and spleen (Table 3) as well as the kidney (not shown). These data show that anti-IFN-γ-treated mice are unable to contain the replication of rickettsiae.

It has been shown that the production of an Ia antigen macrophage inflammatory response is critical for survival of mice following challenge with rickettsiae.[14,17] Using this system we evaluated the effect of monoclonal anti-IFN-γ on the production of Ia antigen bearing macrophages during a rickettsial infection. These studies (Table 4) show that administration of anti-IFN-γ virtually eliminated the Ia bearing macrophage response produced in this infection. Further studies are required to determine if rickettsial replication in this system is unchecked in IFN-γ depleted animals.

Table 3. Effect of Anti-Murine IFN Gamma on Numbers of Rickettsiae in Organs of Treated Mice

Treatment[a]	Day After Infection	$\bar{x}$ Rickettsiae/Field[b]	
		Spleen	Liver
None	5	0.3	ND
	7	0.6	0.1
	8	1.3	1.0
	10	0.4	0.3
Anti-Vero Cell Antibody	5	0.6	0.4
	7	0.6	0.6
	8	1.7	1.8
	10	0.5	0.3
Anti-IFN-γ Antibody	5	5.7	1.1
	7	22.0	5.5
	8	36.0	15.0
	10	1.0	0.7

[a]See footnote to Table 1.
[b]Determined by direct immunofluorescence. Data represent the average number of rickettsiae visualized in 10 high power fields/section. Sections from two animals per time point were prepared and examined.

Table 4. Effect of Anti-Murine IFN Gamma on the Ia Antigen-Bearing Macrophage Influx of Resistant BALB/c Mice Following Infection with the Gilliam Strain of *R. tsutsugamushi*

Treatment[a]	Day After Infection	% Ia Positive Macrophage[b]
PBS	5	27
	7	38
	10	56
Anti-IFN-γ Antibody	5	11
	7	9
	10	26

[a]See footnote to Table 1.
[b]Determined by indirect immunofluorescence using peritoneal cells adherent to glass coverslips. Resident peritoneal cells were 14 ± 3% Ia positive cells.

It is generally thought that IFN-γ is produced by the T-helper cell that is characterized by the presence of the L3T4 surface antigen. To assess the relative importance of this T-cell subpopulation we injected animals with anti-L3T4 antibody produced by the GK.15 hybridoma. The results (Table 5) show that depletion of L3T4 cells from lymphoid organs, as measured by flow cytometry, eliminates the ability of mice to resist an otherwise sublethal, immunizing infection with rickettsiae.

Table 5. Effect of L3T4 Cell Depletion on Resistance to Subcutaneous Infection of Mice with the Karp Strain of *R. tsutsugamushi*

Treatment[a]	% Survival[b]	% L3T4 Cells[c]
PBS	100 (4/4)	29
Anti-L3T4	0 (0/6)	<1.0

[a]Antibody isolated from supernatants of GK.15 hybridoma cultures or phosphate buffered saline was injected in 0.5 ml amounts (250 μg antibody) for three consecutive days.
[b]Two weeks after the last injection animals from each group were infected subcutaneously with 1000 MLD_{50} of Karp rickettsiae.
[c]Determined by flow cytometry at the time of infection using indirect immunofluorescence. Spleen cells (10,000) were counted per group.

DISCUSSION

The data generated using monoclonal antimurine IFN-γ in *in vitro* studies have suggested that IFN-γ is an important molecule in antirickettsial immunity both within the immune response by macrophage activation and also acting on cells outside the immune system.[11-13] These and other studies [6,7,9,10] have led to the conviction that IFN-γ is of critical importance in immunity. The definitive experiments to establish the importance of IFN-γ are now possible using high titered ascites fluid from athymic mice. This material, when administered to mice that are normally resistant, essentially reversed the resistance to *R. conorii* as evidenced by an increase in morbidity and mortality. Although resistance to rickettsial infection has been shown to have a genetic basis[18] or to be associated with macrophage defects,[19,20] it nevertheless depends on the ability of an animal to develop a population of antigen-reactive T-cells.[4] It is now well accepted that innate and acquired resistance to rickettsial infection is critically dependent on the development of a cellular immunity. The data generated in this study clearly establish that an essential aspect of the immune response is the production of IFN-γ.

Also, it is evident from this study that other factors are playing a role in host survival. Even though IFN-γ was not detectable in infected animals approximately 50% of the animals survived the infection, and it must be assumed the rickettsiae were cleared. The data presented in Table 3 would suggest that rickettsiae are being cleared even in anti-IFN-γ-treated mice and further administration of anti-IFN-γ through day 14 had no effect on this clearance (unpublished). It is possible that other lymphokines not related to IFN-γ are active in mechanisms of rickettsiae clearance or nonspecific host factors also are important in rickettsial resistance as suggested by other studies from this laboratory.[21]

We are unable to define a mechanism of action of IFN-γ in this model; however, IFN-γ is critically involved in many aspects of the immune response. One important aspect of IFN-γ is the induction of class II MHC molecules on antigen presenting cells that are necessary for T-cell recognition of antigen. We have shown that the monoclonal antibody used in this study blocks the production of Ia antigen bearing macrophages during an infection of resistant mice with *R. tsutsugamushi*.[17] This is undoubtedly an important aspect of IFN-γ since the Ia molecule is essential for T-cell recognition of antigen and is therefore important in the development of the immune response.

One disadvantage of *in vivo* depletion of mediators is the difficulty in establishing the site of action of the mediator. We have established the critical role of IFN-γ in antirickettsial immunity and established one possible mechanism of action. It is likely that IFN-γ has other important effects *in vivo* such as macrophage activation or effects on the endothelium but this remains to be shown.

In other studies it has been shown that the action of IFN-γ is down regulated by factors produced during acute rickettsial infections.[14] In this system it was shown that relatively high levels of IFN-γ were demonstrable at the site of infection[14] and lymphocytes from spleens of these animals were hyperresponsive in terms of IFN-γ production (unpublished data). Inspite of this macrophages did not express Ia antigens. It was found that high levels of prostaglandin E_2 and corticosteroids were produced during these infections and these substances modulated the effects of IFN-γ. It is not known if other aspects of IFN-γ are also similarly suppressed but this would seem likely.

In summary it is clear from the data presented in this report and in other reports from this laboratory that IFN-γ is a major element in immunity to obligate intracellular rickettsiae. In vivo situations where IFN-γ is neutralized with antibody or the effects on target cells are inhibited by inflammatory factors strongly support this contention. It remains to be shown what the most important in vivo aspect of IFN-γ is, and if all of the observed in vitro actions of IFN-γ occur in vivo.

REFERENCES

1. Shirai, A., P.J. Catanzaro, S.M. Phillips, and J.V. Osterman. 1976. Host defenses in experimental scrub typhus: role of cellular immunity in heterologous protection. Infect. Immun. 14:39.
2. Walker, D.J., and F.W. Henderson. 1978. Effect of immunosuppression on Rickettsia rickettsii infection in guinea pigs. Infect. Immun. 20:221.
3. Kokorin, I.N., E.A. Kabanova, E.M. Shirokova, G.E. Abrosimova, N.N. Rybkina, and V.I. Pushkareva. 1982. Role of T lymphocytes in Rickettsia conorii infection. Acta Virol. 26:91.
4. Jerrells, T.R., and C.S. Eisemann. 1983. Role of T-lymphocytes in production to antigens of Rickettsia tsutsugamushi and other Rickettsia species. Infect. Immun. 41:666.
5. Mosmann, T.R., H. Cherwinski, M.W. Bond, M.A. Giedlin, and R.L. Coffman. 1986. Two types of murine helper T cell clone I. Definition according to profiles of lymphokine activities and secreted proteins. J. Immunol. 136:2348.
6. Palmer, B.A., F.M. Hetrick, and T.R. Jerrells. 1984. Production of gamma interferon in mice immune to Rickettsia tsutsugamushi. Infect. Immun. 43:59.
7. Palmer, B.A., F.M. Hetrick, and T.R. Jerrells, 1984. Gamma interferon production in response to homologous and heterologous strain antigens in mice chronically infected with Rickettsia tsutsugamushi. Infect. Immun. 46:237.
8. MacMillan, J.G., R.M. Rice, and T.R. Jerrells. 1985. Development of antigen specific cell-mediated immune responses after infection of cynomolgus monkeys (Macaca fasicularis) with Rickettsia tsutsugamushi. J. Infect. Dis. 152:739.
9. Unanue, E.R. 1984. Antigen-presenting function of the macrophage. Ann. Rev. Immunol. 2:395.
10. Steeg, P.S., R.N. Moore, H.M. Johnson, and J.J. Oppenheim. 1982. Regulation of murine macrophage Ia antigen expression by a lymphokine with immune interferon activity. J. Exp. Med. 156:1780.
11. Jerrells, T.R., J. Turco, H.H. Winkler, and G.L. Spitalney. 1986. Neutralization of lymphokine-mediated antirickettsial activity of fibroblasts and macrophages with monoclonal antibody specific for murine interferon gamma. Infect. Immun. 51:355.
12. Turco, J., and H.H. Winkler. 1983. Inhibition of the growth of Rickettsia prowazekii in cultured fibroblasts by lymphokines. J. Exp. Med. 157:974.
13. Wisseman, C.L., Jr., and A. Waddell. 1983. Interferon-like factors from antigen- and mitogen-stimulated human leukocytes with antirickettsial and cytolytic actions on Rickettsia prowazekii infected human endothelial cells, fibroblasts, and macrophages. J. Exp. Med. 157:1780.
14. Jerrells, T.R., and C.J. Hickman. 1986. Down regulation of Ia antigen expression on inflammatory macrophages by factors produced during acute infections with R. tsutsugamushi, in, Immune Regulation by Characterized Polypeptides, UCLA Symposia on Molecular and Cellular Biology, Goldstein, G., J.F. Bach, and H. Wigzell, eds., New York, Alan R. Liss, Inc., vol. 41.

15. Spitalney, G.R., and E.A. Havell. 1984. Monoclonal antibody to murine gamma interferon inhibits lymphokine-induced antiviral and macrophage tumoricidal activities. J. Exp. Med. 159:1560.
16. Walker, D.H., and F.W. Henderson. 1978. Effect of immunosuppression on *Rickettsia rickettsii* infection in guinea pigs. Infect. Immun. 20: 221.
17. Jerrells, T.R. 1983. Association of inflammatory I region-associated antigen positive macrophage influx and genetic resistance of inbred mice to *Rickettsia tsutsugamushi*. Infect. Immun. 42:549.
18. Eisemann, C.S., M.J. Nypaver, and J.V. Osterman. 1984. Susceptibility of inbred mice to rickettsiae of the spotted fever group. Infect. Immun. 43:143.
19. Meltzer, M.S., and C.A. Nacy. 1980. Macrophages in resistance to rickettsial infection: susceptibility to the lethal effects of *Rickettsia akari* infection in mouse strains with defective macrophage function. Cell. Immunol. 54:487.
20. Nacy, C.A., and M.S. Meltzer. 1982. Macrophages in resistance to rickettsial infection: strains of mice susceptible to the lethal effects of *Rickettsia akari* show defective macrophage rickettsiacidal activity *in vitro*. Infect. Immun. 36:1096.
21. Jerrells, T.R., and J.V. Osterman. 1982. Role of macrophages in innate and acquired host resistance to experimental scrub typhus infection of inbred mice. Infect. Immun. 37:1066.

EFFECT OF INTERFERONS ON THE ACTIVATION OF MURINE PERITONEAL MACROPHAGES TO INHIBIT THE GROWTH OF *LISTERIA MONOCYTOGENES*

Alison M. Badger, Barbara A. Swift and Barbara J. Dalton

Department of Immunology and Anti-Infective Therapy
Smith Kline and French Laboratories
709 Swedeland Road, Swedeland PA, 19479

INTRODUCTION

Peritoneal macrophages are activated to become antimicrobial *in vivo* by infection with intracellular parasites (1,2) or *in vitro* by lymphokine-containing lymphocyte supernatants (3-7). One component of these mitogen stimulated lymphocyte supernatants, gamma interferon (IFN-γ), has been shown to be responsible for the ability of lymphokine supernatants to activate a variety of macrophage functions, including microbicidal and tumoricidal activity. However, there do appear to be non-interferon components of these supernatants that can render macrophages to become microbicidal (8). Izadkhah et al. (9) first demonstrated that treatment of mice with sera containing IFN-γ was able to increase the survival of mice infected with *Salmonella typhimurium*. More recent studies with pure and recombinant murine IFN-γ (rMuIFN-γ) have demonstrated that this lymphokine can indeed activate macrophages to inhibit the growth of (or kill) several intracellular parasites. IFN-γ treatment (both *in vitro* and *in vivo*) inhibits the intracellular protozoa *Toxoplasma gondii* (10,11) and *Leishmania donovani* (12) and the *in vivo* growth of *Listera monocytogenes* (13). A recent report indicates that the *in vivo* production of IFN-γ is required for the clearance of *Listeria* in infected mice (14). In human studies IFN-γ has been shown to activate peripheral monocytes to kill *Toxoplasma gondii* (15) and *Leishmania donovani in vitro* (12, 16) and a recent study describes the enhanced capacity of these cells to kill *Listeria* (17).

In a preliminary study we previously reported that rMuIFN-γ could activate murine peritoneal macrophages to inhibit the growth of *Listeria* in an *in vitro* assay (18). In the present study we describe that this macrophage-mediated decrease in *Listeria* is probably a growth inhibitory effect rather than a direct killing of the microorganisms; we describe the kinetics of this activation for growth inhibition and the effect of a monoclonal antibody to MuIFN-γ on this activity, as well as comparing the activity of IFN-γ with that of IFN-α/ß. We have also demonstrated that a preparation of rat gamma interferon (rRatIFN-γ) can cross species and activate murine macrophages at concentrations equivalent to rMuIFN-γ.

METHODS AND MATERIALS

Animals

Specific pathogen-free inbred C57Bl/6 male mice were obtained from Charles River Kingston, Stone Ridge N.Y. Within any given experiment mice were matched for age and weight.

Reagents

Paraffin oil was from Arthur H. Thomas Co (Philadelphia, PA). Lipopolysaccharide (LPS) from *E.coli* 0127:B8 (Difco Laboratories, Detroit, MI); Muramyl dipeptide (MDP) (Calbiochem, La Jolla CA). Recombinant *E. coli* derived murine gamma interferon (rMuIFN-γ), specific activity 6 x 10^6 U/mg was provided by Genentech, Inc., South San Francisco, CA; murine alpha/beta interferon (MuIFN-α/ß), specific activity 1x10^8 U/mg was prepared as described previously (19); the preparation of a polyclonal antibody raised against IFN-α/ß has also been described previously (20). A monoclonal antibody to MuIFN-γ was kindly provided by Dr. G.L. Spitalny (Bristol Myers). The activity of this antibody is expressed as antiviral neutralizing units (21). Recombinant rat gamma interferon was kindly provided by Dr. P.H. van der Meide, (TNO, Netherlands). Lymphokine preparations containing macrophage activating activity (MAF) were cell free supernatants from C57Bl/6 spleen cell cultures cultured for 72 hr with Con A (5 µg/ml) as described previously (22).

The murine interferons and MAF preparations were titered for their protective effect on L-929 cells challenged with vesicular stomatitis virus and the rRatIFN-γ for it's protective effect on RATec cells (a rat embryo fibroblast) challenged with EMC virus. *Listeria monocytogenes* (Strain EGD) was provided by the Trudeau Institute. All tissue culture media were obtained from Grand Island Biological Co., (Gibco), Grand Island, New York. Fetal calf serum (FCS) was from Flow Laboratories Rockville, Md. and was heat inactivated (56 ^{o} for 30 min.).

Preparation of macrophages

Peritoneal exudate cells (PEC) were obtained 5-6 days after intraperitoneal injection of 2 ml of paraffin oil. Erythrocytes were lysed by brief (20 sec) hypoosmotic shock and the cells washed three times in Hank's balanced salt solution (HBSS), counted and resuspended in RPMI containing 20% FCS. One ml of cell suspension containing 10^6 cells were added to 24 well flat-bottomed plates (Linbro, McLean, VA). Following a 2 hr incubation at 37 ^{o}C in a humidified 5% CO_2 atmosphere nonadherent cells were removed by washing 3 times. Cell monolayers contained more than 95% macrophages (MØ) as determined by non-specific esterase staining and phagocytic capability. Test compounds were added in 100ul of medium and the cells incubated overnight at 37°C in humidified 5% CO_2. There were no antibiotics included in the media at any time during the harvesting, preparation or activation of the macrophages, or during the assay procedures.

Macrophage-mediated anti-Listeria activity

The procedures used were modifications of those described by Harrington-Fowler (23) and Spitalny and North (24). Macrophage monolayers were infected with 10^5 bacteria in logarithmic growth phase and opsonized with pooled homologous serum (diluted 1-2 in saline). Phagocytosis was allowed to proceed for 40 min. and then the cultures washed 5X with HBSS to remove extracellular bacteria. The zero time count of MØ associated bacteria (a term used to describe any phagocytosed or cell surface bound viable organisms) was determined by plate counts of water lysed, sonicated macrophages scraped from the culture with a rubber policeman. In separate cultures MØ mediated anti-*Listeria* activity was assayed in triplicate culture in which the media was changed at 30 min intervals for 5 hr and then the intracellular count determined. Culture medium was monitored for free bacteria during the incubation period by transferring 100 ul aliquots onto tryptic soy agar plates and determining the number of *Listeria* colonies 48 hr later. To examine the number of phagocytosed microorganisms, 1×10^6 PEC were allowed to adhere to glass coverslips in 24 well flat bottomed plates. These cells were then washed and treated with IFN as described previously and then exposed to 1×10^7 *Listeria* for 20 min. The coverslips were then washed 10x with HBSS, fixed in methanol for 5 min and then stained with Wright's Giemsa stain.

For statistical analysis, treated groups were compared to the control untreated group by Student's t test.

RESULTS

Recombinant murine gamma interferon activates oil elicited peritoneal macrophages to inhibit the growth of macrophage-associated *Listeria*. The most active concentrations in these experiments were found to be 10-20 units/ml and this treatment consistently resulted in a five-fold reduction in the number of *Listeria* and in many experiments a ten-fold reduction was obtained. Table 1 shows the combined results of six different experiments.

Table 1

Recombinant murine gamma interferon activates macrophages to inhibit the growth of *Listeria*

Treatment	Surviving *Listeria*[a] ($\pm$ S.D.)	% change	Significance (p value)
Control	46,431 $\pm$ 11,359[b]		
rMuIFN-γ (10 units/ml)	9,693 $\pm$ 5,262	-80	<.001

a Surviving organisms after 5 hours in culture.

b Pooled results of 6 experiments each having triplicate samples.

Statistical analysis by Student's t test. Treated cultures compared to the untreated control.

We have recently found that concentrations as low as 0.02 - 0.2 units/ml can result in a reduction in surviving bacteria. A representative experiment showing the dose response effect obtained with IFN-γ is shown in Figure 1.

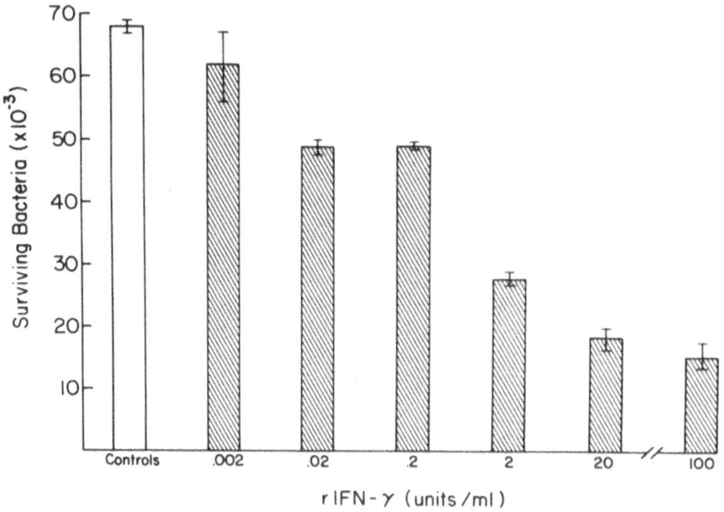

Figure 1. Dose dependent effect of rMuIFN-γ on macrophage mediated inhibiton of Listeria after 5 hour in culture. Cells were incubated overnight in medium or rMuIFN-γ.

Statistically significant inhibitory activity could be obtained with 0.2 units/ml ($p = < .05$) with maximum activity being obtained with 20 units/ml ($p = < .01$).

The effect of interferon in the experimental circumstances described here appears to be an inhibition of the growth rate of the bacteria (although concomitant killing cannot be ruled out). We have compared the numbers of phagocytosed bacteria (zero time count) with the number in the macrophage cultures after 5 hr incubation. On the average there is a ten to twenty fold increase in the bacterial counts in this time period in the control cultures but only a three to four fold increase following macrophage activation by IFN-γ (Table 2). The zero time count of bacteria in the treated MO was either the same or slightly less than the untreated cultures but this was not statistically significant. Microscopic counts of phagocytosed Listeria confirmed the finding there was no significant difference between the phagocytic capacity of IFN-γ treated macrophages and the control cultures. (Table 3).

Table 2

Comparison of *Listeria* growth in control cultures and cultures treated with gamma interferon.

Treatment	Surviving *Listeria* (Mean ± S.D.) Zero time	5 Hours	% Change
Controls	3,914 ± 1,253[a]	34,179 ± 6,408	
rMuIFN-γ (10 units/ml).	2,889 ± 553[NS]	11,195 ± 1,789	-67***

a Pooled results of 4 different exps. each with triplicate samples

Statistical analysis by Student's t test. Treated cultures compared to the untreated controls. N.S. Not significant, *** $p = < .001$

Table 3

Number of infected cells and number of *Listeria*/infected cell in control and IFN-γ treated cultures.

Treatment	% Infected cells	# *Listeria*/infected cell
Control	61 ± 9[a]	2.58 ± 0.16
rMuIFN-γ (10 units/ml)	74 ± 5[NS]	2.66 ± 0.32[NS]

a Mean ± S.D. of three separate counts of 300 cells (900 total).

Statistical analysis by Student's t test. Treated cultures compared to the control: NS Not significant.

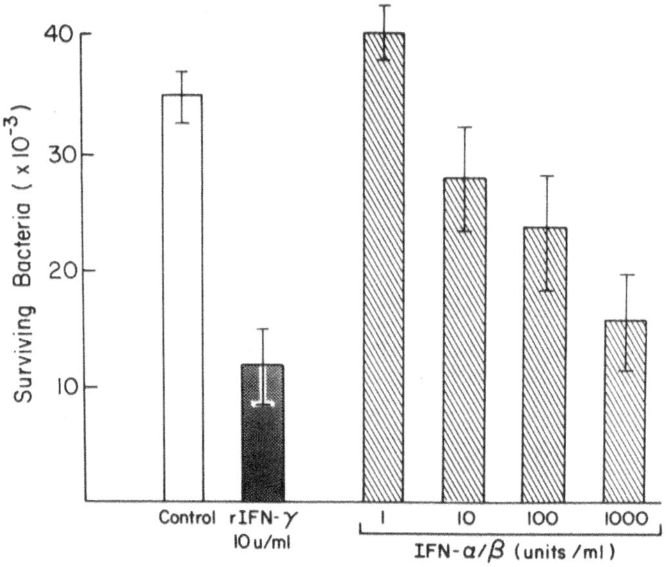

Figure 2. Comparison between rMuIFN-γ and IFN-α/ß on macrophage mediated inhibition of <u>Listeria</u> after 5 hours in culture. Cells were incubated overnight in medium, rMuIFN-γ or IFN-α/ß.
Inhibitory activity was significant for rIFN-γ ($p = < .01$), IFN α/ß at 1000 units/ml ($p = < .01$), and 100 units/ml ($p = < .05$).

Murine alpha/beta interferon also activated macrophages to inhibit <u>Listeria</u> growth (Fig.2); however 100x more IFN-α/ß was required to obtain activity equivalent to that of 10 units of rIFN-γ.

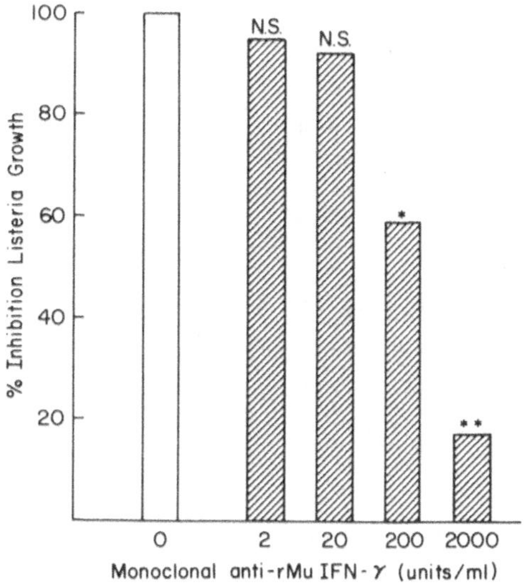

Figure 3. Partial reversal of rMuIFN-γ inhibitory activity with specific monoclonal antibody.

☐ rMuIFN-γ control (20 units/ml).

▨ rMuIFN-γ (20 units/ml) plus antibody.

Significant reversal of IFN activity was obtained with 2000 ($p = <.01$) and 200 ($p = <.05$) neutralizing units of monoclonal antibody.

The activity of IFN-γ was reduced but not eliminated in the presence of specific monoclonal antibodies and it required 2000 antiviral neutralizing units to obtain 80% reversal of activity (Fig. 3).

Table 4.

A polyclonal antibody to IFN-α/ß inhibits the ability of IFN-α/ß to activate macrophages.

Treatment	Surviving *Listeria*[a] (± S.D.)	% change	Significance (p value)
Control	73,467 ± 6,689		
rMuIFN-γ (20 units/ml)	16,633 ± 4,813	-77	<.001
IFN-α/ß (1000 units/ml)	16,167 ± 1,150	-78	<.001
IFN α/ß 1000 units/ml + anti-IFN-α/ß .			
1000 units	66,500 ± 4,616	-9	N.S.
100 Units	58,167 ± 5,558	-21	<.05
10 units	20,067 ± 1,518	-73	<.001
1 unit	17,100 ± 5,205	-77	<.001
Anti IFN-α/b 1000 units/ml	60,433 ± 4,445	-18	<.05

a Surviving organisms after 5 hours in culture.

Statistical analysis by Student's t test. Treated cultures compared to the untreated control.

The activity of IFN-α/ß on the other hand could be completely reversed in the presence of 100 and 1000 viral neutralising units of a polyclonal anti-IFN α/ß antibody (Table 4). In these experiments the antibody and IFN preparations were incubated together for 60 min. prior to their addition to the macrophage monolayers.

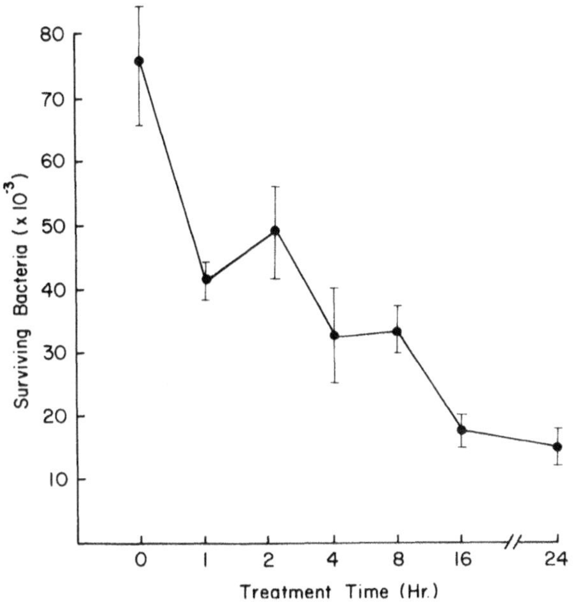

Figure 4. Kinetics of macrophage activation for inhibition of Listeria. Macrophage monolayers were incubated with rMuIFN-γ for the indicated time periods, washed and then incubated for the full overnight period. All the plating assays were carried out at 24 hours. Statistically significant inhibitory activity was obtained following 1-4 ($p = <.05$) and 16-24 ($p= <.001$) hours incubation with IFN.

Experiments designed to determine the kinetics of macrophage activation by rMuIFN-γ resulted in the finding that activity could be demonstrated after only a 60 minute exposure to IFN-γ. The activity increased over the next 4-8 hours with maximal activity usually being obtained after a 16 hour exposure. Figure 4 is a representative experiment of six which gave similar results.

Treatment of macrophages with a preparation of recombinant rat gamma interferon resulted in the finding that this IFN crossed species and was as effective as rMuIFN-γ in this assay system with 20 units/ml giving optimum activity (Table 5). Treatment of macrophages with MDP or LPS did not activate them to inhibit the growth of *Listeria* but resulted in a small but consistent increase in the number of intracellular bacteria compared to the control cultures at the end of the 5 hour incubation period. This increase, although low, was statistically significant and the results of two such experiments are shown in Table 6. In every experiment a lymphokine preparation was included as a positive control. These supernatants were consistently active in this assay at dilutions containing approximately 10-20 units of IFN.

Table 5

Recombinant rat gamma interferon activates murine macrophages to inhibit the growth of *Listeria*

Treatment	Surviving *Listeria*[a] (± S.D.)	% change	Significance (p value)
Control untreated	76,800 ± 6696	-	-
rRat IFN-g (units/ml)			
200	18,067 ± 4,796	-76	<.001
20	22,500 ± 2,784	-69	<.001
2	27,300 ± 3,079	-64	<.001
.2	39,900 ± 1,916	-48	<.001
.02	35,133 ± 7,254	-54	<.001
.002	50,200 ± 6,809	-35	<.05
.0002	75,733 ± 11,756	-1	N.S.

a Surviving organisms after 5 hours in culture.

Statistical analysis by Student's t test. Treated cultures compared to the untreated control. N.S. Not Significant.

There was no significant difference between survivig *Listeria* in the groups treated with 200 and 20 units/ml IFN.

Table 6

Effect of MDP, LK-sup and LPS on macrophage-mediated inhibition of *Listeria* growth.

Treatment	Experiment I Surviving *Listeria*[a] (± S.D.)	Experiment I % Change	Experiment II Surviving *Listeria*[a] (± S.D.)	Experiment II % Change
Control	73,833 ± 11,647		53,833 ± 7,801	
LPS (10 ng/ml)	106,433 ± 2,307	+44*	N.D.	
MDP (20 ug/ml)	N.D.		84,067 ± 6086	+ 56*
LK-sup[b] (1:5)	27,200 ± 5,048	-63***	8,733 ± 378	- 84***

a Surviving organisms after 5 hr in culture.

b Preparation contains approximately 50 units IFN/ml

Statistical analysis by Student's t test. Treated cultures compared to the control: * $p = < .05$, *** $p = < .001$.

DISCUSSION

These results describe the activation of murine peritoneal macrophages by rat and murine interferons to inhibit the growth of *Listeria monocytogenes*. Maximum activity with rMuIFN-γ was obtained with concentrations of 10-20 units/ml although lower concentrations showed varying degrees of activity. A similar activity was shown with a preparation of rat IFN-γ. A partial reversal of the activity of rMuIFN-γ could be obtained when the IFN-γ was preincubated with a monoclonal antibody prior to the macrophage activation step but it required 100 X the antiviral neutralizing units of antibody to obtain an 80% reversal of activity. That a complete reversal of activity was not obtained is not surprising as this phenomenon has been reported by others for reversal of rMuIFN-γ activated B cell proliferation (25) and tumoricidal activity (21). We have also shown that similar activation of macrophages to inhibit *Listeria* can be induced in this cell population by a preparation of IFN-α/ß and that this activity can be totally abrogated with a polyclonal antibody. We have found that 100 fold more IFN-α/ß is required to obtain activity equivalent to that obtained with 10-20 units of IFN-γ.

Additional increases in the concentration of either of these interferons did not result in any additional activity or reversal of activity. These results are in agreement with studies of IFN-activated tumoricidal macrophages where it was demonstrated that at least 100 fold more MuIFN-α/ß than IFN-γ was required to stimulate similar levels of tumoricidal activity in murine macrophages (26-27). We have not been able to demonstrate any synergistic activity for combinations of IFN-γ and IFN-α/ß as has been reported for interferons' antiviral, antiproliferative and natural killer cell enhancing activity (28-30) (data not shown).

Induction of optimal levels of macrophage inhibitory activity by rMuIFN-γ occurred when the macrophages were incubated for 16-24 hrs with the IFN, however considerable inhibition of Listeria growth could be obtained with a 60 minute pulse (Figure 4), and in some experiments a 15 or 30 minute pulse resulted in reduction of Listeria colonies. Extensive washing to ensure removal of the IFN did not abrogate this inhibitory effect. Similar results have been reported by Hoover et al. (16) who demonstrated that human monocytes only required a 30 min pulse with rHuIFN-γ for induction of 70% of maximal activity against Leishmania donovani amastigotes.

There are a number of technical difficulties associated with the in vitro assessment of macrophage mediated antibacterial activity. In most cases, as with the studies reported here, it is not clear whether the macrophages in culture are bactericidal, bacteriostatic or inhibiting the rate of intracellular growth. The inhibition could, in fact, be a combination of these effects. The inhibition of proliferation by activated macrophages as opposed to intracellular killing has recently been addressed by Campbell (31). Although we have not made any special attempts in the experiments reported here to delineate between these activities, there is clearly an inhibition of the growth rate of the bacteria and concomitant killing cannot be ruled out. An additional mechanism which could be involved in the inhibitory activity is that mediated by macrophage secreted products which have been shown to be responsible for some killing of infectious agents including Listeria (32-34).

The inhibitory activity of these activated macrophages is not an artifact due to the internalization of antibiotics used to restrict the growth adherent or unphagocytosed bacteria in the culture medium as has been previously described (35,36). These experiments have been carried out in the absence of antibiotics, this includes the preparation of the adherent cell population, the overnight activation and the Listeria assay. Stained slides of macrophages were prepared following the phagocytosis step in the assay and careful observations of IFN treated cells compared with the controls convinced us that the treatment did not result in an inhibition of phagocytosis as has been suggested by others for interferons under certain circumstances (37).

Our results could not be explained by IFN-mediated depletion of tryptophan as described by Pfefferkorn (38) as increasing concentrations of tryptophan in the culture medium had no effect on the IFN activity (data not shown).

Mononuclear phagocytes may exist in a variety of stages or levels of activation. Even supposedly 'inactive' resident macrophages have been shown to exhibit different activation patterns with regard to their ability to inhibit Listeria growth (39).

Oil elicited macrophages support the growth of Listeria which confirms previous reports (23,40). We have found that there is a ten to twenty fold increase in bacterial cell counts in the control cultures during the 5 hour incubation period and that this is reduced five to ten fold following MØ activation by IFN-γ, IFN-α/ß or lymphokine containing supernatants.

In summary, IFN-α/ß, IFN-γ (murine and rat), and lymphokine-containing supernatants, but not LPS or MDP activate macrophages to inhibit the growth of the intracellular bacterium Listeria monocytogenes. The murine and rat gamma IFNs are more active than the murine alpha/beta IFNs in this respect. The activity of rMuIFN-γ is partially reversible and the activity of MuIFN-α/ß is fully reversible by specific antibody. These data provide further evidence for the role of interferons in the activation of macrophages to control the proliferation of intracellular microorganisms.

REFERENCES

1. G.B. Mackaness, Cellular resistance to infection. J. Exp. Med. 116:381-406 (1962).
2. G.B. Mackaness, The influence of immunologically committed lymphoid cells on macrophage activity in vivo. J. Exp. Med. 129:973-992 (1969).
3. P. Cole, Activation of mouse peritoneal cells to kill Listeria monocytogenes by T-lymphocyte products. Infect. Immun. 12: 36-41 (1975).
4. F.E. Fowles, I.M. Fajardo, J.L. Leiboritch, and J.R. David, The enhancement of macrophage bacteriostasis by products of activated lymphocytes. J. Exp. Med. 138:952-964 (1973).
5. R.W. Godfrey, P.G. Horton, and M.S. Wilder, Time course of antilisterial activity by immunologically activated murine peritoneal macrophages. Infect. Immun. 39:532-539 (1983).
6. T. Jones, and G.P. Youmans, The in vitro inhibition of growth of intracellular Listeria monocytogenes by lymphocyte products. Cell. Immunol. 9:353-362 (1973).
7. J.L. Krahenbuhl, and J.S. Remington. In vitro induction of nonspecific resistance in macrophages by specifically sensitized lymphocytes. Infect. Immun. 4: 337-343 (1971).
8. C.A. Nacy, A.H. Fortier, M.S. Meltzer, N.A. Buchmeier, and R.D. Schreiber, Macrophage activation to kill Leishmania major: activation of macrophages for intracellular destruction of amastigotes can be induced by both recombinant interferon-Y and non-interferon lymphokines. J. Immunol. 135: 3505-3511 (1985).
9. Z. Izadkhah, A.D. Mandel, and G. Sonnenfeld, Effect of treatment of mice with sera containing gamma interferon on the course of infection with Salmonella typhimurium strain LT-2. J. Interferon Res. 1:137-145 (1980).
10. R.E. McCabe, B.J. Luft, and J.S. Remington, Effect of murine interferon gamma on murine Toxoplasmosis. J. Infect. Dis. 150:961-962 (1984).
11. H.W. Murray, G.L. Spitalny, and C.F. Nathan, Activation of mouse peritoneal macrophages in vitro and in vivo by interferon-Y . J. Immunol. 134: 1619-1622 (1985).
12. H.W. Murray, B.F. Rubin, and C.D. Rothermel, Killing of intracellular Leishmania donovani by lymphokine-stimulated human mononuclear phagocytes. Evidence that interferon-Y is the activating lymphokine. J. Clin. Invest. 72:1506-1510 (1983).

13. A.F. Kiderlen, S.H.E. Kaufmann, and M.L. Lohmann-Matthes, Protection of mice against the intracellular bacterium Listeria monocytogenes by recombinant immune interferon. Eur. J. Immunol. 14:904-907 (1984).
14. N.A. Buchmeier, and R.D. Schreiber, Requirement of endogenous interferon-γ production for resolution of Listeria monocytogenes infection. Proc. Natl. Acad. Sci. 82. 7404-7408 (1985).
15. C. Nathan, H.W. Murray, M.E. Wiebe, and B.F. Rubin, Identification of interferon-γ as the lymphokine that activates human macrophage oxidative metabolism and antimicrobial activity. J. Exp. Med. 158:670-689 (1983).
16. D.L. Hoover, C.A. Nacy, and M.S. Meltzer Human monocyte activation for cytotoxicity against intracellular Leishmania donovani amastigotes: induction of microbicidal activity by interferon-γ. Cell. Immunol. 94:500-511 (1985).
17. R. Peck, A one-plate assay for macrophage bactericidal activity. J. Immunol. Methods 82:131-140 (1985).
18. T.P. Koestler, A.M. Badger, D.J. Rieman, R. Greig, and G. Poste, Induction by immunomodulatory agents of a macrophage antigen recognized by monoclonal antibody 158.2 and correlation with macrophage function. Cell. Immunol. 96:113-125 (1985).
19. C.A. Ogburn, K. Berg., and K. Paucker, Purification of mouse interferon by affinity chromatography on anti-interferon globulin sepharose. J. Immunol. 111:1206-1218 (1973).
20. B. Dalton, and K. Paucker, Preparation and absorption of antiserum against mouse L cell interferon. Methods in Enzymology 79:582 (1981).
21. G.L. Spitalny, and E.A. Havell, Monoclonal antibody to murine gamma interferon inhibits lymphokine-induced antiviral and macrophage tumoricidal activities. J. Exp. Med. 159:1560-1565 (1984).
22. A.M. Badger, S.R. Cooperband, and V.J. Merluzzi, The production of proliferation inhibitory factor (PIF) by mouse spleen cells in vitro. J.Immunol. 112:1435-1443 (1974).
23. L., Harrington-Fowler, P.M. Henson, and M.S. Wilder, Fate of Listeria monocytogenes in resident and activated macrophages. Inf. and Immun. 33: 11-16 (1981).
24. G.L. Spitalny, and R.J. North, Destruction of Listeria monocytogenes in vitro. In: Methods for Studying Mononuclear phagocytes. Ed. Adams, D.O., Edelson, P.J. and Hillel, K. Academic Press. 685-691 (1981).
25. J.J. Mond, F.D. Finkelman, C. Sarma, J. Ohara, and S. Serrate, Recombinant interferon-γ inhibits the B cell proliferative response stimulated by soluble but not by sepharose-bound anti-immunoglobulin antibody. J. Immunol. 135:2513-2517 (1983).
26. J.L. Pace, S.W. Russell, P.A. LeBlanc and D.M. Murasko, Comparative effects of various classes of mouse interferons on macrophage activation for tumor cell killing. J. Immunol. 134:977 (1985).
27. W.K. Roberts, and A. Vasil, Evidence for the identity of murine gamma interferon and macrophage activating factor. J. Interferon Res. 2:519-532 (1982).
28. W.R. Fleischmann, J.A. Georgiades, L.C. Osborne, and H.M. Johnson, Potentiation of interferon activity by mixed preparations of fibroblast and immune interferon. Infect. Immun. 26:248-256 (1979).
29. W.R. Fleischmann, Potentiation of the direct anticellular activity of mouse interferons: Mutual synergism and interferon concentration dependence. Cancer Res. 42:869-875 (1982).

30. D.A. Weigent, M.P. Langford, W.R. Fleischmann, and G.J. Standon, Potentiation of lymphocyte natural killing by mixtures of alpha or beta interferon with recombinant gamma interferon. Infect. Immun. 40:35-38 (1983).
31. P.A. Campbell, Are inflammatory phagocytes responsible for resistance to facultative intracellular bacteria Immunol. Today 7(3):70-72 (1986).
32. R.C. Bast, Jr., R.P. Cleveland, B.H. Littman, B. Zbar, and H.J. Rapp, Acquired cellular immunity: extracellular killing of Listeria monocytogenes by a product of immunologically activated macrophages. Cell. Immunol. 10:248-259 (1974).
33. G. Middlebrook, B.J. Salmon, and J.I. Kreisberg, Sterilization of Listeria monocytogenes by guinea pig peritoneal exudate cell cultures. Cell. Immunol. 14: 270-283 (1974).
34. K.K. Sethi, M. Teschner, and H. Brandis, In vitro antilisterial activity of soluble product(s) released from Listeria-immune murine peritoneal macrophages. Infect.Immun. 10:960-962. (1974).
35. D. Adam, F. Staber, B.H.,Belohradsky, and W. Marget, Effect of dihydrostreptomycin on phagocytosis of mouse peritoneal macrophages in vitro. Infect. Immun. 5:537-541 (1972).
36. P. Cole, and J. Brostoff, Intracellular killing of Listeria monocytogenes by activated macrophages (Mackaness system) is due to antibiotic. Nature (London) 256:515-517 (1975).
37. H. Rollag, M. Degre, and G. Sonnenfeld, Effects of interferon-α/ß and interferon-γ preparations on phagocytosis by mouse peritoneal macrophages. Scand. J. Immunol. 20.149-155 (1984).
38. E.R. Pfefferkorn, Interferon-γ blocks the growth of Toxoplasma gondii in human fibroblasts by inducing the host cells to degrade tryptophan. Proc. Nat. Acad. Sci. 81:908-912 (1984).
39. D. Ottendorfer, D. Bitter-Suermann, and U. Hadding, An in vitro system to study Listericidal capacity of macrophages from separate mice: resident macrophages exhibit different activation patterns. Infect. Immun. 49: 685-691 (1985).
40. J. Bennedsen, S. J. Riisgaard, M. Rhodes, and S.O. Larsen, In vitro studies on normal stimulated and immunologically activated mouse macrophages III. Intracellular multiplication of Listeria monocytogenes. Acta Pathol. Microbiol. Scand.Sect.C 85:246-252 (1977).

HUMAN NON-INTERFERON MACROPHAGE ACTIVATING FACTOR: BIOLOGICAL AND BIOCHEMICAL CHARACTERIZATION

John C. Lee, Alison M. Badger, and William J. Johnson

Department of Immunology & Antiinfectives Therapy
Smith Kline & French Laboratories
Philadelphia, PA 19101

ABSTRACT

A HTLV-1 transformed T cell line has been demonstrated to constitutively produce and secrete a lymphokine with macrophage activating properties. This lymphokine was biologically and biochemically distinct from interferon gamma, the interleukins, the colony stimulating factors and lymphotoxin. *In vitro* treatment of human monocytes with the partially purified lymphokine resulted in the acquisition of microbicidal and tumoricidal activities. The activity was associated with a protein with an apparent molecular weight of 55,000 daltons and an isoelectric point of 5.5. The potential for the efficacy of such a lymphokine in activating macrophages *in vivo* provides aspirations for its use in the therapy/prevention of opportunistic infections in immunocompromised hosts.

INTRODUCTION

Activated T lymphocytes of the helper phenotype are known to produce and secrete a number of soluble mediators which affect macrophage functions, including those which inhibit macrophage migration, activate macrophages to become microbicidal and tumoricidal, confer phenotypic changes essential for macrophage differentiation and function in immunoregulation and host defense mechanisms. In particular, the ability of mononuclear phagocytes to generate reactive oxygen intermediates and to kill facultative and obligate intracellular microorganisms and neoplastic cells has been considered a hallmark of the activated state. Furthermore, a large body of evidence has been gathered to define some of the regulatory and effector mechanisms of macrophage activation which have provided objective markers in defining the stages of activation and the signals that induce and regulate activation (1). However, at present, no marker exists for the activated phenotype which is absolutely predictive of microbicidal or tumoricidal activity.

An equally extensive literature has accumulated in regards to agents with the potential to induce the activated state. Much recent work centers on the ability of various cytokines to induce activation. Gamma-interferon, among the many mediators examined, has been demonstrated to be a potent mononuclear phagocyte activator (1-5). However, we (6-10) and others (11-19) have now provided clear evidence for other distinct lymphokines which share similar macrophage activating properties as gamma-interferon. These lymphokines include the colony stimulating factors, in particular the GM-CSF (20), M-CSF (21) and BSF-1 (22). In addition, we have identified an activity constitutively produced by a human T cell line (MT-2) which is unrelated to gamma- interferon as judged by a number of biochemical and serological criteria (6). We have also used a multitude of in vitro assay systems to provide an extensive biological profile of this activity. In this report, we will summarize the biological profile of this activity and provide a rationale for its utility in the therapy or prevention of opportunistic infections in immunocompromised hosts.

Cell Source for Human Non-Interferon Macrophage Activating Factor

Among the many human T cell lines examined for the production of a non-interferon macrophage activating factor, many but not all of the HTLV-1 transformed T cells lines constitutively produce molecule(s) with MAF activity. Other T lymphoma cell lines such as Jurkat, HUT78, CEM, HsB and pertussis antigen specific normal T cell lines did not produce appreciable MAF activity, either constitutively or induced. There was no evidence for the role of viral antigens in the MAF activity detectable in the HTLV-1 infected T cell line culture supernatants. Multiple lymphokine activities such as interferon-gamma, colony stimulating factors and interleukin 2 in various amounts can be detected in such supernatants (23). Of the two cell lines that depicted the most potent activity, MT-2 cell line (24) was examined in detail for the production of non-gamma interferon macrophage activating activity.

Analysis of Lymphokine Activities in MT-2 Cell-Free Culture Supernatant

Cell and virus free culture supernatants were assayed for the presence of interferon (by antiviral activity), interleukin 2 (by proliferation of CTLL-20 cells), and tumoricidal inducing activity. None of the cell lines examined produced appreciable amounts of IL-2 constitutively while there were variable levels of antiviral activity, indicative of the presence of interferon. The antiviral activity detected was due primarily to interferon-gamma, as determined by its neutralization by specific antibodies. There was no clear correlation of levels of interferon activity detected and MAF activity suggesting that the MAF activity might be mediated by a non-interferon related molecule(s). The MAF activity in MT-2 culture supernatant was further analyzed to identify its biological and biochemical nature. First, it was considered unlikely that the MAF activity detected in MT-2 cell supernatants was due to HTLV virions or to soluble viral antigens. Supernatants obtained from all of the cell lines tested contained comparable amounts of virally derived proteins, yet significant MAF activity was detected in supernatants from only seven of the cell lines. The MAF activity was not likely to be due to the small amounts of LPS because the level of LPS as assessed by the limulus lysate agglutination assay revealed insignificant amounts of LPS (< 0.1 ng/ml). Furthermore, the activity was not neutralized by the addition of polymyxin B sulfate (40 μg/ml) which had the capacity to neutralize $\leq$ 5 ng of LPS. The activity was not related to gamma-interferon since the activity was not adsorbed to an affinity column of specific antibody to gamma interferon and a monoclonal antibody to gamma interferon did not neutralize the activity.

Biochemical Characterization of MT-2 Derived Non-Interferon MAF

To further characterize the biochemical properties of the mediator(s) associated with MAF activity produced by MT-2 cells, cell-free culture supernatants were subjected to differential ammonium sulfate precipitation, ion-exchange and molecular sieving chromatography, and isoelectric focusing. The majority of MAF activity was associated with proteins precipitable between 30 to 80% ammonium sulfate. Gel filtration analysis of ammonium sulfate concentrated MT-2 MAF activity eluted between molecular weight markers of 68 kD and 45 kD (nominal molecular weight of bovine serum albumin and ovalbumin, respectively). Linear regression analysis allowed the tentative assignment of the molecular weight (Mr) of MT-2 MAF to be 55 kD. Isoelectric focusing analysis of MT-2 MAF demonstrated that MAF activity had an apparent isoelectric point of 5.5. The active fractions were further subjected to DEAE-ion exchange chromatography and this purification step was adequate to separate interferon-gamma and IL-2 activity from MAF activity, which eluted at 0.12 M salt in a linear salt gradient. The MAF activity was relatively stable under acidic conditions (1 M acetic acid) and at 100°C for 2 minutes. The activity was abrogated, however, by treatment with trypsin or pronase. The activity was not removed by treatment with Concanavalin A sepharose or 0.2 M mercaptoethanol.

Biological Properties of MT-2 MAF

Initially, the bioassay employed for the detection and identification of MT-2 MAF was the tumoricidal assay using human blood monocytes as effector cells and the human melanoma A375 cell line as the target cells. We have extended our studies to other activities mediated by this lymphokine in activating human monocytes. These include the production of reactive oxygen intermediates (9,25), the production of secretory proteins such as interleukin 1 (10), and the killing of intracellular microorganisms.

Lack of Relationship of MT-2 MAF to Other Lymphokine/Cytokines

Aside from gamma interferon, a number of defined lymphokine/cytokines have also been suggested to have macrophage activating activities. For example, the colony stimulating factors, CSF-1 (M-CSF) and CSF-2 (GM-CSF), had been reported to activate human monocytes to kill tumor cells (20,21). It was important, therefore, to establish the relationship between MT-2/MAF and the known macrophage activating proteins. Highly purified MT-2/MAF was devoid of the following activities: antiviral activity, colony stimulating activity, T cell growth or activating activity, and direct cytotoxic effect on tumor necrosis factor/lymphotoxin sensitive target cells. Biochemically, CSF-1 is the only known cytokine which shares major resemblance to that of MT-2/MAF. Using a specific and sensitive radioimmne assay for CSF-1, however, no CSF-1 was detectable. (Personal communication, E.R. Stanley). In fact, we have tested commercially available purified recombinant human GM-CSF as well as G-CSF, and have found them to be inactive in our tumoricidal and superoxide induction assays. Furthermore, we also found human BSF-1 to be inactive.

Implications for the Use of Human Non-Interferon Macrophage Activating Factors as Anti-Infective Therapy in Immunocompromised Hosts

Despite the considerable advances in the management of infectious diseases, infections remain a major cause of death in acquired immunodeficiency disease syndrome and other immunocompromised hosts and constitute a serious impediment to cancer treatment and organ transplantation. The appearance of new pulmonary infiltrate, in conjunction with fever, is recognized as one of the most common and serious complications to occur among immunosuppressed and myelosuppressed patients. For example, pneumonia may develop in as many as 80% of patients with acute leukemia, especially during periods of relapse and up to half of the patients will perish with unresolved pneumonia. Because of the complexity of the immunocompromised host, it seems unlikely that any single therapeutic or preventative modality will be uniformly successful. Therefore, in addition to the development of new antimicrobial agents, current investigations are focused on methods to enhance the depressed nonspecific host defenses as adjuvants to antimicrobial therapy in immunocompromised patients. Among the many immunomodulatory agents being studied, none holds more promise than the lymphokines which stimulate mononuclear phagocytes to kill pathogenic microorganisms and/or neoplastic cells. Included in this group are gamma-interferon, and the non-interferon macrophage activating factors such as the activity described here as well as granulocyte-macrophage colony stimulating factor. In preliminary _ex vivo_ studies, it has been demonstrated that the intratracheal delivery of recombinant rat gamma interferon activates rat alveolar macrophages to become both tumoricidal and microbicidal (Badger et al, unpublished observations). Thus, it is envisioned that with the advent of advanced drug delivery systems and the availability of highly purified recombinant derived macrophage activating factor, it will be possible to deliver the molecules to the infection site via the intratracheal or nasal route of administration.

REFERENCES

1. D.O. Adams and T.A. Hamilton, The cell biology of macrophage activation, _Ann. Rev. Immunol._ 2:283-318 (1984).
2. C.F. Nathan, H.W. Murray, M.E. Weibe, and B.Y. Rubin, Identification of interferon-gamma as the lymphokine that activates human macrophage oxidative metabolism and antimicrobial activity, _J. Exp. Med._ 158:670-689 (1983).
3. C.F. Nathan, T.J. Predergast, M.E. Wiebe, E.R. Stanley, E. Platzer, H.G. Remold, K. Welte, B.Y. Rubin, and H.W. Murray, Activation of human macrophages. Comparison of other cytokines with interferon-gamma, _J. Exp. Med._ 160:600-605 (1984).
4. R.D. Schreiber, Identification of gamma-interferon as a murine macrophage-activating factor for tumor cytotoxicity, _Contemp. Top. Immunobiology_ 13:171-198 (1984).
5. J. Le, W. Prensky, Y.K. Yip, Z. Chang, T. Hoffman, H.C. Stevenson, I. Balazs, J.R. Sadlik, and J. Vilcek, Activation of human monocyte cytotoxicity by natural and recombinant immune interferon, _J. Immunol._ 131:2821-2826 (1984).
6. R.D. Schreiber, J.L. Pace, S.W. Russell, A. Altman, and D.H. Katz, Macrophage activating factor produced by a T cell hybridoma: physicochemical and biosynthetic resemblance to γ-interferon, _J. Immunol._ 131:826-832 (1983).
7. J.C. Lee, L. Rebar, P. Young, F.W. Ruscetti, N. Hanna, and G. Poste, Identification and characterization of a human T cell-line derived lymphokine with MAF-like activity distinct from interferon-gamma, _J. Immunol._ 136:1322-1328 (1986).
8. J.C. Lee, Constitutive production of a non-interferon macrophage activating factor by HTLV-transformed T cells, _Lymphokine Research_ 5(S1):S127-S132 (1986).
9. J.C. Lee, A.M. Badger, W.J. Johnson, C.P. Sung, and P. Horan, Human non-gamma interferon macrophage activating factor (MT-2/MAF) elicits multiple and cross-species effects on macrophage activation, _Proceedings of the Sixth International Congress of Immunology_ (1986) (abstract).
10. J.C. Lee, L. Rebar, J. Laydon, B. Dalton, and P.L. Simon, Induction of interleukin-1 as an indicator for monocyte activation by macrophage activating factor (MT-2/MAF), _Lymphokine Research_ 6:61 (1987) (abstract).

11. D.L. Hoover, D.S. Finbloom, R.M. Crawford, C.A. Nacy, M. Gilbreath, and M.S. Meltzer, A lymphokine distinct from interferon-gamma that activates human monocytes to kill Leishmania donovani in vitro, J. Immunol. 136:1329-1333 (1986).
12. E.S. Kleinerman, R. Zicht, P.S. Sarin, R.C. Gallo, and I.J. Fidler, Constitutive production and release of a lymphokine with macrophage-activating factor activity distinct from gamma-interferon by a human T-cell leukemia virus-positive cell line, Cancer Res. 44:4470-4475 (1984).
13. P.W. Andrew, A.D.M. Rees, A. Scoging, N. Dobson, R. Mathews, J.T. Whitthall, A.R.M. Coates, and D.B. Lowrie, Secretion of a macrophage-activating factor distinct from interferon-gamma by human T cell clones, Eur. J. Immunol. 14:962-964 (1984).
14. M.S. Meltzer, M. Gilbreath, C.A. Nacy, and R.D. Schreiber, Macrophage activation factor from EL-4 cells distinct from murine gamma interferon (IFN), Fed. Proc. 44:1697 (1985) (abstract).
15. Y. Buchmuller, W.Y. Weiser, and H.G. Remold, Partial purification and characterization of a human lymphokine which induces anti-leishmanial activity in mouse macrophages, Cell. Immun. 90:242-250 (1985).
16. C.M. Jones, C.A. Prince, M.P. Langford, and J.P. Hester, Identification of a human monocyte cytotoxicity-inducing factor from T cell hybridomas produced from Sezary cells, J. Immunol. 137: 571-577 (1986).
17. S. Gregory, R.S. Kornbluth, H. Helin, H.G. Remold, and T.S. Edgington, Monocyte procoagulant inducing factor: A lymphokine involved in the T cell-instructed monocyte procoagulant response to antigen, J. Immunol. 137:3231-3239 (1986).
18. S. Hinuma, K. Sugamura, K. Tsukamoto, and Y. Hinuma, Constitutive production of phagocytosis inducing factor(s) in a monocyte/macrophage lineage cell line (THP-1) by retrovirus-transformed human T cell lines, Microbiol. Immunol. 28:935-947 (1984).
19. J.B. Margolick, J.L. Ambrus, Jr., D.J. Volkman, and A.S. Fauci, Human T4+ lymphocytes produce a phagocytosis-inducing factor (PIF) distinct from interferon-α and interferon-γ, J. Immunol. 136:546-554 (1986).
20. K.H. Grabstein, D.L. Urdal, R.J. Tushinshi, D.Y. Mochizuki, V.L. Price, M.A. Cantrell, S. Gillis, and P.J. Conlon, Induction of macrophage tumoricidal activity by granulocyte-macrophage colony-stimulating factor, Science 232-506 (1986).
21. M.K. Warren, and P. Ralph, Macrophage growth factor CSF-1 stimulates human monocyte production of interferon, tumor necrosis factor, and colony stimulating activity, J. Immunol. 137:2281-2285 (1986).
22. R.M. Crawford, D.S. Finbloom, J. Ohara, W.E. Paul, and M.S. Meltzer, B cell stimulatory factor-1 (interleukin 4) activates macrophages for increased tumoricidal activity and expression of Ia antigens, J. Immunol. 139:135-141 (1987).
23. S.A. Salahuddin, P.D. Markham, S.G. Lindner, J. Gotenberg, M. Popovic, H. Hemmit, P.S. Sarin, and R.C. Gallo, Lymphokine production by cultured human T cells transformed by human T-cell leukemia-lymphoma virus-I, Science 223:703-707 (1984).
24. I. Myoshi, I. Kuibonishi, S. Yoshimoto, R. Akagi, Y. Ohtsuki, Y. Shiraishi, K. Nagata and Y. Hinuma, Type C virus particles in an end T cell line derived by co-cultivating normal human cord leukocytes and human leukemia cells, Nature 294:770-771 (1981).
25. E. Pick, and D. Mizel, Rapid microassays for the measurement of superoxide and hydrogen peroxide production by macrophages in culture using an automatic enzyme immunoassay reader, J. Immunol. Methods 46:211-226 (1981).

REGULATION OF MACROPHAGE EFFECTOR FUNCTION BY B CELL STIMULATORY FACTOR-1 (BSF-1)

Robert M. Crawford, David S. Finbloom, Junichi Ohara, William E. Paul and Monte S. Meltzer

Walter Reed Army Institute of Research, Washington, DC 20307-5100, and National Institutes of Health, Bethesda, MD 20205

INTRODUCTION

Macrophages that accumulate during immune responses *in vivo* acquire a broad range of changes not present in the steady-state tissue macrophage or in cells from sterile, irritant-induced inflammatory reactions. These immunologically activated macrophages display increased levels of certain cell membrane components (Ia antigen, Fc receptors) and become cytotoxic to tumor and microbial target cells. Characterization of the lymphokines (LK) that regulate the activated macrophage, macrophage activation factors or MAF, remains one of the more controversial areas in immunology. Twenty years or even 10 years ago, there was a single, albeit uncharacterized MAF: migration inhibitory factor or MIF. This apparently simple situation rapidly evolved into a labyrinth of multiple LK factors, each with its own acronym: MIF, MAF, SMAF, MCF, MCIF, MCIF2 and others (1). Hope for resolution of this puzzle was provided by recent reports that recombinant gamma interferon (IFN) *alone*, induces many of the changes in macrophages that occur during immunologic activation. Indeed, several groups of investigators now propose IFN as the only MAF (2,3). But macrophage activation is not that simple. MAF physicochemically and biologically distinct from IFN have been described in both murine and human assay systems (4-8). Of special interest is the recent report that recombinant human GM-CSF activates peripheral blood monocytes to kill tumor target cells (9).

B cell stimulatory factor-1 (BSF-1) was initially defined as a LK cofactor with anti-IgM antibodies that initiated entry into S phase of resting B lymphocytes. Experiments with antibody affinity-purified or recombinant BSF-1 now show this LK to have wide ranging effects on both B and T cells. That macrophage cell lines also display large numbers of BSF-1 receptors, suggests that this LK may also affect macrophage function (10).

INDUCTION OF MACROPHAGE-MEDIATED TUMOR CYTOTOXICITY BY PURIFIED OR RECOMBINANT LYMPHOKINES

Macrophages from proteose-peptone induced peritoneal exudates were treated with dilutions of highly purified or recombinant murine LK and cultured with radiolabeled tumor cells (Figure 1). Cells treated with $\leq$ 250 units/ml recombinant IL-2 or partially purified IL-3 had little or no tumoricidal activity. In contrast, macrophages exposed to recombinant GM-CSF or antibody affinity-purified BSF-1 each developed significant cytotoxic activity. That recombinant murine GM-CSF induced macrophage-mediated tumor cytotoxicity (50% maximum cytotoxicity at 100 units GM-CSF/ml) confirms similar findings with recombinant human GM-CSF and peripheral blood monocytes (9). The observation that highly purified BSF-1 activated murine macrophages for tumor cytotoxicity was novel. In this experiment, 50% maximum cytotoxicity was induced in macrophages by about 20 units BSF-1/ml.

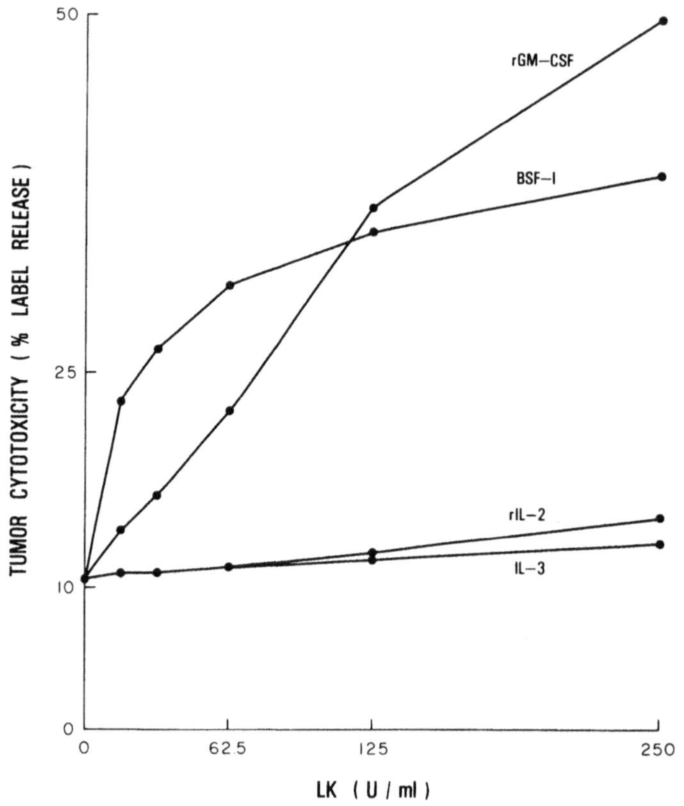

Figure 1. Tumor cytotoxicity by BSF-1, GM-CSF, IL-2 or IL-3 treated macrophages.

The titer of MAF activity in antibody affinity-purified BSF-1 for induction of macrophage-mediated tumor cytotoxicity was not affected by 5 ug/ml polymyxin B. This antibiotic inhibits the binding of lipid A to cell membranes on an equimolar basis. That polymyxin B did not affect BSF-1 activity on macrophages suggested little or no role for contaminant bacterial endotoxins in this system. Both antibody affinity-purified and recombinant BSF-1 induced macrophage tumoricidal activity: the titer of MAF activity in each BSF-1 preparation was identical. Neither antibody affinity-purified nor recombinant BSF-1 was directly toxic to the tumor target cells through

500 units/ml. The concentration of BSF-1 that induced 50% maximum tumor cytotoxicity was 38 ± 4 units/ml for 7 separate experiments.

INDUCTION OF MACROPHAGE-MEDIATED TUMOR CYTOTOXICITY BY COMBINATIONS OF DIFFERENT LYMPHOKINES

It was clear from the preceding experiments that MAF activity was a property of more than one LK: IFN, GM-CSF and BSF-1 each activated macrophages for tumor cytotoxicity. Indeed, it is also likely that during immune responses *in vivo*, macrophages are simultaneously exposed to multiple LK activation signals. To determine the influence of BSF-1 as a MAF under these

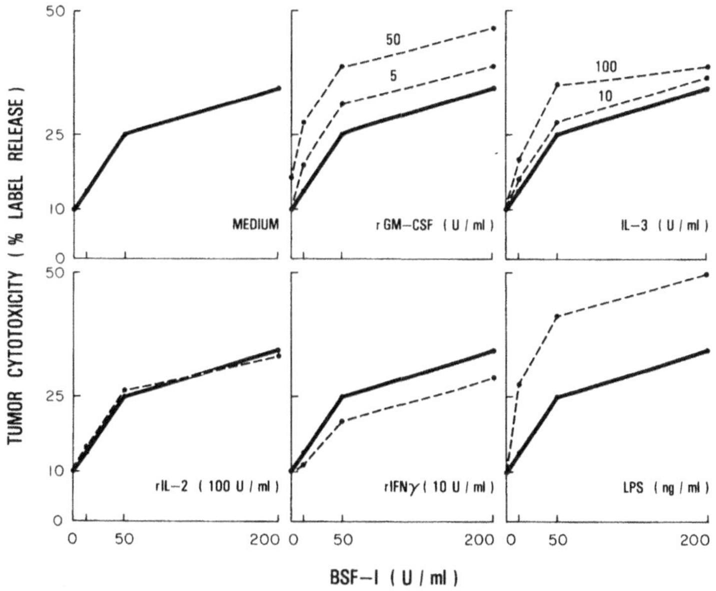

Figure 2. BSF-1 induced macrophage tumoricidal activity: effects of coincident treatment with other LK or LPS.

conditions, we treated macrophages with different concentrations of BSF-1 and any one of several other defined LK (Figure 2). Again, BSF-1 alone (heavy solid line) activated macrophages for tumoricidal activity: 50% maximum cytotoxicity was evident at about 40 units/ml. Further increases in the level of tumor cytotoxicity by BSF-1 activated macrophages were induced by addition of IL-3 (2 fold increase at 100 units IL-3/ml), GM-CSF (5 fold increase at 50 units GM-CSF/ml) and LPS (10 fold increase at 1 ng LPS/ml). No effect on the BSF-1 dose-response was evident with the addition of IL-2. Most surprisingly, IFN (a potent MAF by itself) actually inhibited by about 50% the induction of macrophage-mediated tumor cytotoxicity by BSF-1.

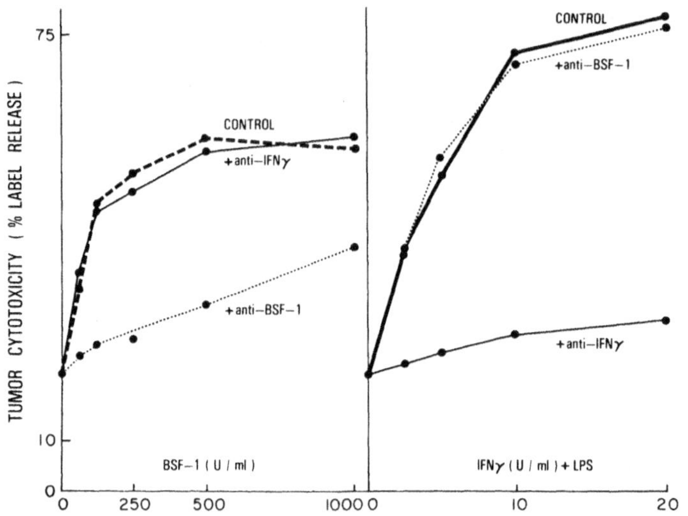

Figure 3. Inhibition of MAF activity by BSF-1 or IFN with specific neutralizing antibodies.

INHIBITION OF MAF ACTIVITY IN BSF-1 AND IFN BY NEUTRALIZING ANTIBODIES

The rat monoclonal anti-murine BSF-1, 11B11, neutralizes recombinant or antibody affinity-purified BSF-1 in the fluid phase (11). Ascitic fluid of the 11B11 hybridoma raised in nude mice had a neutralizing titer for BSF-1 dependent B cell proliferation of about 500 units BSF-1/mg protein. A similar neutralizing titer was evident for the IL-2 dependent T cell lines, CT6 or HT2: proliferative responses of these T cell lines were sustained by BSF-1 in the absence of added IL-2 (10). MAF activity induced by BSF-1 was neutralized by the 11B11 monoclonal anti-BSF-1 in fluid phase (Figure 3); an identical concentration of 11B11 antibody had no effect on macrophage-mediated tumor cytotoxicity induced by IFN or GM-CSF. Moreover, rabbit polyclonal anti-IFN had no effect on macrophage tumoricidal activity induced by BSF-1. Thus, MAF activity induced by either IFN or BSF-1 was specifically inhibited by the appropriate antibody. No functional cross-reactivity could be demonstrated by these assays.

BSF-1 INDUCTION OF MACROPHAGE Ia ANTIGEN AND Fc RECEPTOR EXPRESSION

Bone marrow-derived macrophages, $\geq$ 95% macrophages at 7 days, bind increased amounts of radioiodinated murine IgG immune complexes after 24 hr treatment with 10 units IFN/ml: IFN-treated cells bound 2470 $\pm$ 200 (mean $\pm$ sem for triplicate wells) cpm versus 1100 $\pm$ 120 cpm for untreated control cells. In the same experiment, equal numbers of bone marrow-derived macrophages treated with 100 units BSF-1/ml bound 3560 + 340 cpm, a 3-fold increase above control levels. In 3 subsequent experiments, the maximum Fc-dependent binding of radiolabeled immune complexes to BSF-1 treated bone marrow-derived macrophages was always significantly more than the maximum bound by equal numbers of IFN-treated cells.

About 5 to 10% of peritoneal macrophages from proteose peptone-induced inflammatory reactions express Ia antigen (Ia^k) by fluorescence microscopy. Further incubation of these cells in 20 units IFN/ml for 72 hrs increased the number of Ia-positive macrophages to 63 $\pm$ 6% (mean $\pm$ sem for triplicate cultures) versus 12 $\pm$ 5% for untreated control cultures. In the same experiment, proteose peptone-elicited macrophages treated with 200 units BSF-1/ml were 48 $\pm$ 7% Ia positive after 3 days in culture. An irrelevant Ia antigen (Ia^d) remained at baseline levels with all treatments. Thus by fluorescence microscopy, macrophage Ia antigen expression was markedly increased by both IFN and BSF-1.

DISCUSSION

The preceding data clearly document BSF-1 regulation of macrophage function: recombinant or affinity-purified BSF-1 induced macrophage-mediated cytotoxicity against tumor target cells; BSF-1 also induced increased expression of Ia antigen and Fc-IgG receptors on macrophage plasma membranes. Each of these responses is induced by recombinant IFN, the prototypic MAF. Furthermore, most of these responses are also induced by recombinant GM-CSF. Thus IFN, BSF-1 and GM-CSF are each MAF that ostensibly induce identical changes in macrophage function. LK regulation of macrophage effector function is not only complex but redundant, why? One explanation for redundancy in the regulation of macrophage function is safety. There are many, well-documented examples for subversion of host immunity by infectious agents. Multiple and distinct signals that control reactions vital to host survival provide a failsafe mechanism against pathologic change.

But redundancy in MAF may also occur for other reasons. Different MAF may act on certain macrophage subpopulations. Even with a single MAF, variation in response is evident with cells from different body compartments. The level of tumoricidal activity induced by IFN in inflammatory macrophages is more than 10-fold greater than that induced in an equal number of resident peritoneal cells. Yet, the number of IFN receptors/cell for inflammatory and resident macrophages are comparable. The number of macrophages able to be infected with *Rickettsia tsutsugamushi* in resident and inflammatory cell populations are equal. Small amounts of IFN ($\leq$ 10 u/ml) added to infected cell cultures activates macrophages to kill the intracellular bacteria. In contrast to tumoricidal activity, no difference in IFN dose-response is detected between resident and inflammatory cell populations for induction of this microbicidal activity. Similarly, macrophages infected with amastigotes of *Leishmania major* also respond to IFN and develop microbicidal activity. In this case, microbicidal activity induced in the resident macrophage population is more than 10-fold greater than that induced in inflammatory macrophages (12).

Different MAF may be released by distinct T cell subpopulations. Recent experiments document selective release of LK by certain T cell subsets or after treatment with immunosuppressive agents (13). Moreover, T cells that accumulate in lesions of leishmaniasis or leprosy may have a relatively selective defect in production of certain LK (14). Different MAF may appear at different times during the evolution of an immune response or be operative only within certain body compartments. In this context, it should be noted that IFN is acid labile but BSF-1 resists degradation at low pH. Finally, different MAF may interact with each other to amplify and/or suppress the ultimate macrophage effector response.

The true pathophysiologic role for each MAF can only be assessed in the intact host. These studies are difficult, but experiments such as those reported by Schreiber and colleagues with anti-IFN and murine listeriosis document that they are not impossible (15). Potentially, identification of relevant MAF in infectious or neoplastic disease provides a basis for rational immunotherapeutic intervention.

REFERENCES

1. M.S. Meltzer, R.M. Crawford, D.S. Finbloom and C.A. Nacy. 1987. Lymphokine macrophage activation factors for induction of nonspecific, macrophage-mediated cytotoxicity against tumor cell and microbial targets, In: "Biological Response Modifiers and Cancer Research," J.W. Chiao, ed., Marcel Dekker, Inc., New York (in press).
2. C.F. Nathan, H.W. Murray, M.E. Wiebe and B.Y. Rubin. 1983. Identification of interferon-gamma as the lymphokine that activates human macrophage oxidative metabolism and antimicrobial activity, J. Exp. Med. 158:670.
3. L.P. Svedersky, C.V. Benton, W.H. Berger, E. Rinderknecht, R.N. Harkins and M.A. Palladino. 1984. Biological and antigenic similarities of murine interferon-gamma and macrophage activating factor, J. Exp. Med. 159:812.
4. M.S. Meltzer, W.R. Benjamin and J.J. Farrar. 1982. Macrophage activation for tumor cytotoxicity, induction and macrophage tumoricidal activity by lymphokines from EL-4, a continuous T cell line, J. Immunol. 129:2802.
5. E.S. Kleinerman, R. Zicht, P.S. Sarin, R.C. Gallo and I.J. Fidler. 1984. Constitutive production and release of a lymphokine with macrophage-activating factor activity distinct from gamma-interferon by a human T-cell leukemia virus-positive cell lines, Cancer Res. 44:4470.
6. C.A. Nacy, A.H. Fortier, M.S. Meltzer, N.A. Buchmeier and R.D. Schreiber. 1986. Macrophage activation to kill *Leishmania major*: activation of macrophages for intracellular destruction of amastigotes can be induced by both recombinant interferon-gamma and non-interferon lymphokines, J. Immunol. 135:3505.
7. D.L. Hoover, D.S. Finbloom, R.M. Crawford, C.A. Nacy, M.G. Gilbreath and M.S. Meltzer. 1986. A lymphokine distinct from interferon-gamma activates human monocytes to kill *Leishmania donovani* in vitro, J. Immunol. 136:1329.
8. J.C. Lee, L. Rebar, P. Young, F.W. Ruscetti, N. Hanna and G. Poste. 1986. Identification and characterization of a human T cell line-derived lymphokine with MAF-like activity distinct from interferon-gamma, J. Immunol. 136:1322.
9. K.H. Grabstein, D.L. Urdal, R.J. Tushinshi, D.Y. Mochizuki, V.L. Price, M.A. Cantrell, S. Gillis and P.J. Conlon. 1986. Induction of macrophage tumoricidal activity by granulocyte-macrophage colony-stimulating factor, Science 232:506.
10. W.E. Paul and J. Ohara. 1987. B cell stimulatory factor-1/interleukin 4, Ann. Rev. Immunol. in press.
11. J. Ohara and W.E. Paul. 1985. Production of a monoclonal antibody to and molecular characterization of B-cell stimulatory factor-1, Nature 315:333.
12. C.A. Nacy, C.N. Oster, S.L. James and M.S. Meltzer. 1984. Microbicidal effector reactions of activated macrophages against intracellular and extracellular parasites, Cont. Topics Immunobiol. 14:147.
13. T.R. Mosmann, H. Cherwinski, M.W. Bond, M.A. Giedlin and R.L. Coffman. 1986. Two types of murine helper T cell clone. I. Definition according to profiles of lymphokine activities and secreted proteins, J. Immunol. 136:2348.

14. R.L. Modlin, F.M. Hofman, D.A. Horwitz, L.A. Husmann, S. Gillis, C.R. Taylor and T.H. Rea. 1984. In situ identication of cells in human leprosy granulomas with monoclonal antibodies to interleukin 2 and its receptor, J. Immunol. 132:3085.
15. N.A. Buchmeier and R.D. Schreiber. 1985. Requirement of endogenous interferon-gamma production for resolution of Listeria monocytogenes infection, Proc. Natl. Acad. Sci. 82:7404.

IDENTIFICATION AND CHARACTERIZATION OF A NON-INTERFERON ANTILEISHMANIAL MACROPHAGE ACTIVATING FACTOR (ANTILEISHMANIAL MAF)

Anthony Van Niel, Susan E. Zacks, John R. David, Heinz G. Remold, and Weishui Y. Weiser

Department of Medicine, Harvard Medical School and Department of Rheumatology and Immunology, Brigham and Women's Hospital Boston, Massachusetts 02115

INTRODUCTION

Macrophages, the final effector cells in many cellular immune responses are capable of destroying a variety of intracellular pathogens such as viruses, fungi, chlamydia, rickettsiae and leishmania (1,2) as well as neoplastic cells (3). However, the biochemical identity of macrophage activating factor (MAF), and therefore the elucidation of its mechanism of action on macrophages have remained ill-defined. In part, this has been due to the limited amounts of MAF produced under conventional conditions, amounts insufficient to achieve a full biochemical purification of this factor. In addition, conventional culture supernatants of activated T cells normally contain a heterogeneous mixture of lymphokines, such as interferon-gamma (IFN-gamma), granulocyte macrophage colony stimulating factor (GM-CSF) and macrophage migration inhibitory factor (MIF) that can all affect the functions of macrophages. Although both human and murine interferon-gamma have been attributed to be the lymphokines to activate macrophages for enhanced oxidative and antimicrobial activity (4-7), numerous reports also demonstrated the existence of non-IFN-gamma MAFs (8-12).

The data reported here show that antileishmanial MAF, a human lymphokine which is elaborated by stimulated T-CEMA cells (cells from a T-cell hybridoma) and is distinguishable from IFN-gamma, is also a potent activator of cultured human monocyte-derived macrophages and induces the intracellular killing of *Leishmania donovani* by these cells.

MATERIALS AND METHODS

Parasites. Promastigotes of *L. donovani* were obtained from the World Health Organization, Geneva, Switzerland and were maintained in vitro at 26°C in tissue culture flask containing Schneider's drosophila medium (GIBCO Laboratories, Grand Island, NY), 20% heat-inactivated fetal calf serum (FCS), and 5 ng/ml gentamycin (M.A. Bioproducts, Walkersville, MD). The parasites were subcultured by weekly passage at 1:10 dilution.

Cells. Human peripheral blood was obtained from healthy volunteers. Mononuclear cells isolated by Ficoll-Hypaque density centrifugation were suspended at 2.5 x 10^6 cells/ml in medium 199 (M.A. Bioproducts) containing 15% heat-inactivated FCS, 2 mM L-glutamine (GIBCO Laboratories), and 5 ng/ml gentamycin and seeded on top of 4 glass coverslips in a 35 mm petri dish (Falcon Labware, Oxnard, CA). After 2 hours of incubation at 37°C the nonadherent cells were removed by washing, and the remaining cells were incubated for 10-12 days in a 5% CO_2 atmosphere to obtain monocyte-derived macrophages. After 10 days, the monolayers consisted of 95-97% macrophages, as determined by morphology and esterase staining.

Production and partial purification of antileishmanial MAF. A human T-cell hybridoma line, T-CEMA, constructed through the fusion of cells from a HAT-sensitive T-cell line (CEM-WH4) with T-cells from human peripheral blood (13) was used as the source of the lymphokines. For the production of lymphokines, T-CEMA cells at 1 x 10^6/ml were cultured in serum free medium consisting of RPMI 1640, 2 mM L-glutamine, 10 ng/ml phorbol myristate acetate (PMA, Sigma Chemical Co.), and 10 µg/ml concanavalin A (Con A, Miles Laboratories, Inc., Naperville, IL). After 48 hr of incubation at 37°C in a humidified 95% air, 5% CO_2, incubator, supernatants were removed and concentrated. The material from 500 ml supernatant was chromatographed on a precalibrated Sephadex G-100 column (2.5 x 100 cm). Fractions containing antileishmanial activity were collected, concentrated and isoelectrofocused (IEF) on LKB 8102 ampholine eletrofocusing equipment (LKB producter, Bromma, Sweden) using ampholines with an isoelectric point range of 2.5 to 6.0, stabilized in a sucrose density gradient as previously described (14). After 24 hr of IEF at 6 W, the gradient was drained into tubes containing 0.5 mg of human serum albumin (Sigma Chemical Co.) in 0.5 ml of water. After measuring the pH, tubes were pooled to yield 11 fractions which were dialyzed and concentrated before use.

Infection of monocyte-derived macrophages. Promastigotes of *L. donovani* at the stationary growth phase were used to infect macrophages which have been pretreated with various dilutions of antileishmanial MAF or IFN-gamma. The parasite to cell ratio was approximately 10:1 in all experiments. After 2 hours of incubation at 37°C, the uningested parasites were removed by washing, and the cultures were reincubated in fresh medium. Coverslips were removed at 2, 24, 48 and 72 hr, washed in phosphate buffered saline, and stained with Diff-Quick stain (American Scientific Products, McGaw Park, IL); the number of intracellular parasites was determined by microscopy. From each coverslip, 3-4 randomly selected areas were examined; each consisted of 100 cells.

MIF assay. MIF activity was assayed as described (13) employing human peripheral blood monocytes as indicator cells in an agarose droplet assay system. Briefly, 1 µl of monocytes in the agarose mixture was dispensed into the center of each microtiter well using a 50 µl repeating dispenser. Samples to be tested were added to wells at 100 µl per well. The size of each agarose droplet was measured. After overnight incubation at 37°C, the total area of migration including the original agarose droplet was again measured and the migration was calculated. The percentage of inhibition (%I) was derived as (1-average area of migration in MIF-containing sample/ average area of migration in control sample) x 100. Inhibition of greater than 20% was considered to be significant.

Antiviral activity of IFN-gamma. The antiviral activity of human IFN-gamma was determined in human fibroblasts (GM 2767, Institute for Medical Research, Camden, NJ) using vesicular stomatitis virus as previously described (14). The sensitivity of this assay was approximately 0.5 U/ml. The titer of IFN-gamma was also assessed by RIA-IFN-gamma assay (Centocor, Malvern, PA). The neutralizing activity of polyclonal and monoclonal anti-IFN antibodies (Meloy Laboratories, Springfield, VA) was titrated by their ability to abrogate antiviral activity in vitro.

RESULTS

Identification of antileishmanial MAF from a human T-cell hybridoma line, T-CEMA. Various concentrations of PMA and Con A-stimulated supernatants from 8 human T-cell hybridomas were screened for antileishmanial MAF activity. After 1-3 days of pretreatment, macrophages were challenged for 2 hours with promastigotes of L. donovani. Uningested parasites were removed by washing, the medium was replaced, the percentage of cells infected and the number of parasites/100 macrophages were enumerated in stained preparations of cover slips. Among the 8 T-cell hybridoma lines tested, supernatant from T-CEMA was found to contain the best and the most reproducible

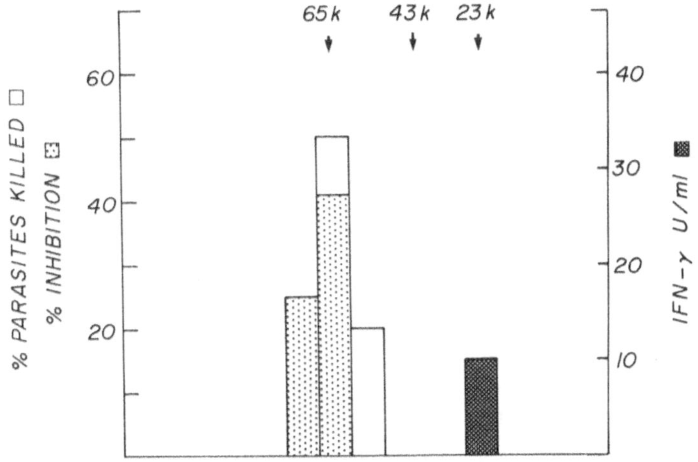

Figure 1. Lymphokine activities of T-CEMA supernatants after Sephadex G-100 chromatography

a. Antileishmanial activity was assessed 48 hours after infection by counting and comparing the number of parasites/100 macrophages in both control and MAF treated cultures.
b. MIF activity was measured by agarose droplet method and expressed as % inhibition.
c. The titer of IFN-gamma was determined by antiviral activity and based on parallel assay of NIH human IFN-alpha standard.

antileishmanial activity. Supernatants from T-CEMA cells were also examined for MIF activity and for the presence of IFN-gamma. The former was determined by agarose droplet MIF assay, whereas the latter was determined by antiviral activity. It was found that, in addition to antileishmanial activity, supernatants from T-CEMA cells also contain MIF activity and low titers of IFN-gamma.

In order to examine the molecular weight of these mediators and to investigate whether the different activities can be seperated, supernatants derived from stimulated T-CEMA cells were subjected to Sephadex G-100 chromatography. Fractions were pooled and tested for all three activities. As can be seen in Figure 1, antileishmanial MAF and MIF but not IFN-gamma cochromatograph and share the same apparent mw of 65,000. The IFN-gamma with an apparent mw of less than 23,000 is thus separated from the antileishmanial MAF and MIF by gel chromatography.

It was also found that mRNA obtained from PMA and Con A-stimulated T-CEMA cells hybridized with cDNA probe of recombinant GM-CSF. Therefore, antileishmanial MAF was examined for colony stimulating activity using KG-1 cells (15). However, no colony stimulating activity could be detected (Experiments kindly performed by Dr. S.C. Clark). Furthermore, treatment of antileishmanial MAF with anti-GM-CSF antiserum was unable to diminish the antileishmanial activity of this lymphokine.

Antileishmanial MAF and MIF share the same isoelectric point. To establish the isoelectric point of antileishmanial MAF and to examine whether antileishmanial MAF could be dissociated from MIF, fractions containing both activities obtained after gel chromatography were subjected to IEF. Fractions with a pH range of 0.3 to 0.5 were pooled and analyzed for antileishmanial and MIF activities. The results of two experiments are listed in Table 1.

IFN-gamma has been demonstrated to activate macrophages for intracellular killing of *L. donovani* (5). To further establish the non-interferon identity of this antileishmanial MAF, antileishmanial MAF obtained from gel chromatography and IEF was examined for the presence of IFN-gamma by antiviral assay and by RIA-IFN assay. No IFN was detected by either method. In addition, treatment of antileishmanial MAF with monoclonal as well as polyclonal anti-IFN-gamma antibodies could not reduce the biologic activity of antileishmanial MAF.

Antileishmanial MAF can be distinguished from MIF by monoclonal anti-MIF antibody. Since antileishmanial MAF and MIF were found to cochromatograph and to cofocus, fractions containing both activities were preincubated with monoclonal anti-MIF antibody for 30 min at 37°C (Exp. 1, Exp. 2) or subjected to elution from anti-MIF bound protein A Sepharose column (Exp. 3) before being employed to activate human monocyte derived macrophages for intracellular killing of *L. donovani* in order to investigate whether these two lymphokines could be dissociated from each other antigenically. The

Table 1. Distribution of antileishmanial activity and MIF activity after isoelectric focusing

pH	Antileishmanial Activity % Parasites Killed		MIF Activity % Inhibition	
2.0-2.4	0	0	14	17
2.4-2.9	0	0	0	13
2.9-3.3	0	0	0	0
3.3-3.6	0	0	0	0
3.6-4.0	0	0	0	0
4.0-4.3	0	0	0	10
4.3-4.6	0	0	0	0
4.6-5.0	0	8	0	0
5.0-5.3	7	2	19	11
5.3-5.6	56	41	48	59
5.6-6.1	5	6	12	0

Table 2. Antileishmanial MAF is not neutralized by monoclonal anti-MIF antibody

Treatment	Antileishmanial Activity % Parasites Killed Exp. 1	Exp. 2	Exp. 3	MIF Activity % Inhibition Exp. 1	Exp. 2	Exp. 3
MAF + anti-MIF	37 ± 5	48 ± 3	37 ± 2			
MAF only	43 ± 4	51 ± 3	39 ± 4			
MIF + anti-MIF				-5	-7	-8
MIF only				48	39	42

data presented are percent of parasites killed in treated cultures 48 hours after infection as compared to that of parasites in untreated cultures. MIF activity before and after treatment with anti-MIF antibody was assayed simultaneously. As can been seen in Table 2, anti-MIF antibody has no effect on antileishmanial MAF.

DISCUSSION

Supernatants derived from 10 ng/ml PMA and 10 ug/ml Con A-stimulated T-cell hybridoma, T-CEMA, have been found to contain antileishmanial MAF, MIF and antiviral activities. The objectives of this study are to establish the identity of the antileishmanial activity and to investigate whether the antileishmanial activity is induced exclusively by IFN-gamma (5) or can also be mediated by a lymphokine distinct from IFN-gamma.

In the present study, we have shown that a lymphokine, antileishmanial MAF, which is distinct form IFN-gamma can also activate human peripheral blood monocyte-derived macrophages to exhibit enhanced intracellular killing of L. donovani. This antileishmanial MAF, which has an apparent mw of 65,000 and pI of 5.3-5.6 is dissociated from IFN-gamma by gel chromatography and by isoelectric focusing. Although this antileishmanial MAF shares the same molecular weight and isoelectric point with MIF, it can be separated from the latter by elution from an anti-MIF bound protein A Sepharose column.

Recently, the contribution of highly active NK-cells which are present in small numbers in monocyte preparations to extracellular cytotoxicity has gained increasing attention (16). This finding is important because target cells which have been employed in tumor killing assays were found to be susceptible to NK-cell killing. We have, however, circumvented this problem by assessing intracellular killing associated exclusively with macrophages.

mRNA derived from stimulated T-CEMA cells was found to hybridize with cDNA probe of GM-CSF, a mediator that differentiates and expands cells of granulocyte and macrophage lineage (15,17). Since GM-CSF has been shown to alter the physiology of mature neutrophils (18) and eosinophils (19) and to activate macrophages for extracellular killing of tumor cells (12), fractions containing antileishmanial activity was also assayed for colony stimulating activity. However, no CSF activity was detected nor could treatment of antileishmanial MAF with anti-GM-CSF antiserum abrogate any antileishmanial activity. In the context of GM-CSF, it is of note that other studies have also addressed the process of macrophage activation by GM-CSF. It was demonstrated by Handman and Burgess (20) that conditioned medium from mouse spleen cells containing GM-CSF activity was able to enhance ingestion and killing of L. tropica by mouse macrophages. On the other hand, Ralph et al., (21) also using conditioned medium from mouse spleen cells, reported that GM-CSF does not play a role in the induction of tumoricidal and microbicidal activity of mouse macrophages.

In summary, we have shown that a non-interferon lymphokine is also able to induce intracellular killing of L. donovani by monocyte-derived macrophages. Our findings, together with the findings of others add to the growing body of evidence that IFN-gamma is not the only lymphokine capable of activating macrophages but that IFN-gamma is one of several MAFs which may function independently or synergistically in controlling infection and combatting neoplastic growth.

SUMMARY

A non-interferon lymphokine elaborated from PHA and Con A-stimulated human T-cell hybridoma, T-CEMA, has been found to activate monocyte-derived macrophages for the intracellular killing of L. donovani (antileishmanial MAF). This T-cell hybridoma derived antileishmanial MAF which has an apparent mw of 65,000 and pI of 5.3-5.6, contains neither antiviral activity nor colony stimulating activity. Furthermore, antileishmanial MAF is not neutalized by anti-MIF, anti-IFN-gamma or anti-GM-CSF antibodies.

REFERENCES

1. Nacy, C.A., C.N. Oster, S.L. James, and M.S. Meltzer. 1984. Activation of macrophages to kill Rickettsiae and Leishmania: Dissociation of intracellular microbicidal activities and extracellular destruction of neoplastic and helminth targets. Contemporary Topics in Immunobiology. 13:146.
2. Murray, H.W. 1984. Macrophage activation: Enhanced oxidative and antiprotozoal activity. Contemporary Topics in Immunobiology 13:97.
3. Adams, D.O., and T.A. Hamilton. 1984. The cell biology of macrophage activation. Ann. Rev. Immunol. 2:283.
4. Murray, H.W., and D.M. Cartelli. 1983. Killing of intracellular Leishmania donovani by human mononuclear phagocytes. Evidence for oxygen-dependent and -independent leishmanicidal activity. J. Clin. Invest. 72:32.
5. Nathan, C.F., H.W. Murray, M.E. Wiebe, and B.Y. Rubin. 1983. Identification of interferon-gamma as the lymphokine that activates human macrophage oxidative metabolism and antimicrobial activity. J. Exp. Med. 158:670.
6. Murray, H.W., G.L. Spitalny, and C.F. Nathan. 1985. Activation of mouse peritoneal macrophages in vitro and in vivo by IFN-gamma. J. Immunol. 134:1619.
7. Rothermel, C.D., B.Y. Rubin, E.A. Jaffe, and H.W. Murray. 1986. Oxygen-independent inhibition of intracellualr Chlamydia psittaci growth by human monocytes and interferon-gamma-activated macrophages. J. Immunol. 137:689.
8. Gately, C.L., S.M. Wahl, and J.J. Oppenheim. 1983. Characterization of hydrogen peroxide-potentiating factor, a lymphokine that increases the capacity of human monocyte and monocyte-like cell lines to produce hydrogen peroxide. J. Immunol. 131:2853.
9. Buchmuller, Y., W.Y. Weiser, and H. Remold. 1985. Partial purication and characterization of a human lymphokine which induces antileishmanial activity in mouse macrophages. Cell. Immunol. 90:242.
10. Lee, J.C., L. Rebar, P. Young, F.W. Ruscetti, N. Hanna, and G. Poste. 1986. Identification and characterization of a human T-cell line-derived lymphokine with MAF-like activity distinct from interferon-gamma. J. Immunol. 136:1322.

11. Hoover, D.L., D.S. Finbloom, R.M. Crawford, C.S. Nacy, M. Gilgreath, and M.S. Meltzer. 1986. A lymphokine distinct from interferon-gamma that activates human monocytes to kill Leishmania donovani in vitro. J. Immunol. 136:1329.
12. Grabstein, K.H., D.L. Urdal, R.J. Tushiuski, D.Y. Mochizuki, V.L. Price, M.A. Cantrell, S. Gillis and P. Conlon. 1986. Induction of macrophage tumoricidal activity by granulocyte-macrophage colony-stimulating factor. Science 232:506.
13. Weiser, W.Y., H.G. Remold, and J.R. David. 1985. Generation of human hybridomas producing migration inhibitory factor (MIF) and of murine hybridomas secreting monoclonal antibodies to human MIF. Cell. Immunol. 90:167.
14. Weiser, W.Y., H.G. Remold, L.H. Block, and J.R. David. 1984. Dissociation of human interferon-gamma like activity from migration inhibitory factor. Cell. Immunol. 88:109.
15. Wong, G.G., J.S. Witek, PA. Temple, K.M. Wilkens, A.C. Leary, D.P. Luxenberg, S.S. Jones, E.L. Brown, R.M. Kay, E.C. Orr, C. Shoemaker, D.W. Golde, R.J. Kaufman, R.M. Hewick, E. Wang, and S.C. Clark. 1985. Human GM-CSF: Molecular cloning of the complementary DNA and purification of the natural and recombinant proteins. Science 228:810.
16. Koren, H.S., and R.B. Herberman. 1985. The current status of human monocyte mediated cytotoxicity against tumor cells. J. Leukocyte Biol. 38:441.
17. Burgess, A.W., and D. Metcalf. 1980. The nature and action of granulocyte-macrophage colony stimulation factor. Blood 56:947.
18. Gasson, J.C., R.H. Weisbart, S.E. Kaufman, S.C. Clark, and R.M. Hewick. 1984. Purified human granulocyte-macrophage colony-stimulating factor: Direct action on neutrophils. Science 226:1339.
19. Silberstein, D.S., W.F. Owen, J.C. Gasson, J.F. Dipersio, D.W. Gold, J.C. Bina, R. Soberman, K.F. Austen, and J.R. David. 1986. Enhancement of human eosinophil cytotoxicity and leukotriene synthesis by biosynthetic (recombinant) granulocyte-macrophage colony-stimulating factor. J. Immunol. 137:3290.
20. Handman, E., and A.W. Burgess. 1979. Stimulation by granulocyte-macrophage colony-stimulating factor of Leishmania tropica killing by macrophages. J. Immunol. 122:1134.
21. Ralph, P., C.A. Nacy, M.S. Meltzer, N. Williams, I. Nakoinz, and E.J. Leonard. 1983. Colony-stimulating factors and regulation of macrophage tumoricidal and microbicidal activities. Cell. Immunol. 76:10.

LYMPHOKINE-INDUCED MACROPHAGE RESISTANCE TO INFECTION WITH *LEISHMANIA MAJOR*

Miodrag Belosevic, Charles E. Davis, Monte S. Meltzer, and Carol A. Nacy

Department of Immunology, Walter Reed Army Institute of Research, Washington, D.C. 20307-5100

INTRODUCTION

Leishmania are obligately intracellular protozoan parasites whose host cell within infected humans and experimental animals is the macrophage. Development of an effective immune response to these organisms presents a unique immunologic predicament: the cell that sustains parasite viability within the host is also the central effector cell for induction of immune responses and expression of cytotoxic effector reactions. Once the parasite is inside a macrophage, it is protected from many of the humoral host defense mechanisms that develop during infectious diseases. Resolution of infection, then, is primarily dependent upon extraordinary alterations in the intracellular environment of the macrophage that lead to death of the parasite, or elimination of the infected cell itself (4,8,9). An alternative approach for intervention in the cycle of infection with *Leishmania* is the development of macrophages resistant to infection with the parasite. Macrophages from animals that are undergoing a vigorous immune response to an infectious agent ingest fewer obligate or facultatively intracellular pathogens in vitro than macrophages from uninfected mice (8,14). In fact, this decreased uptake of parasites, which we call "resistance to infection", has been observed in activated macrophages obtained from mice infected with *Mycobacterium bovis* strain BCG, as well as macrophages from *L. donovani*-infected mice that were resolving systemic disease (5,14).

The observations of enhanced resistance to infection by in vivo activated macrophages can be reproduced in vitro by treatment of cells with the soluble mediators released by antigen or mitogen-stimulated spleen cells (lymphokines, LK). These LK dramatically alter the capacity of *Leishmania major* to infect and replicate within macrophages. At least two different phenomena account for the increase in parasite-free macrophages observed in cultures treated with LK before exposure to the amastigote forms of *L. major*: (a) an initial alteration in macrophage-parasite interaction that results in fewer infected macrophages shortly (1 to 2 hr) after exposure to the parasites (LK-induced resistance to infection), and (b) destruction of residual intracellular organisms over 24-72 hr (LK-induced intracellular killing) (7).

LK-induced decrease in susceptibility of macrophages to infection with *L. major* is a persistent change in macrophage phenotype: cells resist infection through 96 hr after treatment with LK (12). Not only is this change persistent, but it is also nonspecific. Macrophages treated with LK resist infection with several antigenically diverse microorganisms (leishmania, rickettsia, legionella and mycobacteria) whose survival depends upon rapid entry into cells (1-3,5,6,11,13,14): these organisms have evolved unique mechanisms to facilitate their uptake into cells, and each must be metabolically active for infection to occur. Activated macrophages that resist infection with metabolically active intracellular pathogens remain phagocytic, and avidly ingest latex beads, erythrocytes, nonviable _Candida_, and complement or immunoglobulin-coated particles (10). They do not, however, ingest dead leishmania or rickettsiae. It is interesting to note that resistance to infection is also not observed with the _Chlamydia_, another obligate intracellular microorganism; the infectious EB particle of _Chlamydia_, however, is metabolically inert. It is possible that the mechanism of resistance to infection disrupts the metabolic integrity of certain intracellular parasites, and thus compromises the essential parasite-facilitated entry into cells. Since resistance to infection also occurs with macrophages activated in vivo, LK that induce resistance to infection have strong potential for use as prophylactic immunomodulating agents for defense against a variety of pathogenic microorganisms.

In this report, we show that the induction of macrophages resistant to infection by _L. major_ is absolutely dependent upon the cooperation of gamma-interferon (IFN) and other macrophage activation factors which are antigenically and physicochemically distinct from IFN.

RESISTANCE TO INFECTION

To evaluate LK-induced resistance to infection, we developed a cell pellet culture system that permits quantitative determination of the percent infected macrophages. Resident peritoneal macrophages from untreated C3H/HeN mice exposed to conventional LK (culture fluids of PPD-stimulated spleen cells from BCG-infected mice) develop the capacity to resist infection with _L. major_ (Fig. 1):

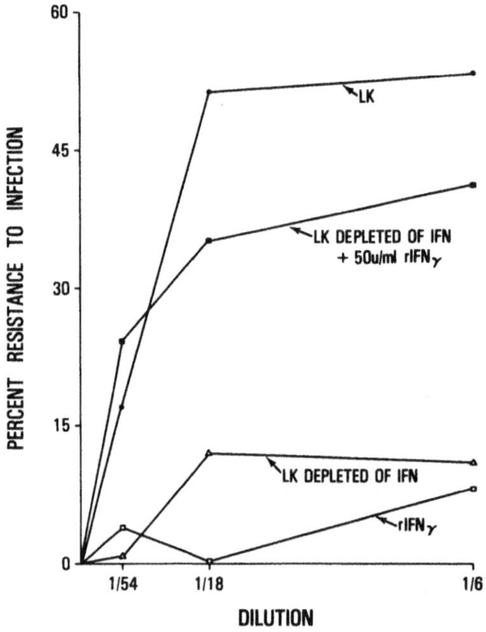

Fig. 1. Peritoneal macrophages treated with LK or IFN for induction of resistance to infection with amastigotes of _L. major_.

A minimum of 4 hr LK treatment of cells before addition of parasites is required for expression of this activated macrophage effector function. Once initiated, this effector activity persists for up to 96 hrs. Typically, LK-induced resistance to infection is manifest by 40% to 60% fewer infected macrophages than that found in control cultures. Removal of IFN from LK by immunoaffinity chromatography completely abolished the capacity of LK to induce resistance to infection (Fig. 1). The addition of recombinant IFN (5 to 50 U/ml), itself ineffective in induction of this effector activity, restored capacity of the inactive IFN-depleted LK to induce resistance to infection (Fig. 1). Thus resident peritoneal macrophage resistance to infection with L. major requires at least 2 LK activities: one activity is IFN, the other is antigenically distinct from IFN.

The resident peritoneal cells of the preceding experiment were about 50% macrophages. It is possible that the other cell types in these cultures influence development of LK-induced macrophage resistance to infection. To determine whether the induction of this effector activity by LK occurred via direct action on macrophages, we used two approaches: (a) T-lymphocytes (40% of resident peritoneal cell populations) were removed using anti-Thy 1.2 antibody and complement before the addition of LK. Removal of these cells did not affect the capacity of LK to induce macrophage resistance to infection, and (b) the capacity of LK to induce resistance to infection in macrophages derived from 7 day bone marrow cultures (greater than 98% macrophages) was assessed. As shown in Fig. 2, bone marrow macrophages in the absence of any other contaminating cell types developed the capacity to resist infection with L. major when treated with LK. Again, IFN or LK depleted of IFN were each ineffective for induction of resistance to infection, but the IFN-reconstituted LK was as potent as the unfractionated material.

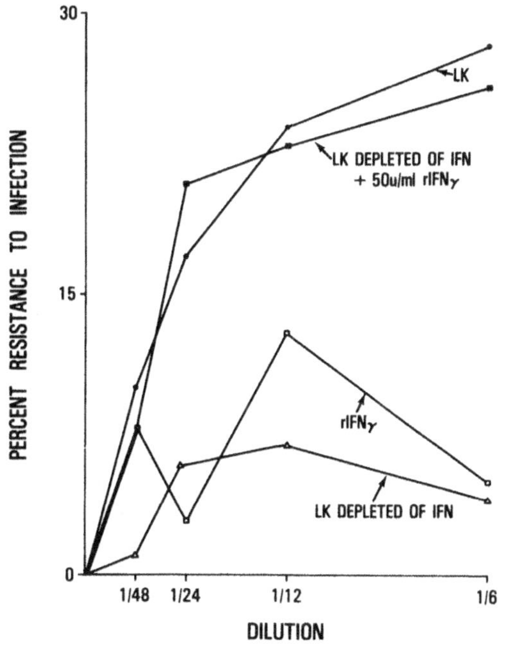

Fig. 2. Bone marrow macrophages (day 7 in culture) treated with LK or IFN for induction of resistance to infection with amastigotes of L. major.

Thus, by both experimental approaches, induction of macrophage resistance to infection was a result of the direct action of LK on macrophages, and was not dependent upon contaminant T lymphocytes. It should be noted that capacity of bone marrow macrophages to resist infection with amastigotes (30% resistance to infection) was consistently lower than that of peritoneal macrophages (40% to 60% resistance to infection).

COOPERATION OF LK FOR INDUCTION OF MACROPHAGE RESISTANCE TO IFNECTION

LK activation of macrophages for a number of effector functions occurs as a multi-step reaction: LK activation signals induce certain undefined quantitative changes in macrophage function that can be further amplified by second activation signals. These second signals can be supplied by endogenous (found in LK) or exogenous (bacterial lipopolysaccharides, lectins) factors. A hallmark of this sequential activation of macrophages is that signal sequence is critical: cells exposed to activation agents in the incorrect sequence do not develop the effector activity. To further define the interaction between the two endogenous factors in LK, IFN and the non-IFN LK, for induction of macrophage resistance to infection with L. major, we analyzed the time course for development of this effector activity (Fig. 3). Treatment of macrophages with IFN followed by IFN-depleted LK, or vice versa, induced macrophage resistance to infection as early as 1 hr after addition of second signal, and activity was maximal 4 to 8 hrs after completion of the sequential treatment. The ability of macrophages to resist infection was similar when the second signal was either IFN or IFN-depleted LK. Induction of resistance to L. major infection, then, is a cooperative process between IFN and another LK factor(s) antigenically and physicochemically distinct from IFN, and is not dependent upon signal sequence.

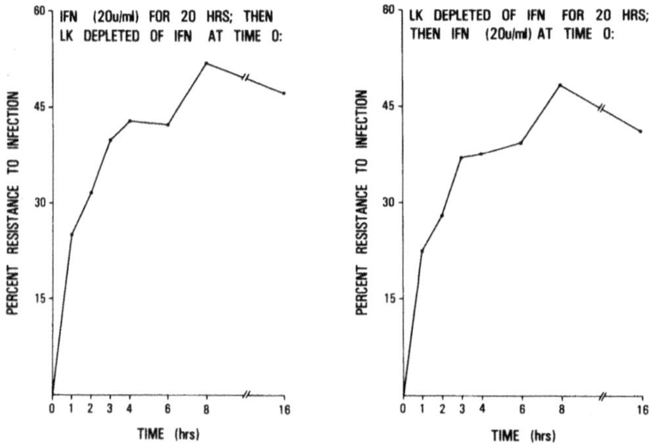

Fig. 3. Left panel: Resident peritoneal macrophages were treated for 20 hr with IFN, washed, then treated for 1 to 16 hr with LK depleted of IFN prior to addition of amastigotes. Right panel: Resident peritoneal macrophages were treated for 20 hr with LK depleted of IFN, washed, and then treated with IFN for 1 to 16 hr prior to addition of amastigotes. 95% confidence limits for replicate control cultures in this experiment was 15% resistance to infection.

LK THAT INDUCE RESISTANCE TO INFECTION

LK-induced resistance to infection is not very different in concept from the phenomenon of viral interference, the first described activity of interferons. Thus, it was a surprise that no activity for resistance to infection was detected in peritoneal or bone marrow-derived macrophages treated with recombinant IFN alone. Even more surprising, however, was that the high titers of LK activity for induction of this effector function were completely abrogated by treatment with anti-IFN immunoaffinity chromatography (Figs. 1,2), even though recombinant IFN at all concentrations tested failed to induce resistance to infection. We resolved this apparent paradox in the following manner: active spleen cell-derived LK that contained about 50 U/ml IFN was treated with anti-IFN immunoaffinity chromotography. All IFN activity was removed in the eluate, as determined by ELISA, and the once active LK now failed to induce resistance to infection. The inactive LK was fractionated by polyacrylamide gel chromatography (P-100). To each inactive fraction (open circles, Fig. 4) we then added 50 U/ml recombinant IFN (closed circles, Fig. 4). The addition of IFN completely restored LK activity for resistance to infection.

LK that induce resistance to infection elute from sizing gels with an apparent Mr of 55,000 and 37,000 in the presence of IFN. We are presently characterizing these non-IFN LK that cooperate with IFN for induction of this macrophage effector activity (see chapter by Nacy et al., this volume).

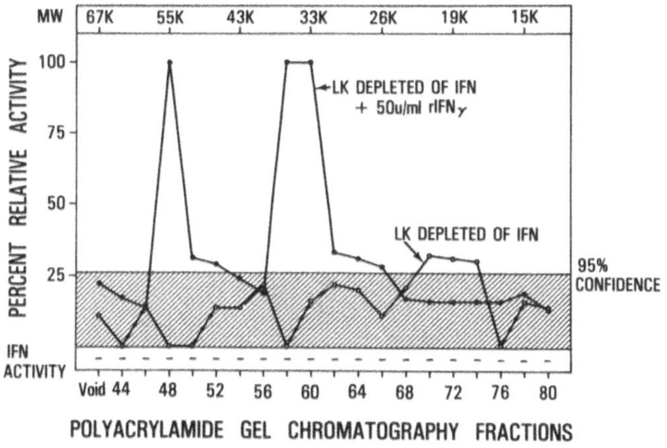

Fig. 4. Resident peritoneal macrophages were treated with 1/6 concentration of fractions of IFN-depleted LK alone (open circles) or with fractions + 50 U/ml IFN (closed circles) for 6 hr, washed, and infected with amastigotes of L. major for 2 hr. Results are expressed as percent relative activity of individual fractions compared to a dose response of active unfractionated LK. Shaded area represents the 95% confidence level for replicate control cultures. IFN activity of individual fractions was monitored by ELISA.

SUMMARY

Resistance to infection is an effector activity of macrophages that is induced by the cooperation of several molecularly distinct factors in LK: IFN and another nonIFN macrophage activation factor. Unlike many other effector activities of activated macrophages, signal sequence is not critical for induction of resistance to infection. Nor is the activation of macrophages for resistance to infection dependent upon the presence of T lymphocytes in the culture vessel: T cell-depleted peritoneal cell cultures and bone marrow-derived macrophages both develop resistance to infection with *L. major* in the presence of LK that contains IFN. Further characterization of this activity of activated macrophages will include the identification of LK that cooperate with IFN for induction of resistance to infection, and characterization of the LK-induced changes in macrophage function that mediate this resistant state.

REFERENCES

1. Blanden, R.V., M.J. Lefford, and G.B. Mackaness. 1969. J. Exp. Med. 129:1079.
2. Hoff, R. 1975. J. Exp. Med. 142:299.
3. Horwitz, M.A., and S.C. Silverstein. 1981. J. Exp. Med. 154:1618.
4. Meltzer, M.S., and C.A. Nacy. 1980. Cell. Immunol. 54:487.
5. Millar, H.C., and D.W. Twohy. 1969. J. Parasitol. 55:200.
6. Nacy, C.A., and M.S. Meltzer. 1979. J. Immunol. 123:2544.
7. Nacy, C.A., M.S. Meltzer, E.J. Leonard, and D.J. Wyler. 1981. J. Immunol. 127:2381.
8. Nacy, C.A., and M.S. Meltzer. 1982. Infect. Immun. 36:1096.
9. Nacy, C.A., A.H. Fortier, M.G. Pappas, and R.R. Henry. 1983. Cell. Immunol. 177:298.
10. Nacy, C.A., C.N. Oster, S.L. James, and M.S. Meltzer. 1984. Cont. Topics Immunobiol. 14:147.
11. Nyka, W. 1956. Am. Rev. Tuberc. 73:251.
12. Oster, C.N., and C.A. Nacy. 1984. J. Immunol. 132:1494.
13. Panosian, C.B., and D.J. Wyler. 1983. J. Infect. Dis. 148:1049.
14. Pappas, M.G., and C.A. Nacy. 1983. Cell. Immunol. 80:222.

IN VITRO PRODUCTION OF COLONY-STIMULATING FACTORS BY LISTERIA-IMMUNE SPLEEN CELLS

D. Mitchell Magee and Edward J. Wing

University of Pittsburgh School of Medicine

Montefiore Hospital, Pittsburgh PA 15213

INTRODUCTION

The survival of mice during Listeria monocytogenes infection is dependent on the efficiency of the early phases of host defenses. These early host defenses consist primarily of the production of bone marrow-derived monocytes and granulocytes and their accumulation at the site of infection. Two important parameters that are believed to affect the production of leukocytes during early infection are the number of leukocyte progenitors in bone marrow and the secretion of colony-stimulating factors (CSFs). At least four discrete CSFs, as determined by an in vitro colony forming assay, have been described: macrophage CSF (M-CSF), granulocyte CSF (G-CSF), granulocyte-macrophage CSF (GM-CSF), and multi-CSF (IL-3) (1). CSFs not only help to regulate the production of phagocytic cells, but also affect the function of mature phagocytes. For example, macrophages stimulated by CSFs secrete increased levels of oxygen reduction products (2) and have increased anti-tumor activity (3,4).

In previous studies from this laboratory we analyzed changes in serum concentrations of M-CSF during infection by Listeria (5,6). M-CSF levels rose within 24 hr after infection and remained elevated for 7 - 14 days before returning to normal. These levels paralleled the bacterial load in the tissues. In immune mice, M-CSF levels rose earlier than in non-immune mice and then decreased rapidly. This rapid increase in M-CSF levels in immune animals suggests that there is a level of immune control over CSF production. Additionally, others have shown that splenectomy ablates the

CSF response during listeriosis (7). From these and other data, we postulated that CSFs are produced during immune reactions and that splenic lymphocytes are either directly or indirectly responsible for their production. We designed experiments, therefore, to determine which CSFs are produced by spleen cells during in vitro immune stimulation and which cell types are responsible for their production.

MATERIALS AND METHODS

Supernatant Production

C57Bl/6J mice were inoculated with either 0.1 LD_{50} *Listeria* or saline. Seven days later single cell suspensions were prepared from spleens; SAL = saline cells, and IMM = *Listeria*-immune cells. In some experiments, the cells were passed over nylon wool to enrich for T lymphocytes (8). Cells were cultured in RPMI 1640 medium, supplemented with fetal bovine serum and antibiotics, with or without heat-killed *Listeria* (HKL). The supernatants (S) were harvested at the designated time, filtered, and stored at -20° C until assay.

Colony-Forming Assay

Various amounts of S were placed into 35 mm culture dishes with 1 x 10^5 bone marrow cells in McCoy 5A medium supplemented with antibiotics, 15% fetal bovine serum, amino acids, and 0.3% agar (9). Cells were cultured for 7 days at 37° C in a humidified atmosphere containing 7.5% CO_2. Colonies consisting of greater than 50 cells were scored with a dissecting microscope. Colony-stimulating activity (CSA)/ml was calculated by multiplying the colonies per plate by the inverse of the S dilution used. Colony cell type was determined by microscopic examination of colonies from the whole cultures that had been fixed, dried, and stained with Mayer's hematoxylin. In some assays, purified anti-M-CSF was added to the S to bind M-CSF and thus determine the relative proportion of M-CSF in the S (10). M-CSF was also directly measured by a double-antibody radioimmunoassay (RIA) (9).

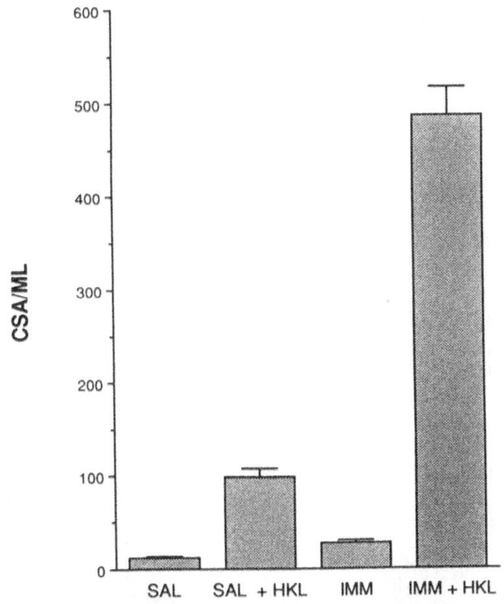

FIGURE 1. Saline (SAL) or Listeria-immune cells (IMM) were incubated with or without heat-killed Listeria (HKL) for 96 hours. Supernatants (S) were harvested and assayed for colony-stimulating activity (CSA) in the bioassay. Results are expressed as total CSA/ml ± the standard error of the mean (SEM) of S from six consecutive experiments. Analysis of variance showed that IMM cells stimulated with antigen produced significantly higher CSFs levels than SAL cells. There was no difference between groups of cells incubated without antigen.

RESULTS

Production of Colony-Stimulating Factors

Initial experiments were performed to assess the capacity of IMM and SAL cells to produce CSFs in response to HKL. Stimulation of IMM cells led to secretion of large amounts of CSF as determined by the analysis of the S (Figure 1). SAL cells produced low levels of CSFs when stimulated with HKL. Neither group of cells produced CSFs when cultured without

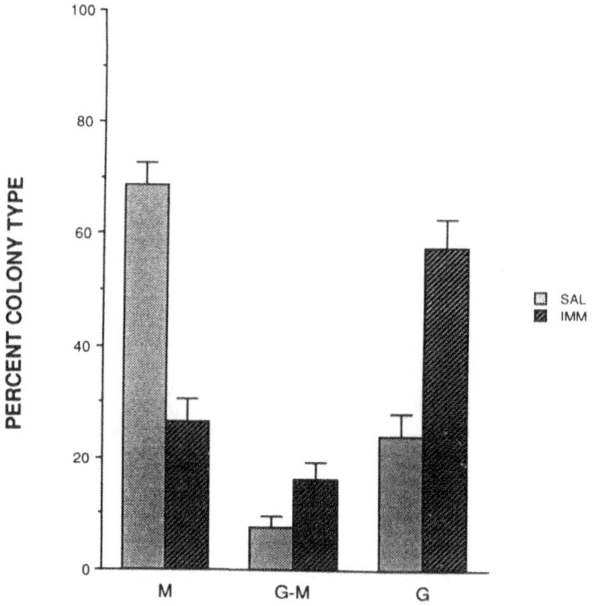

FIGURE 2. Colony cell type was assessed by performing differential counts of colonies from three of the assays presented in Figure 1. The percentage, ± SEM, of either macrophage (M), mixed granulocyte-macrophage (G-M), or granulocyte colonies (G) is presented.

Table 1. M-CSF by RIA

Experiment #	SALINE	IMMUNE
1	36	121
2	0	143
3	24	207
4	40	295
5	6	199
6	18	39

M-CSF was measured by a specific RIA from the S that were assayed in Figure 1. Data are expressed as units of M-CSF/ml, where one unit is defined as that amount of M-CSF that induces the formation of one colony as extrapolated from the linear portion of the dose response curve.

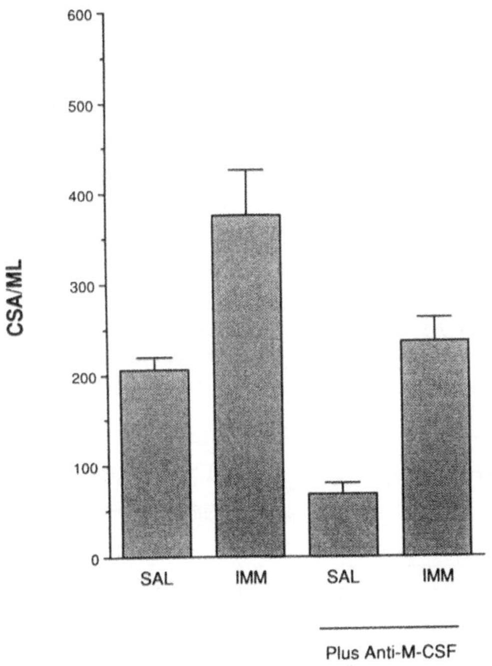

FIGURE 3. Anti-M-CSF antibodies were added to S prior to performance of the bioassay. The results are expressed as the mean CSA ± SEM of two experiments on some of the S presented in Figure 1. The amount of antibody added was sufficient to inhibit 50% of the activity of L-cell conditioned media (M-CSF) containing 1000 units/ml CSF activity. Normal rabbit serum was used as a control and did not affect the CSA in the S.

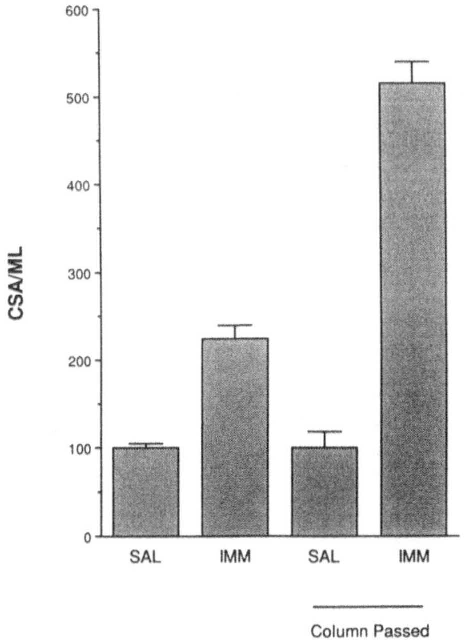

FIGURE 4. Populations of cells were placed directly into culture or passed over nylon wool columns before culture with HKL. The results are expressed as the mean CSA/ml ± SEM of two experiments.

stimulation. However, both groups of cells produced low levels (approximately 100 units/ml of CSA) of CSFs in response to an unrelated antigen, heat-killed Salmonella typhimurium (data not shown). There was a moderate amount of variation in total CSA detected from experiment to experiment.

Types of Colony-Stimulating Factors Produced

The types of CSFs that were secreted during stimulation were estimated by performing microscopic examination of the colonies that formed in the bioassay (from the experiment described in Figure 1). Additionally, M-CSF was measured directly by a specific RIA and by incorporating anti-M-CSF antibodies into the supernatants before performing the bioassay. There were both qualitative and quantitative differences in the CSFs produced by the IMM and SAL cells. The types of colonies produced by the S from IMM cells were 26% macrophage, 16% granulocyte-macrophage, and 58% granulocyte. SAL cell S produced 58% macrophage, 8% granulocyte-macrophage, and 24% granulocyte colonies (Figure 2). Measurement of M-CSF directly showed that more M-CSF was produced by IMM cells than SAL cells (Table I). Estimation of the specific proportion of M-CSF in the supernatants was determined by adding specific M-CSF antibodies to the supernatants before bioassay. As seen in Figure 3, anti-M-CSF antibodies blocked approximately 60% of the activity in the SAL supernatants and 40% in the IMM supernatants. Normal rabbit IgG had no effect on the CSF activity of the supernatants (data not shown).

Determination of the Cell Types Producing CSFs

To determine the cell types responsible for the production of CSFs, whole splenic cell populations were passed over nylon wool columns to enrich for the T-lymphocyte populations. Column-purified IMM cells produced significantly more CSFs than non-column passed cells, (Figure 4). Passage of SAL cells over nylon wool had minor effects on CSF production. Nylon wool passage routinely raised the Thy 1.2 positive population from 30% - 40% to 60% - 80%. This suggested that T-lymphocytes may be a major producer of CSFs.

DISCUSSION

In these studies we showed that the production of CSFs by spleen cells had at least two components. The first was a nonspecific, low level, secretion that occurred when nonimmune spleen cells were cultured with either heat-killed Listeria or Salmonella. The primary CSF detected in these supernatants was M-CSF. These results may be analogous to the data derived from experiments in which injection of muramyl dipeptide derivatives (11) or endotoxin (12) increased serum levels of CSF. The second type of production was characterized by an increase in the total amount of CSFs secreted. There was generally a three to five fold increase in secretion of CSFs after antigenic stimulation. Also, there was a shift in the types of CSFs secreted. The CSFs from the immune-driven reactions led primarily to the formation of granulocyte colonies.

The spleen is considered a source of all four major CSFs and T cells can produce at least GM-CSF and IL-3 (13). In the experiments described above, the relative contribution of these specific CSFs to the overall colony-stimulating activity is difficult to estimate based solely upon the type of colony produced. All of these CSFs can lead to the formation of granulocyte, macrophage, or mixed colonies; the percentage of the type of colony formed depends on the concentration of the specific CSFs. For example, M-CSF which produces mainly macrophage colonies, can cause the formation of a low percentage of either granulocyte or granulocyte-macrophage colonies (13). The results of our experiments showed that nonspecific CSF production was primarily M-CSF. In immune reactions, M-CSF was produced in larger amounts than in the nonspecific production, but did not account for the majority of the CSA. In vitro immune reactions, therefore, lead to the secretion of multiple species of CSFs.

Several investigators over the past few years have studied the role of the two major lymphocyte subpopulations (helper and cytotoxic) in host resistance to *Listeria*. Studies using either whole immune spleen cells depleted of specific subpopulations or *Listeria*-specific T-lymphocyte clones have shown that both helper and cytotoxic subsets are needed for optimal protection (14-19). Since T-lymphocytes play a central role in host resistance to *Listeria*, splenic lymphocytes were assessed for their ability to produce CSFs in response to listerial antigens. The first experiments were performed with spleen cells that had been passed over nylon wool to enrich for the T-lymphocyte population. The production of CSFs by immune cells was increased approximately two fold by column passage. This increase corresponded to the increased percentage of T-lymphocytes in the splenic population. In preliminary experiments to further characterize the contribution of T-lymphocytes, different T cell subsets were isolated and studied for their ability to produce CSFs. The L3T4 T-lymphocyte subpopulation apppears to be responsible for the majority of the CSF production (unpublished data).

The production of CSFs during *Listeria* infection may contribute to host defenses in two ways. First, the rise in CSF levels could increase the production of phagocytic cells in the bone marrow and other hematopoietic sites. The increased production of both granulocytes and monocytes would make more cells available for migration into the infective foci. The presence of infiltrating granulocytes and monocytes is believed to be a critical factor in limiting the early multiplication of bacteria. Second, many of the CSFs have been shown to activate effector functions of both granulocytes and monocytes (2,3,4). The two mechanisms of CSF production, nonspecific and immune, may act in concert during the host defenses against *Listeria*. The production of CSFs in a nonspecific manner would most affect the early, T-lymphocyte-independent, phases of host resistance. This early response may provide a mechanism for control of bacterial replication until the immune, T-lymphocyte-dependent, mechanisms become activated. Thus, the ability of these molecular species to increase both the numbers of available phagocytes and to increase their effector functions would be advantageous to the host.

SUMMARY

In this series of experiments we have shown that there are at least two mechanisms of CSF production by spleen cells in vitro: nonspecific secretion of CSF by nonimmune cells and immune, antigen-driven production by specific T-lymphocytes. M-CSF was mainly produced in the nonspecific reaction. The immune production by T-lymphocytes consisted of increased CSF production and secretion of multiple species of CSFs.

ACKNOWLEDGMENTS

These studies were supported by grants from the National Institutes of Health (RO1 CA 15237, RO1 CA 33035, and RO1 AI 20638).

REFERENCES

1. D. Metcalf, The molecular biology of granulocyte macrophage colony-stimulating factors, Blood. 67:257 (1986).
2. E.J. Wing, N.M. Ampel, A. Waheed, and R.K. Shadduck, Macrophage colony-stimulating factor (M-CSF) enhances the capacity of murine macrophages to secrete oxygen reduction products, J. Immunol. 135:2052 (1985).
3. E.J. Wing, A. Waheed, R.K. Shadduck, L. S. Nagle, and K Stephenson, Effect of colony-stimulating factor on murine macrophages: Induction of anti-tumor activity, J. Clin. Invest. 69:270 (1982).
4. K.H. Grabstein, D.L. Urdal, R.J. Tushinski, D.Y. Mochizuki, V.L. Price, M.A. Cantrell, S. Gillis, and P.J. Conlon, Induction of macrophage tumoricidal activity by granulocyte-macrophage colony-stimulating factor, Science. 232:506 (1986).
5. E.J. Wing, A. Waheed, and R.K. Shadduck, Changes in serum colony-stimulating factor and monocyte progenitor cells during *Listeria monocytogenes* infection in mice, Infect. Immun. 45:180 (1984).

6. E.J. Wing, L. C. Barczynski, A. Waheed, and R.K. Shadduck, Effect of Listeria monocytogenes infection on serum levels of colony-stimulating factor and number of progenitor cells in immune and nonimmmune mice, Infect. Immun. 49:325 (1985).

7. P.R. Wood, A.M. Young, J.L. McKimm-Breschkin, and C. Cheers, Effect of splenectomy on the production of interferon and colony-stimulating factor in Listeria monocytogenes infected mice, Infect. Immun. 46:860 (1984).

8. A.C. Weinblatt, S.N. Vogel, and D.L. Rosenstreich, Adherence to nylon- or rayon-wool columns, in "Manual of macrophage methodology: collection, characterization, and function," H.B. Herscowitz, H.T. Holden, J.A. Bellanti, and A. Ghaffar eds., Marcel Dekker, New York (1981).

9. F. Boegel, A. Waheed, and R.K. Shadduck, Evaluation of radioimmunoassay and in vitro colony forming assay techniques for determination of colony-stimulating factor and inhibitory activity in murine serum and tissue, Blood. 58:1141 (1981).

10. R.K. Shadduck, and D. Metcalf, Preparation and neutralization characteristics of an anti-CSF antibody, J. Cell Physiol. 86:247 (1975).

11. A. Gallelli, P. Lefrancier, and L. Chedid, Colony-stimulating activity induced by synthetic muramyl dipeptides: Variation with chemical structure and association with anti-infectious activity, Infect. Immun. 46:495 (1984).

12. E.J. Wing, and R.K. Shadduck, Colony-stimulating factor, in "Biological response modifiers," P.F. Torrence, ed., Academic Press, New York (1985).

13. D. Metcalf, The colony-stimulating factors, in "The hemopoietic colony stimulating factors," Elsevier, Amsterdam (1984).

14. S.H.E. Kaufmann, M.M. Simon, and H. Hahn, Specific Lyt 123 T cells are involved in protection against Listeria monocytogenes and delayed-type hypersensitivity to listerial antigens, J. Exp. Med. 150:1033 (1979).

15. S.H.E. Kaufmann, and H. Hahn, Biological functions of T cell lines with specificity for the intracellular bacterium Listeria monocytogenes in vitro and in vivo, J. Exp. Med. 155:1754 (1982).

16. R.J. Kearns, and E.C. DeFreitas, In vitro propagation of antigen-specific T lymphocytes that adoptively transfer resistance to Listeria monocytogenes, Infect. Immun. 40:713 (1983).

17. H. Naher, U. Sperling, and H. Hahn, H-2K restricted granuloma formation by Ly-2^+ cells in antibacterial protection to facultative intracellular bacteria, J. Immunol. 134:569 (1985).

18. S.H.E. Kaufmann, E. Hug, U. Vath, and I. Muller, Effective protection against Listeria monocytogenes and delayed-type hypersensitivity to listerial antigens depend on cooperation between specific L3T4^+ and Lyt 2^+ cells, Infect. Immun. 48:263 (1985).

19. S.H.E. Kaufmann, E. Hug, and G. DeLibero, Listeria monocytogenes-reactive T lymphocyte clones with cytolytic activity against infected target cells, J. Exp. Med. 164:363 (1986).

EFFECT OF TUMOR NECROSIS FACTOR ON GROWTH OF *TRYPANOSOMA MUSCULI* IN VIVO AND IN VITRO

Patricia A.L. Kongshavn[1] and Esfandiar Ghadirian

Departments of Physiology and Medicine and Montreal General Hospital Research Institute, McGill University, Montreal, Quebec, Canada

Trypanosoma musculi, a natural parasite of mice, produces a self-limiting infection which lasts for approximately 3 weeks and comprises an early growth phase, a plateau phase and an elimination phase (1). The mechanism of protection which controls the early growth of the parasite, leading to the plateau phase, is not well understood but is known to be highly sensitive to ionizing radiation. Macrophages of the reticuloendothelial system also become activated at this time (2). We have shown recently that elimination of parasitaemia and termination of the infection depends on an effector mechanism involving a thermolabile, anti-trypanosomal IgG2a antibody, complement component C3 and an effector cell, possibly a macrophage (3,4).

Tumor necrosis factor (TNF) (5), or cachectin (6), is a product of activated macrophages which has not only been shown to have anti-tumor properties but also to play a protective role in some parasitic infections. Thus TNF has been reported to inactivate certain species of malarial parasites and to inhibit intracellular multiplication of *T. cruzi* in cultured macrophages (7,8). In fact, cachectin was first observed in rabbits infected with *T. brucei* that were shown to develop cachexia, with an associated suppression of peripheral lipoprotein lipase activity (9). Because macrophages appear to play a role both in the early control of parasitaemia and possibly in the elimination phase, we considered it of interest to study the effect of human recombinant TNF (r-TNF) on *T. musculi*.

Human r-TNF was kindly provided by Dr. H.M. Shepard (Genentech Inc., South San Francisco, Ca).

THE EFFECT OF TNF ON THE COURSE OF *T. MUSCULI* INFECTION

C57BL/6 mice inoculated with 10^4 *T. musculi* on day 0 were treated with intravenous injections of 10^3 or 10^4 units (U) TNF in saline every

[1] Correspondence to: P.A.L. Kongshavn
Department of Physiology, McGill University
3655 Drummond Street
Montreal, Quebec H3G 1Y6
Canada

2-3 days and the parasitaemia was determined at various time intervals. The parasite and methods used have been reported previously (10). As shown in Table 1, over the early course of infection parasitaemia was elevated in the TNF-treated mice. This was apparent by day 7 post-infection (p.i.) and showed its maximal effect on day 14 at the time of peak parasitaemia. A dose of 10^4 U TNF produced a greater effect than when 10^3 U were given, and 10^2 (data not shown) had no effect.

In another experiment, mice were treated later in infection, giving 10^5 or 10^3 U TNF on days 10, 12, 14 and 17 p.i. It was observed that the parasties were eliminated more rapidly in the TNF-treated groups. Thus, by day 19 p.i., mice receiving 10^5 U TNF were cleared of parasitaemia, as were 3 out of 4 mice receiving 10^3 U TNF. In contrast, parasitaemia was still high in 3 out of 4 mice that had not been treated with TNF (Table 2).

THE EFFECT OF TNF ON GROWTH OF *T. MUSCULI* IN VITRO

T. musculi were separated from heparinized blood taken from ex-sanguinated infected A/J strain mice by washing the blood 5-6 times with phosphate glucose saline (PGS), using slow speed centrifugation, and decanting the supernatant containing the parasites. They were resuspended in RPMI 1640 culture medium supplemented with 20% fetal calf serum (FCS), 5×10^{-5} M 2-mercaptoethanol and antibiotics (50 μg/ml Gentamycin) at an approximate concentration of 50×10^4 *T. musculi* per ml. Four to six cultures of 200 μl parasites/well were set up for each time point in 96-well plates and TNF (or saline as a control) was added. The plates were incubated at 37°C in a humidified chamber containing 5% CO_2, and the parasite number was enumerated daily, using a 5 μl sample taken from each well. In experiment 3, TNF was added daily. The results (Table 3) show that, in the presence of TNF in the cultures, trypanosome multiplication is inhibited significantly. This direct anti-trypanosomal activity of TNF could be due to an inhibition of parasite replication and/or a trypanocidal action of this monokine. In experiment 1, in addition to using 10^5 U TNF, other cultures were treated with 10^2 U TNF and similar results obtained (data not shown). In experiments 2 and 3, concentrations of 10^1 - 10^5 U TNF were tested and, again, the results did not differ significantly between the TNF-treated groups. Therefore, only the results using 10^3 U TNF are given. Presumably, all doses of TNF tried are in the range above which a dose-response would be observed.

THE EFFECT OF TNF ON GROWTH OF *T. MUSCULI* IN VITRO IN PRESENCE OF PERITONEAL EXUDATE CELLS

T. musculi separated from the blood were cultured in 96-well plates as before, at an initial concentration of either 20×10^4/ml (Table 4, experiment 1) or 1×10^4/ml (Table 4, experiment 2). Peritoneal exudate cells (PEC), elicited by injection of thioglycollate 3 days previously, were added to all wells at a final concentration of 10^6/ml. When the initial parasite density was low (experiment 2), the trypanosomes multiplied to a much greater extent in the presence of TNF. When the initial number of parasites present in the culture was higher (experiment 1), the trypanosome population reached peak numbers more rapidly, and declined sooner, in the cultures containing TNF. This situation resembles that seen in the in vivo experiments. Thus, in the presence of PEC, TNF has an effect on parasite growth which is opposite to that seen when mouse cells are absent from the cultures.

Table 1. Effect of TNF on course of parasitaemia

Day of Infection	Dose of TNF (U)[a]		
	10^4	10^3	0
7	1.1 ± 0.4[b]	0.8 ± 0.2	1.0 ± 0.1
10	27.5 ± 9.4	18.0 ± 10.0	5.0 ± 2.0
14	50.7 ± 9.9*	31.6 ± 11.0*	5.3 ± 1.7
17	26.1 ± 10.6*	27.7 ± 13.5*	0.12± 0.07
18	17.3 ± 7.4	19.2 ± 11.2	0.8 ± 0.4
19	4.6 ± 2.9	11.9 ± 9.2	0.3 ± 0.1
20	0.5 ± 0.3	5.1 ± 4.9	0
21	0	0	0

[a]Given on days 0, 3, 5, 7, 10, 12, 14, 17 post-infection
[b]*T. musculi* x 10^6 per ml blood. Mean of 4 mice ± 1 s.e.m.
*TNF-treated vs. non-TNF treated mice, $P < 0.05$ (Student t test).

Table 2. Effect of TNF given late in infection on elimination of parasites

Day of Infection	Dose of TNF (U)[a]		
	10^5	10^3	0
16	> 100[b,c]	> 100[b]	> 100[b]
18	0,0,0,1	0,0,3,50	0,6,150,150
19	0,0,0,0	0,0,0,16	0,1,50,50
21	0[b]	0[b]	0[b]

[a]Given on days 10, 12, 14, 17 p.i.
[b]All values
[c]*T. musculi* x 10^4 per ml blood (individual values)

Table 3. Effect of TNF on growth of *T. musculi* in cell free cultures

Day of	Experiment 1		Experiment 2		Experiment 3	
incubation	TNF[a]	Saline	TNF[b]	Saline	TNF[c]	Saline
0	43.0 ± 2.0[d]	43.0 ± 2.0	34.0 ± 3.0	34.0 ± 3.0	43.0 ± 3.5	43.0 ± 3.5
1	42.0 ± 7.1*	72.7 ± 4.0	22.0 ± 1.6*	51.0 ± 10.0	25.5 ± 3.5	58.5 ± 13.4
2	73.2 ± 7.7*	116.0 ± 7.4	45.0 ± 2.2	65.2 ± 10.3	26.2 ± 2.8*	59.3 ± 9.5
3	84.0 ± 8.5	109.6 ± 7.9	41.0 ± 12.9	95.0 ± 25.6	8.5 ± 1.8*	27.8 ± 2.2
4	84.8 ± 9.0*	142.8 ± 6.4	38.2 ± 7.0	55.0 ± 6.3	1.7 ± 0.3*	13.5 ± 3.3
6	ND[e]	ND	25.5 ± 2.6	52.5 ± 16.3	ND	ND
7	83.8 ± 7.0	88.9 ± 8.2	ND	ND	ND	ND
9	55.2 ± 3.4	56.7 ± 3.9	ND	ND	ND	ND

[a] 10^5 U TNF added to cultures on day 0
[b] 10^3 U TNF added to cultures on day 0
[c] 10^3 U TNF added to cultures daily from day 0
[d] *T. musculi* x 10^4/ml. Mean of 4-6 cultures ± 1 s.e.m.
[e] ND = not done.
*Values for cultures containing TNF vs. control cultures, $P < 0.05$ (Student t test).

SUMMARY

The effect of r-TNF on T. musculi is complex. When trypanosomes are incubated in culture with this monokine, TNF exerts a direct anti-trypanosomal effect (Table 3). Similarly, if mice are treated with TNF during the later stages of infection, after the parasitaemia has stabilized, it hastens the elimination of the trypanosomes (Table 2). When TNF is given to mice from the early stage of infection onwards, it enhances the growth of the parasites (Table 1). (This enhanced early growth probably masks any subsequent anti-trypanosomal effect of TNF exerted later in infection). The ability of TNF to promote parasite multiplication is observed even more clearly in in vitro experiments, when peritoneal exudate cells are added to the T. musculi cultures (Table 4). It is conceivable, therefore, that the enhancing effect of TNF in vivo is mediated via a cell present in thioglycollate-induced peritoneal exudate, which mostly comprises macrophages.

In summary, the results of these experiments suggest that r-TNF exerts a direct anti-trypanosomal effect while simultaneously promoting the growth of the parasite through an indirect effect mediated via the host's cells, possibly the macrophages.

ACKNOWLEDGEMENTS

This work was supported by grant 5448 from the Medical Research Council of Canada.

We gratefully acknowledge the expert technical assistance of Ms. Isabelle Rajotte.

Table 4. Effect of TNF on growth of T. musculi in cultures containing peritoneal exudate cells (10^6/ml)

Day of incubation	Experiment 1: 10^3 U TNF[a]	Experiment 1: Saline	Experiment 2: 10^3 U TNF[a]	Experiment 2: Saline
0	18.5 ± 2.8[b]	18.5 ± 2.8	1.0 ± 1.0	1.0 ± 1.0
1	22.2 ± 7.5	17.8 ± 2.5	1.8 ± 0.6	1.5 ± 0.3
2	45.8 ± 8.4*	12.2 ± 1.3	4.0 ± 0.4	2.5 ± 0.9
3	118.2 ± 29.0	73.0 ± 22.0	9.5 ± 1.5*	4.0 ± 0.4
4	125.0 ± 16.6	106.0 ± 18.0	23.7 ± 5.2	10.2 ± 2.3
6	108.0 ± 17.5	152.5 ± 15.0	71.8 ± 17.7*	18.0 ± 1.8
7	106.8 ± 20.3	119.5 ± 17.8	107.5 ± 12.0*	18.5 ± 2.2
8	97.8 ± 17.6	99.0 ± 15.6	86.2 ± 11.2*	22.0 ± 4.2

[a]TNF added daily to cultures
[b]Mean of quadruplicate cultures x 10^4
*TNF vs. saline $P < .05$ (Student t test)

REFERENCES

1. Viens, P., Targett, G.A.T., Leuchars, and Davies, A.J., 1974. The immunological response of CBA mice to Trypanosoma musculi. I. Initial control of the infection and the effect of T-cell deprivation. Clin. Exp. Immunol., 16:279.
2. Rapattoni, W., Ghadirian, E., and Kongshavn, P.A.L., 1984. Importance of cellular mechanisms in controlling murine trypanosomiasis. Abst. #7, 21st National RES Meeting.
3. Wechsler, D.S., and Kongshavn, P.A.L., 1985. Characterization of antibodies mediating protection and cure of Trypanosoma musculi infection in mice. Infect. Immun., 48(3):787.
4. Wechsler, D.S., and Kongshavn, P.A.L., 1986. Heat-labile IgG2a antibodies effect cure of Trypanosoma musculi infection in C57BL/6 mice. J. Immunol. 137:2968-2972.
5. Carswell, E.A., Old, L.J., Kassel, R.L., Green, S., Fiore, N., and Williamson, B., 1975. An endotoxin-induced serum factor that causes necrosis of tumors. Proc. Natl. Acad. Sci. USA, 72:3666.
6. Beutler, B., Greenwald, D., Hulmes, J.D., Chang, M., Pan, Y.-C.E., Mathison, J., Ulevitch, R., and Cerami, A., 1985. Identity of tumor necrosis factor and the macrophage-secreted factor cachectin. Nature, 316:552.
7. Taverne, J., Dockrell, H.M., and Playfair, J.H.L., 1981. Endotoxin-induced serum factor kills malarial parasites in vitro. Infect. Immun., 33:83.
8. De Titto, E.H., Catterall, J.R., and Remington, J.S., 1986. Activity of recombinant tumor necrosis factor on Toxoplasma Gondii and Trypanosoma cruzi. J. Immunol., 137:1342.
9. Beutler, B., and Cerami, A., 1987. Cachectin and tumour necrosis factor as two sides of the same biological coin. Nature, 320:588.
10. Wechsler, D.S., and Kongshavn, P.A.L., 1984. Cure of Trypanosoma musculi infection by heat-labile activity in immune plasma. Infect. Immun. 44(3):756.

MECHANISMS OF IMMUNOLOGICAL UNRESPONSIVENESS IN THE SPECTRA OF LEPROSY AND LEISHMANIASIS

Barry R. Bloom, Vijay Mehra, Johanne Melancon-Kaplan, Marianella Castes*, Jacinto Convit*, Patrick J. Brennan~, Thomas H. Rea+ and Robert L. Modlin+

Albert Einstein College of Medicine, Bronx, NY; *Institute of Dermatology, Caracas, Venezuela; ~Colorado State Univ., Fort Collins, CO; and +University of Southern California, Los Angeles, CA.

Leprosy and cutaneous leishmaniasis share a number of important characteristics[1,2]. They are both chronic granulomatous diseases; both affect the skin and both present a spectrum of clinical manifestations. In the case of leprosy, there is a remarkable correlation between the clinical and histopathological spectrum, and cell-mediated immune responsiveness to antigens of *M. leprae*. At the tuberculoid pole, patients have few lesions which contain rare organisms and are able to mount strong T-cell-mediated immune responses to *M. leprae* antigens *in vitro* and *in vivo*. In contrast, at the lepromatous end of the spectrum, patients have disseminated skin lesions containing large numbers of acid-fast bacilli and are selectively unresponsive to antigens of *M. leprae*. In American cutaneous leishmaniasis, the spectrum is somewhat less well defined, more variable clinically and less predictable at the histopathologic level. The disease ranges from a single defined lesion containing few amastigotes in localized cutaneous leishmaniasis (LCL) to diffuse cutaneous leishmaniasis (DCL) which, like lepromatous leprosy, is characterized by disseminated granulomata containing macrophages laden with amastigotes and immune unresponsiveness to leishmanial antigens. There are other clinical forms of cutaneous leishmaniasis including the highly destructive mucocutaneous (espundia) form, and a verrucous form, the pathogenesis of which are not entirely predictable from histopathology and molecular immunological data. In addition, in different parts of the world systemic forms of visceral leishmaniasis (kala-azar) occur in Asia, and a mild local form, Oriental Sore, exists in the Middle East primarily. Antibody levels appear to be elevated in both lepromatous leprosy and in diffuse cutaneous leishmaniasis, indicating that antibodies are unlikely to play a major role in protection.

Because most patients with lepromatous leprosy and diffuse cutaneous leishmaniasis are clearly able to exhibit cell-mediated immunity to common recall antigens, such as tuberculin PPD, Candida, and SKSD, the mechanism of selective or specific unresponsiveness at the level of cell-mediated immunity is of importance in understanding the pathogenesis of these conditions, as well as of more general immunological interest.

Immunological Unresponsiveness in Lepromatous Leprosy

The immunologically most challenging question in lepromatous leprosy concerns the mechanisms which govern the specific unresponsiveness of patients to antigens of *M. leprae*[3]. This is particularly puzzling when the available evidence indicates that antibodies to *M. tuberculosis* or BCG are capable of cross-reacting with most of the known protein and glycoprotein antigens of *M. leprae*. To reconcile these observations we formulated the hypothesis that there may be one or a small number of unique antigens associated with *M. leprae* capable of inducing active suppression of the responses of potentially reactive helper T cells. In order to initiate these studies, it was necessary to have an *in vitro* model for the study of suppression in man, particularly in circumstances where it was virtually impossible to obtain HLA-A,B,C,D-matched lymphocytes from patients with discordant forms of leprosy. We reasoned that if there were indeed *M. leprae*-induced suppressor cells that could block the expansion of potentially reactive specific T_H cells and/or block the effector activity of already sensitized T cells, we might be able to detect them by their ability to depress the polyclonal expansion of T-cells of helper phenotype induced by mitogens such as Concanavalin A (Con A). Initially we developed an assay system measuring lepromin-induced suppression of Con A used at sub-optimal doses for lymphocyte stimulation[4]. As shown in Figure 1, significant lepromin-induced suppression was observed in 84% of patients with lepromatous and borderline leprosy, but no suppressive activity could be detected in patients with tuberculoid leprosy or in lepromin-positive contacts or normal donors.

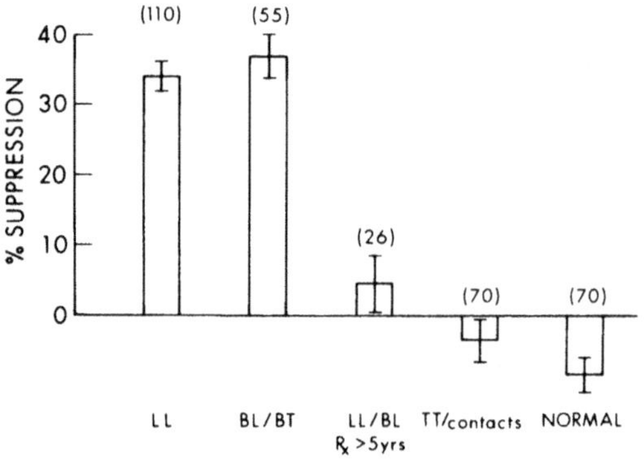

Fig. 1. Lepromin Induced Suppression of Con A responses in Leprosy (From Ref.3)

Two cells types were found to mediate lepromin-induced *in vitro* suppression[4]: adherent cells with monocytic properties were found to be present in some of the patients; and non-adherent suppressor cells were found to be present in the majority of patients. A number of laboratories have confirmed the existence of monocyte or macrophage suppressor cells in leprosy and identified suppressor activity in soluble extracts from these cells[5,6,7]. It is our impression that macrophage-induced *in vitro* suppression of mitogen responses is related to the bacillary load and extent of disease; in recent studies of lepromatous patients early in the course of their disease, the frequency of macrophage suppressors appears to be less, although virtually all retain non-adherent suppressor cells and remain unresponsive to *in vitro* stimulation with lepromin. A second concern is how to reconcile the non-specific *in vitro* suppressor activity of the monocytes with the exquisite specificity of the unresponsiveness *in vivo*.

Consequently, we have directed our attention primarily to characterizating the lymphocyte population involved in the antigen-induced suppression. In studies using the fluorescence-activated cell sorter (FACS) we were able to establish that T cells from lepromatous patients added to peripheral blood of normal donors in the presence of lepromin induced significant suppression of Con A responses[8]. When these T cells were further fractionated by FACS, we observed that the suppressor activity was contained within a 20% subset identified by the OKT5 monoclonal antibody or a 30% subset contained within the OKT8 subset. It should be noted that these experiments were only possible because we had chosen a mitogen system in which proliferative responses could be assessed at 72 hours, an early time point at which any confounding effects due to mixed lymphocyte reactions are avoided. Nonetheless, because most T cell interactions are genetically restricted by the MHC, it was quite puzzling to us that such a high frequency of suppression was detected after mixing putatively allogeneic cells, until we found that essentially 50% of the T8 subset from patients with lepromatous leprosy are HLA-DR (Ia) positive and Fc-receptor positive as well. The fact that a very high percentage of the T8 cells from lepromatous donors express MHC class II antigens makes it possible for them to present antigen to other T cells from the same donor[9]. We have recently shown that DR^+ T8 suppressor cells (and clones) present alloantigens in mixed lymphocyte reactions very effectively[10].

T Suppressor Cells in the Spectrum of Cutaneous Leishmaniasis

Similar *in vitro* studies have been carried out in patients with American cutaneous leishmaniasis in Caracas, Venezuela[11,12]. The results clearly indicate that lymphocyte proliferative responses to leishmanial antigens were present in patients with localized cutaneous leishmaniasis and significantly augmented in mucocutaneous leishmaniasis. Patients with diffuse cutaneous leishmaniasis demonstrated a complete absence of specific immune responsiveness both *in vivo* and *in vitro* (Table 1).

Table 1. T cell responses of patients with leishmania induced with *L. braziliensis* promastigote antigens. (From ref. 12).

Patients	Stimulation Index
LCL	3.8 ± 0.8
MCL	18.4 ± 6.0
DCL	1.1 ± 0.2
Controls	2.6 ± 0.4

These patients were further analyzed for antigen-induced suppression of Con A responses using killed promastigote antigens. The results clearly indicated that a significant leishmanial antigen-induced suppression of in vitro Con A responses was found in patients with diffuse cutaneous leishmaniasis but not in localized or mucocutaneous forms (Table 2). Indeed, a significant inverse correlation was found between the degree of suppression and specific antigen-induced lymphocyte proliferation. While the phenotype of the cell responsible for the leishmania-induced suppression remains to be clarified, there is a striking parallelism in the in vitro suppressor activity of immunologically unresponsive patients with diffuse cutaneous leishmaniasis and lepromatous leprosy.

Specificity of T Suppressor Cells in Lepromatous Leprosy

Our initial attempts to establish the antigen specificity of the suppression in vitro were confounded by the finding that a variety of cultivable mycobacteria had the ability to induce suppression of mitogen responses of some normal PPD-negative individuals from non-endemic areas, and hence the specificity of T suppressor cell induction in lepromatous leprosy was problematic. We were fortunate in obtaining monoclonal antibodies specific for several species of human Interferon alpha which were capable of eliminating the in vitro suppression induced by all of the cultivable mycobacteria tested in normal individuals (Fig. 2).

Table 2. Suppression of T cell responses to Con A of patients with leishmaniasis induced by L. brasiliensis promastigote antigens. (From Ref. 12)

Patients	Percent suppression
LCL	16.2 ± 6.6
MCL	5.1 ± 11.1
DCL	39.1 ± 6.1
Controls	15.1 ± 2.7

Yet these antibodies to Interferon failed to eliminate the suppression induced by lepromin or M. leprae in cells of patients with lepromatous leprosy[3]. These experiments formally established that the suppression was specific for antigens of M. leprae.

To test our suppressor hypothesis, it became necessary to search for a unique antigen associated with M. leprae. Hunter and Brennan had recently discovered a novel phenolic glycolipid, the terminal trisaccharide of which was unique to M. leprae[13,14]. When this material was incorporated into liposomes, it was found to induce suppression of mitogen responses in lepromatous patients almost as well as intact lepromin[15].

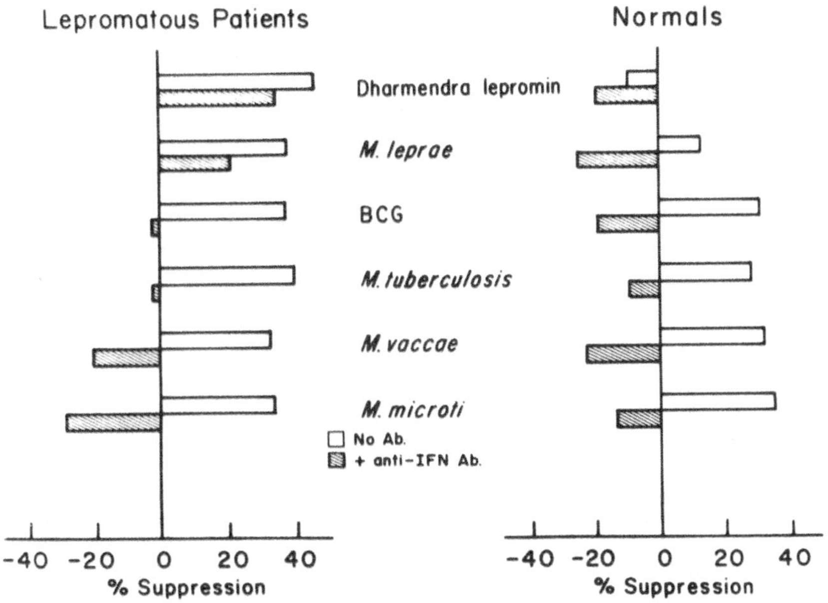

Fig. 2. Specificity of T cell suppression using various mycobacterial antigen in culture containing antibodies to IFN alpha (shaded). From Ref. 3.

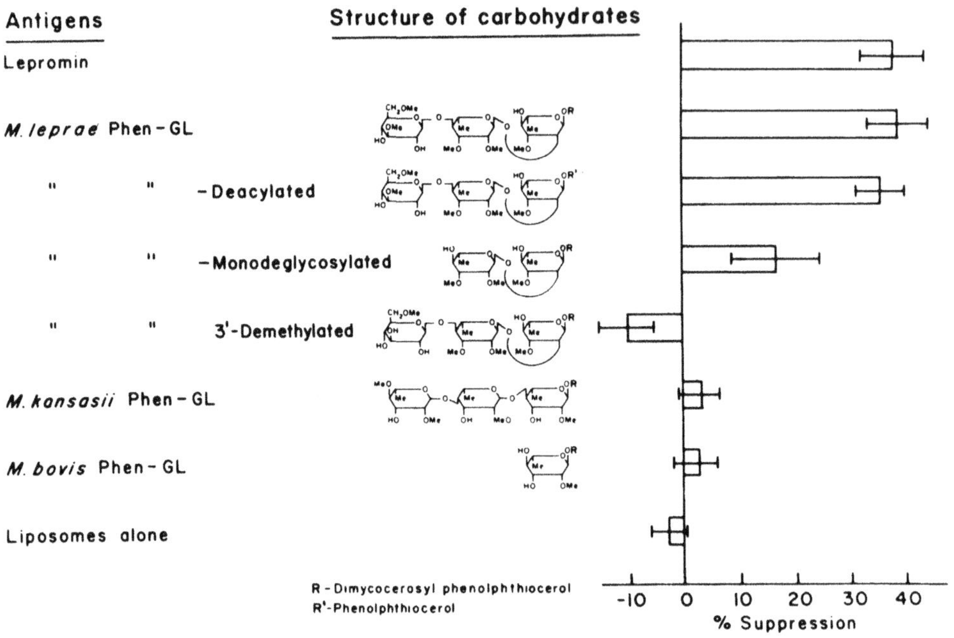

Fig. 3. Structural Requirements for Induction of T Cell Suppression in vitro by Phenolic glycolipid I. (From Ref.15)

Chemical modification to remove the mycolic acid side-chains, (deacylated phenolic glycolipid) had no effect on the suppression; removal of the terminal dimethylglucose diminished suppressor activity; removal of the 3'-methyl group eliminated suppression; and glycolipid homologs from M. bovis and M. kansasii containing the phthiocerocerol backbone associated with different terminal sugars were not suppressive (Fig. 3). A significant portion of the suppression induced by M. leprae and all of that induced by the phenolic glycolipid could be eliminated by a monoclonal antibody to the terminal disaccharide. Finally, recent observations indicate that chemically synthesized disaccharide conjugated to bovine serum albumin is fully capable of inducing the suppressor response in vitro. We believe that these experiments provide some of the best documented evidence that T cells, in this case T suppressor cells, are capable of recognizing carbohydrate epitopes.

One caveat in interpretation is required. Recent studies by Baker indicate that, in the classical system of induction of specific unresponsiveness to pneumococcal polysaccharides in mice, which appears to be exquisitely carbohydrate-specific and mediated by T-suppressor cells, indicate that the suppressor T cells recognized an immunoglobulin idiotype to the poly-saccharide, rather than the carbohydrate antigen itself[16]. In the case of the T8 suppressor cells in leprosy, 50% of which express Fc receptors, in spite of repeated washing and even cell sorting, it is formally not possible for us to exclude the possibility that small amounts of idiotypic antibodies against the phenolic glycolipid may be carried on the Fc receptors and be the determinants recognized by other suppressor cells. We have, however, been unable to induce in vitro suppression using murine or human monoclonal antibodies against the phenolic glycolipid.

Suppressive Determinants in Leishmania

It is of great interest to us that in a murine model a glycoconjugate derived from the *Leishmania major* receptor for macrophages has been reported to be a suppressogenic, disease-promoting antigen in cutaneous leishmaniasis. Mitchell and Handman have shown that a membrane-bound glycolipid is a receptor used by the parasite in attachment to macrophages[17]. The membrane- associated form of the glycolipid can protect mice against cutaneous leishmaniasis, whereas a water-soluble glycoconjugate derived from this lipid has been found to increase the size and persistence of cutaneous leishmaniasis in genetically resistant C57Bl/6 mice. While the structural characterization of the glycoconjugate has not yet been completed, there is a striking parallelism with the immunological effects of the phenolic glycolipid antigen of *M. leprae* would suggest that a glycolipid moiety may well be involved in activating suppressor cells in leishmaniasis. Finally, it may not be without interest that virtually all tumor-associated antigens identified to date

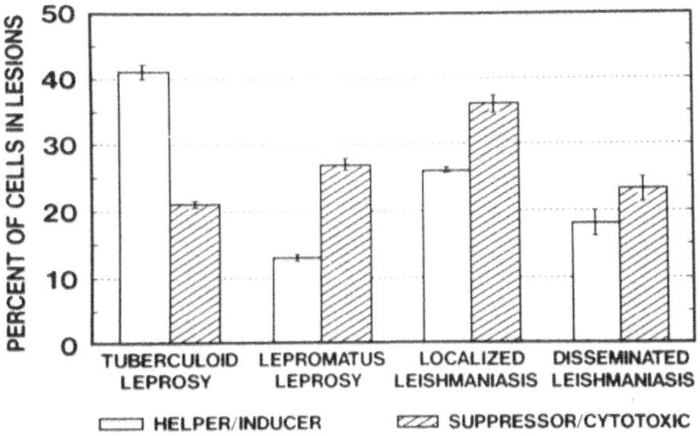

Fig. 4. T cell subsets in lesions of leprosy or leishmania

with monoclonal antibodies have been found to be glycolipids, and not recognized by T-cells of helper or cytotoxic phenotype. By analogy with the glycolipids of these bacterial pathogens, one wonders whether the tumor glycolipids may be involved in suppressing some cellular immune responses to tumors.

Relationship Between Suppressor Activity in vitro to the Disease State in vivo

If the *in vitro* studies on T8 suppressor cells have relevance to the unresponsiveness *in vivo*, then one would predict that in lesions of lepromatous leprosy and diffused cutaneous leishmaniasis $T8^+$, Dr^+ cells would predominate, while in tuberculoid lesions and localized cutaneous leishmaniasis reaction sites, $T4^+$ cells would predominate. Substantial evidence has accumulated in a number of laboratories that the majority of lymphocytes in tuberculoid lesions are $T4^+$, whereas $T8^+$ cells predominate in lepromatous lesions[18,19,20,21,22,23].

In addition, T8 cells predominate in lesions of diffuse cutaneous leishmaniasis[24]. Unexpectedly, however, the T4:T8 ratio in localized cutaneous leishmaniasis is not greatly dissimilar to that in lepromatous leprosy, yet the disease, while persisting, remains quite localized presumably due to immunologic attack (Fig. 4). Modlin, et al[24] were able to establish that, while the phenotypes of cells from skin lesions were similar in both cases, in lepromatous leprosy there were virtually no identifiable IL-2^+ cells whereas there were a significant number found in localized cutaneous leishmaniasis. IL-2 receptor positive (TAC^+) cells were found in roughly equal proportions in both types of lesions[25] (Fig. 5).

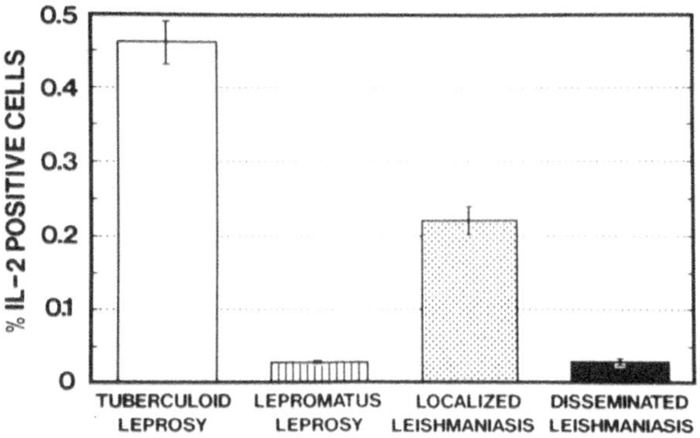

Fig. 5. IL-2 Positive T cells in lesions of leprosy and leishmania

These results suggested that the phenotype of cells present in lesions was less informative than their functional activity, particularly production of appropriate lymphokines. Further, in the case of tuberculoid leprosy and of localized cutaneous leishmaniasis, in which significant numbers of IL-2^+ cells can be detected, there is clearly a local immune response capable of restricting the dissemination of the pathogens. However, both these conditions are associated with tissue injury; in tuberculoid leprosy nerve damage is prominent, and in localized cutaneous leishmaniasis, ulceration at the site of infection is frequent. We and others have suggested that the high levels of local cell-mediated immunity results in production of lymphokines which activate macrophages and cause secretion of proteases, including collagenase and elastase, may cause bystander tissue injury[26].

Human T Suppressor Clones and their MHC Restriction

While very efficient methodology has been developed to permit the isolation of antigen specific T helper clones and cytotoxic T lymphocyte clones in mice and in man, it has been exceedingly difficult to establish continuous cloned cell lines of antigen-specific suppressor cells. In the mouse, T-T hybrid cell lines have been developed which are reported to have antigen-specific suppressor activity, some of which also produce soluble suppressor factors. However, studies at the molecular level have failed to account for the genetic restriction across I-J and, in the majority of cases, the immunoglobulin beta genes are either not rearranged or are deleted, raising questions about their mechanism of antigen recognition[27].

The critical test of the suppressor T cell hypothesis was whether cells actually infiltrating lesions of lepromatous leprosy patients could be shown to manifest antigen-induced suppressive activity that was similar to that observed from the cells of peripheral blood of such patients. Techniques were developed to isolate, FACS-sort these cells into subsets and establish them as short-term lines[9] and then as single cell clones[28]. In most cases, these cells were established by maintaining them in IL-2 with appropriate feeder cells, since the presence of antigen seemed to inhibit their ability to proliferate. In any case, one third of the T8 lines from lepromatous lesions, but none from tuberculoid lesions could be triggered by M. leprae to suppress mitogen responses (Fig. 6).

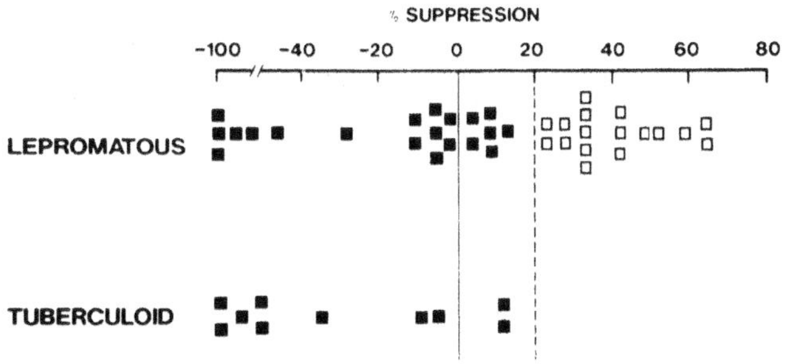

Fig. 6. Suppression of Con A responses by T_8 cell lines obtained directly from leprosy lesions

Six T8 clones from lepromatous lesions have been obtained, and studied for their ability to induce *in vitro* suppression. Two clones have been carefully characterized and found to be able to suppress Con A responses of peripheral mononuclear cells of MHC Class II matched donors stimulated with Con A. Of particular interest was the fact that these two clones were capable of suppressing the response of T4 antigen-specific helper T cell clones to lepromin, and that this suppression was MHC Class II restricted. These T8 clones could only suppress the proliferative responses of MHC Class II-matched cells but not of cells solely matched for MHC Class I antigen. A T4 clone that did not respond to lepromin was included in every experiment to control for the addition of cells to the assay and for possible competition for available IL-2 and it invariably failed to suppress (Fig. 7).

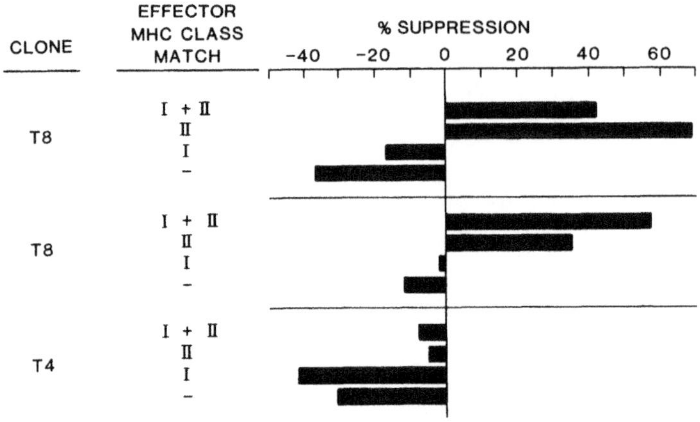

Fig. 7. MHC Class II Restriction of T8 suppressor cell lines obtained from lepromatous lesions.

We believe that these studies provide strong evidence for the first instance of functional suppressor cells within lesions in human disease, and that these T8 suppressor cells are MHC Class II-restricted. We fully appreciate that there may be other types of suppressor cells, e.g. suppressor inducers, anti-idiotypic suppressors, in addition to the antigen-specific probable effector-suppressor cells described here. Secondly, it is quite possible that mechanisms other than suppression may be involved in the failure of patients with leishmaniasis and leprosy to fully respond. Thirdly, suppressor cells have been found in the peripheral blood and lesions of borderline patients[3,18,29], indicating that there is a quantitative interaction between antigen-responsive helper cells and antigen-specific suppressor cells that is likely to be involved in the final clinical manifestations of disease.

Even if one accepts that T suppressor cells are a major determinant in regulating the evolution of disease within the spectrum of leprosy and leishmaniasis in any individual patient, it still remains totally unclear what factors determine the predominant development of T suppressor cells in a very small percentage of people infected with the pathogens. It is unclear whether this is a matter of genetic or environmental predisposition of the individual, variation of the genetics in the parasite, the route of infection, or subversion of the antigen-presenting capability of the macrophages, or dendritic cells or Langerhans cells leading to suppressor dominance.

In no system are the mechanisms by which suppressor cells act to block specific antigen responses are known. It is unclear whether they are involved in depressing IL-2 or IFN-gamma production, by blindfolding, vetoing or killing T helper cells, or by killing or blocking the function of antigen-presenting cells. These are fundamental questions related to the understanding of immunological tolerance, and we believe that these two diseases provide unique opportunities for gaining insight into these mechanisms in man.

Implications of Suppressor Mechanisms for Vaccines Against Leprosy and Leishmaniasis

Even in the most highly endemic areas of the world, incidence rates for leprosy are seldom more than 1-5 per thousand, and for cutaneous leishmaniasis are likely to be even lower. In addition, in the case of leprosy, there is a latent or incubation period averaging 5 years between the putative time of infection and patent manifestation of clinical disease. These two factors impose formidable constraints on any vaccine strategy. In any endemic population, there is a proportion of apparently normal individuals who have been infected with *M. leprae* and are already developing lepromatous disease, and therefore already unable to respond appropriately to antigens of the pathogen.

A major breakthrough in designing an appropriate vaccine strategy was the demonstration that a mixture of live BCG + killed *M. leprae* was capable of converting lepromin-negative lepromatous patients to lepromin skin test positivity. Between 60% and 80% of such individuals markedly improved their histopathological status and many have remained free of disease (Table 3)[30,31,32,33].

Table 3. Clinical and immunological changes in leprosy patients and contacts after vaccination.

	Active		Inactive		Indeterminate	Contacts
	LL	BL	LL	BL		
Clinical Changes	57.0%	76.0%	NA	NA	51%	NA
Positive Reaction	20.4%	58.6%	31.8%	62.5%	95%	100%

We have had an opportunity in a blind study, to examine *in vitro* suppressor T cell activity in 10 patients prior and subsequent to immunotherapy against leprosy using BCG + killed *M. leprae*[3]. The results indicated that in 10 of 10 such patients, the *in vitro* suppressor activity that we measure was reduced to normal levels following successful immunotherapy.

Thus, if it is possible to overcome unresponsiveness in patients who already have active lepromatous leprosy using the combined vaccine, it should be possible as well to immunize an endemic population with such a vaccine as well and prevent disease. Those individuals who have not yet been infected would be identified and immunized against *M. leprae* antigens. Those individuals who have been infected and are incubating the lepromatous form of the disease would in essence be vaccinated immunotherapeutically, presumably overcoming tolerance so that they too would develop appropriate cell-mediated immunity and eliminate their infection.

It is gratifying to know that under the sponsorship of the Venezuelan government and the IMMLEP Committee of WHO, a controlled, blinded prophylactic trial is being carried out to evaluate the effectiveness of killed *M. leprae* + BCG versus BCG alone in 68,000 contacts of lepromatous patients in Venezuela. Under the auspices of LEPRA and IMMLEP at WHO, a second control blinded trial of a total population of 125,000 people in

Malawi comparing killed M. leprae + BCG versus BCG has recently been undertaken. This is a population in which recent case-controlled and cohort data indicate that BCG vaccination alone in this population engenders at least 50% protection against leprosy, and the possibility will be tested that the combined vaccine might be even more effective[34].

Finally, Convit and his associates have recently adopted a similar strategy for therapeutic vaccination of patients with American cutaneous leishmaniasis. While in essence, over 95% of such patients ultimately respond to multiple cycles of pentavalent antimonial treatment, the incidence of side effects, many of them severe, is greater than 50%. In contrast, when killed leishmanial promastigotes are admixed with BCG, 3 vaccinations over a 9 month period are sufficient to bring about a 95% cure rate, with fewer than 7% side effects, all of them minor. It is crucial to unravel the immunological mechanisms involved in protection, particularly since these patients do give positive Montenegro skin tests, and to examine particularly the effects of vaccine therapy on leishmanial suppressor cells.

The recent advances in monoclonal antibodies, development of specific T cell clones and recombinant DNA technology provide tools for identifying and producing protective antigens[35,36,37]. In the case of leprosy and leishmaniasis, it is important, perhaps best using T cell clones, to identify those antigens required for induction of T helper and T killer cell responses that are likely to be important in protection[38,39]. It is similarly important to identify those antigens or epitopes involved in inducing T cell suppression. And in both cases, it is important to learn to what extent those determinants are a property of the antigens, or depend on genetic polymorphisms in T cell receptors and MHC Class I and Class II antigens in the populations. Only with this knowledge will it be possible, with any degree of certainty, to develop recombinant vaccines as useful as the present ones, but hopefully significantly less expensive. Because of the unique adjuvant properties of mycobacteria, it is our objective to develop a recombinant mycobacterial multivaccine vehicle, particularly BCG, capable of expressing recombinant genes for antigens from a variety of pathogens to which T cell immunity is critical for protection.

Acknowledgement

Supported by NIH Grants AI 22187, 22553, 07118, 02111 and 23545, from the UNDP/World Bank/ WHO Special Programme for Research and Training in Tropical Diseases (IMMLEP) and Special Programme for Vaccine Development (IMMTUB), the Hartford Foundation, the Irvington House Institute for Medical Research.

References

1. J. Convit, Leprosy and leishmaniasis. Similar clinical-immunological-pathological models. Ethiop. Med. J. 12:187-195 (1974).

2. D.P. Humber, ed., Immunological Aspects of Leprosy, Tuberculosis and Leishmaniasis. Excerpta Med. Intl. Cong. Ser. 574, pp. 312, (1981).

3. B.R. Bloom, and V. Mehra, Immunological unresponsiveness in leprosy. Immunol. Rev. 80:5-28 (1984).

4. V. Mehra, L.H. Mason, J.P. Fields and B.R. Bloom, Lepromin-induced suppressor cells in patients with leprosy, J. Immunol. 123:1813-1817 (1979).

5. I. Nath, J.J. Van Rood, N.K. Mehra and M.C. Vaidya, Natural suppressor cells in human leprosy: the role of HLA-D-identical peripheral lymphocytes and macrophages in the in vitro modulation of lymphoproliferative responses. Clin. Exp. Immunol. 42:203-210 (1980).

6. Salgame, P.R., P.R. Mahadevan and N.H. Antia, Mechanism of immunosuppression in leprosy: presence of suppressor factor(s) from macrophages of lepromatous patients, Infect. Immun. 40:1119-1126 (1983).

7. I. Nath, J. Jayaraman, M. Sathish, L.K. Bhutani and A.K. Sharma, Inhibition of interleukin-2 production by adherent cell factors from lepromatous leprosy patients. Clin. Exp. Immunol. 58:531-538 (1984).

8. V. Mehra, L.H. Mason, W. Rothman, E. Reinherz, S.F. Schlossman and B.R. Bloom, Delineation of a human T cell subset responsible for lepromin-induced suppression in leprosy patients, J. Immunol., 125:1183-1188 (1980).

9. V. Mehra, J. Convit, A. Rubinstein and B.R. Bloom, Activated suppressor T cells in leprosy, J. Immunol. 129:1946-1951 (1982).

10. R.L. Modlin, V. Mehra, L. Wong, Y. Fujimiya, W-C. Chang, D.A. Horwitz, B.R. Bloom, T.H. Rea and P.K. Pattengale, Suppressor T lymphocytes from lepromatous leprosy skin lesions, J. Immunol. 137:2831-2834 (1986).

11. M. Castes, A. Agnelli, O. Verde and A.J. Rondon, Characterization of the cellular immune response in American cutaneous leishmaniasis, Clin. Immunol. Immunopathol. 27:176-186 (1983).

12. M. Castes, A. Agnelli and A.J. Rondon, Mechanisms associated with immunoregulation in human American cutaneous leishmaniasis. Clin. Exp. Immunol. 57:279-286 (1984).

13. S.W. Hunter, and P.J. Brennan, A novel phenolic glycolipid from Mycobacterium leprae possibly involved in immunogenecity and pathogenicity, J. Bacteriol. 147:728-735 (1984).

14. S.W. Hunter, T. Fujiwara and P.J. Brennan, Structure and antigenicity of the major specific glycolipid antigen of Mycobacterium leprae, J. Biol. Chem. 257:15072-15078 (1981).

15. V. Mehra, P.J. Brennan, E. Rada, J. Convit and B.R. Bloom, Lymphocyte suppression in leprosy induced by unique M. leprae glycolipid, Nature 308:194-196 (1984).

16. P.J. Baker, Homeostatic control of antibody responses: a model based on the recognition of cell-associated antibody by regulatory T cells, Transplant. Rev. 26:3-20 (1975).

17. G.F. Mitchell, and E. Handman, The glycoconjugate derived from a Leishmania major receptor for macrophages is a suppressogenic, disease-promoting antigen in murine cutaneous leishmaniasis. Parasite. Immunol. 8:255-263 (1986).

18. W.C. van Voorhis, G. Kaplan, E.N. Sarno, M.A. Horwitz, R.M. Steinman, W.R. Levis, N. Nogueira, L.S. Hair, C.R. Gattass, B.A. Arrick, and Z.A. Cohn, The cutaneous infiltrates of leprosy: cellular characteristics and the predominant T-cell phenotypes. N. Engl. J. Med. 307:1593-1597 (1982).

19. R.L. Modlin, F.M. Hofman, C.R. Taylor and T.H. Rea, T lymphocyte subsets in the skin lesions of patients with leprosy, J. Am. Acad. Dermatol. 8:182-189 (1983).

20. R.L. Modlin, F.M. Hofman, P.R. Meyer, O.P. Sharma, C.R. Taylor and T.H. Rea, In situ demonstration of T lymphocyte subsets in granulomatous inflammation: leprosy, rhinoscleroma and sarcoidosis. Clin. Exp. Immunol. 51:430-438 (1983).

21. R.L. Modlin, J.F. Gebhard, C.R. Taylor and T.H. Rea, In situ characterization of T lymphocyte subsets in the reactional states of leprosy, Clin. Exp. Immunol. 53:17-24 (1983).

22. R.B. Narayanan, S. Laal, A.K. Sharma, L.K. Bhutani, and I. Nath. Differences in predominant T cell phenotypes and distribution pattern in reactional lesions of tuberculoid and lepromatous leprosy, Clin. Exp. Immunol., 55:623-628 (1984).

23. J. Longley, A. Haregewoin, T. Yemaneberhan, T. van Diepen, T. Warndorff, J. Nsibami, D. Knowles, K.A. Smith and T. Godal, In vivo responses to Mycobacterium leprae: antigen presentation, interleukin-2 production, and immune cell phenotypes in naturally occurring leprosy lesions, Int. J. Lepr. 53:385-394 (1985).

24. R.L. Modlin, F.J. Tapia, B.R. Bloom, M.E. Gallinoto, M. Castes, A.J. Rondon, T.H. Rea and J. Convit, In situ characterization of the cellular immune response in American cutaneous leishmaniasis. Clin. Exp. Immunol. 60:241-248 (1985).

25. R.L. Modlin, F.M. Hofman, D.A. Horwitz, L.A. Husmann, S. Gillis, C.R. Taylor and T.H. Rea, In situ identification of cells in human leprosy granulomas with monoclonal antibodies to interleukin 2 and its receptor, J. Immunol. 132:3085-3090 (1984).

26. W. Cammer, B.R. Bloom, W.T. Norton, and S. Gordon, Degradation of basic protein in myelin by proteases secreted by stimulated macrophages: A possible mechanism of inflammatory demyelination. Proc. Nat. Acad. Sci. 75:1554-1558 (1978).

27. M. Kronenberg, J. Goverman, R. Haars, M. Malissen, E. Kraig, L. Phillips, T. Delovitch, N. Suciu Foca and L. Hood, Rearrangement and transcription of the beta-chain genes of the T-cell antigen receptor in different types of murine lymphocytes. Nature. 313:647-653 (1985).

28. R.L. Modlin, H. Kato, V. Mehra, E.E. Nelson, X-d. Fan, T.H. Rea, P.K. Pattengale and B.R. Bloom, Genetically restricted suppressor T-cell clones derived from lepromatous leprosy lesions,. Nature. 322:459-461 (1986).

29. T.H.M. Ottenhoff, D.G. Elferink, P.R. Klaster and R.R.P. de Vries, Cloned suppressor T cells from a lepromatous leprosy patient suppress Mycobacterium leprae reactive helper T cells, Nature. 322:462-464 (1986).

30. J. Convit, M.E. Pinardi, G. Rodriguez Ochoa, M. Ulrich, J.L. Avila and M. Goihman, Elimination of Mycobacterium leprae subsequent to local in vivo activation of macrophages in lepromatous leprosy by other mycobacteria, Clin. Exp. Immunol. 17:261-265 (1974).

31. J. Convit, N. Aranzazu, M. Pinardi and M. Ulrich, Immunological changes observed in indeterminate and lepromatous leprosy patients and Mitsuda-negative contacts after the inoculation of a mixture of Mycobacterium leprae and BCG, Clin. Exp. Immunol. 36:214-220 (1979).

32. J. Convit, N. Aranzazu, M. Ulrich, M.E. Pinardi, O. Reyes and J. Alvarado, Immunotherapy with a mixture of Mycobacterium leprae and BCG in different forms of leprosy and in Mitsuda-negative contacts, Int. J. Lepr. 50:415-424 (1982).

33. J. Convit, N. Aranzazu, M. Zuniga, M. Ulrich, M.E. Pinardi, Z. Castellazzi and J. Alvarado, Immunotherapy and immunoprophylaxis of leprosy, Lepr. Rev. 4760:47-60 (1983).

34. P.E.M. Fine, J.M. Ponnighaus, N. Maine, J.A. Clarkson and L. Bliss. Lancet ii: 499-502, 1986.

35. H.D. Engers, M. Abe, B.R. Bloom, V. Mehra, W. Britton, T.M. Buchanan, S.K. Khanolkar, D.B. Young, O. Closs, T. Gillis, M. Harboe, J. Ivanyi, A.H.J. Kolk, and C.C. Shepard, Workshop: Results of a World Health Organization-Sponsored Workshop on Monoclonal Antibodies to Mycobacterium leprae. Inf. & Immun. 48:603-605 (1985).

36. R.A. Young, V. Mehra, D. Sweetser, T. Buchanan, J. Clark-Curtiss, R.W. Davis and B.R. Bloom, Genes for the major protein antigens of the leprosy parasite Mycobacterium leprae, Nature, 316:450-452 (1985).

37. A.S. Mustafa, H.K. Gill, A. Nerland, W.J. Britton, V. Mehra, B.R. Bloom, R.A. Young, and T. Godal, Human T-cell clones recognize a major M. leprae protein antigen expressed in E. coli. Nature. 319:63-66 (1986).

38. A.S. Mustafa, H.K. Gill, A. Nerland, W.J. Britton, V. Mehra, B.R. Bloom, R.A. Young and T. Godal, Human T-cell clones recognize a major M. leprae protein antigen expressed in E. coli. Nature. 319:63-66 (1986).

39. T.H. Ottenhoff, P.R. Klatser, J. Ivanyi, D.G. Elferink, M.Y. de Wit, and R.R. de Vries, Mycobacterium leprae-specific protein antigens defined by cloned human helper T cells, Nature, 319:66-68 (1986).

PARTIAL CHARACTERIZATION OF SUPPRESSOR FACTORS IN SPLEEN CELL CULTURE SUPERNATANTS OF MYCOBACTERIUM LEPRAEMURIUM-INFECTED MICE

L. Richard[1], A. Forget[2], and R. Turcotte[1]

[1] Institut Armand-Frappier, Université du Québec, Ville de Laval, Québec, [2]Faculté de Médecine, Université de Montréal, Québec

INTRODUCTION

The presence of suppressor cells (macrophage-like and T lymphocytes) have been demonstrated in the spleen of mice infected with Mycobacterium lepraemurium (M.lm) (1, 2). These suppressor cells depressed several in vitro immune functions, such as the lymphoblastic responses to polyclonal mitogens (2, 3), to alloantigens (4) and to specific antigens (5), the generation of cytotoxic T-cell response and the expression of natural killing activity (Lemieux et al., unpublished results). Recently, we have found that splenic T-cell subpopulations from M.lm-infected mice, when adoptively transferred to syngeneic mice, can depress the induction and/or the expression of the delayed-type hypersensitivity (DTH) to M.lm antigens (6).

The present paper deals with the kinetics of in vitro production of soluble suppressor factors by spleen cells from leprous mice and with some of their biological and physicochemical properties.

MATERIALS AND METHODS

Induction of suppressor cells

Female mice of the inbred strain C57BL/6 (Charles River Breeding Labs, Mass. USA) were infected i.v. with 1 X 10^7 bacilli of the Hawaiian strain of M. lepraemurium (M.lm). Eight to 10 weeks later, suppressor cells were detected, as shown by the ability of infected spleen cells to depress the blastogenic responses of normal spleen cells to polyclonal mitogens and to mycobacterial antigens (2).

Separation of spleen cells

Adherent cells from infected and age-matched control mice were isolated on plastic petri dishes after a one-h incubation at 37°C. The plastic nonadherent cells were also separated into Ig^+ and Ig^- cells (enriched T lymphocytes) using a panning technique (7). Plastic nonadherent cells were also separated into antigen-specific and -nonspecific cells on plastic petri dishes coated with water-soluble mycobacterial antigens.

Spleen cells (whole or separated populations) at a density of 1 X 10^7/ml of serum-free and mitogen-free RPMI-1640 medium were incubated at 37°C in a humidified atmosphere of 5% CO_2. At various times thereafter, supernatants were harvested, filtered through 0.22-μm pore-size membranes and stored at -20°C until testing for suppressor activity or using in passive transfer experiments.

Assessement of suppressor activity

The suppressor activity in crude and fractionated culture supernatants was evaluated by their ability to depress thymidine incorporation into mitogen- and mycobacterial antigen-stimulated normal spleen cells (8). All experiments were carried out in triplicate and the results expressed as percentage of suppression according to the formula: percentage of suppression = 1 - (cpm-M.lm/cpm-normal) X 100, where cpm-M.lm and cpm-normal represent the mean incorporation by normal splenocytes in the presence of supernatants, respectively, from M.lm-infected and normal spleen cells.

Passive transfer of suppressor factors-containing supernatants

One ml of crude supernatants from infected or normal mice (as controls) was inoculated i.v. into syngeneic mice just prior to or 5 weeks after footpad infection with 1 X 10^7 M.lm bacilli. Normal recipient mice were challenged 5 weeks later in the opposite footpad with a sonicated M.lm extract (6) to study the effects of suppressor factors on the induction of DTH whereas, infected recipient mice were challenged 24 h after the transfer of supernatants to study their effects on the expression of DTH. The footpad thickness was measured with a dial-gauge calipers prior to and 24 and 48 h after the challenge and expressed in 0.1 mm units.

Isoelectric focusing of suppressor factors

Culture supernatants (20-times concentrated on Amicon PM-10 membranes) were fractionated by preparative flat-bed isoelectric focusing in a pH gradient from 3.0 to 10.0. After dialysis against RPMI medium and lyophilization, each fraction was tested for suppressive activity as described above.

RESULTS

Kinetics of secretion of suppressor factors

Spleen cells from C57BL/6 mice infected with M.lm 9 weeks earlier released into the culture supernatants suppressor factors (SF) that depressed the blastogenic responses to mycobacterial antigens ("specific" SF) and to polyclonal mitogens (nonspecific SF) (Fig. 1-A). The release of "specific" SF occurred at 4 to 8 h after the initiation of cultures; they reached a maximum level at 12 h and then disappeared rapidly during the next 12 h to reappear again at 32 h. In contrast, the nonspecific SF started to be produced after 12 h of incubation and their activity remained relatively low till the end of the observation period.

At 12 weeks post-infection (Fig. 1-B), the nonspecific suppressive activity appeared earlier and was larger than that observed at 9 weeks. It should be noted that both "specific" and nonspecific SF seemed to be released in a cyclic manner of about 8-h duration.

Nature of suppressor factors-producing cells

Spleen cells from mice infected 9 weeks earlier were separated into different populations and incubated at a density of 1 X 10^7/ml (5 X 10^5/ml, in the case of antigen-specific cells) during 15 h for the production of SF. As shown in Table 1,

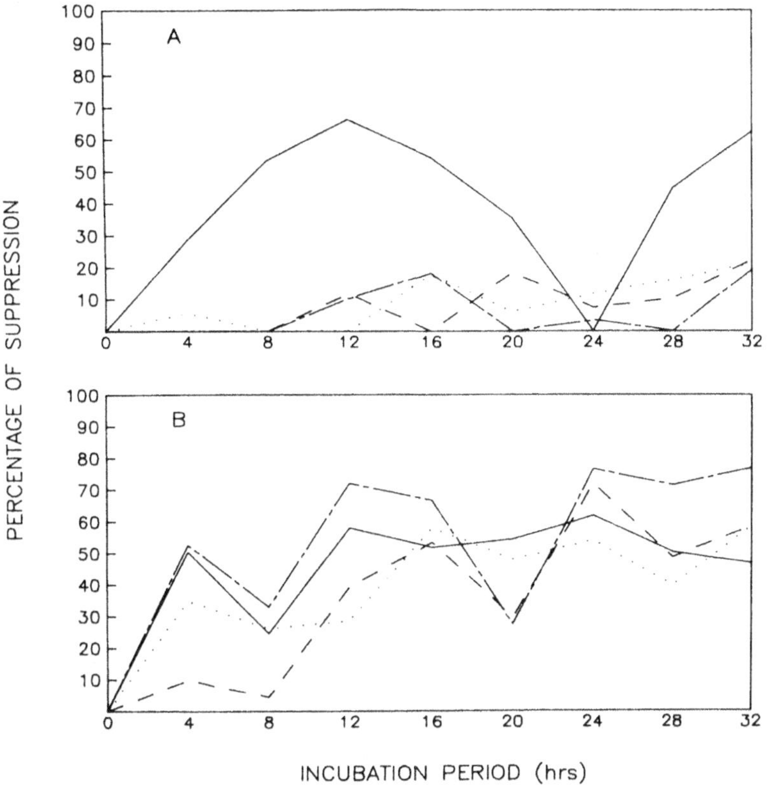

Fig. 1. Kinetics of production of suppressor factors in spleen cell cultures from mice infected 9 weeks (A) and 12 weeks (B) earlier with M. lepraemurium. The (———) represents the inhibition of the response to Mycobacterial antigens; the (—— –), the response to LPS; the (– – – –), the response to PHA; and the (··········), the response to Con A.

the response to Con A was depressed whatever the origin of culture supernatants whereas, the responses to PHA, LPS and mycobacterial antigens were depressed only by supernatants originating from unseparated cells, T lymphocytes and antigen-specific cell populations. Both "specific" and nonspecific SF were secreted by the antigen-specific cells. Moreover, high suppressive activities were produced by these cells if one considers that a relatively low number of cells was incubated.

Suppression of DTH by passive transfers of suppressor factors

Crude supernatants obtained from spleen cell cultures of mice infected 9 weeks earlier were passively transferred into syngeneic mice prior to and 5 weeks after infection with M.lm in order to investigate whether SF regulated the induction and the expression of DTH to M.lm antigens. No suppressive effect on the induction of DTH (Table 2) and on the intensity of the granulomatous reaction at the site of infection (unshown data) was found. In contrast, both the expression of DTH (Table 2) and the intensity of the local granulomatous reaction were depressed to a significant extent.

TABLE 1. Suppressive activity of culture supernatants obtained from spleen cell populations of M.lm-infected mice[a].

Origin of culture supernatants	% Inhibition of $^{3}H(TdR)$ incorporation in spleen cells stimulated with:			
	PHA	Con A	LPS	Myco. Ag.
Whole spleen cells	35	24	6	38
Enriched T cells[b]	52	16	0	54
Surface Ig^{+} cells[b]	0	12	0	0
Plastic adherent cells	0	9	0	0
Ag-specific cells[c]	8	41	7	38
Ag-nonspecific cells[c]	0	28	0	0

[a] Mice infected 9 weeks earlier were used.
[b] Surface Ig^{+} cells were recovered from plastic petri dishes coated with affinity purified anti-mouse IgG + IgM (H + L) anti-serum; the enriched T cells being the corresponding surface Ig^{-} population.
[c] Ag-specific and ag-nonspecific cells refer to cells that respectively, did and did not adhere to mycobacterial antigen-coated petri dishes.

TABLE 2. Effects of suppressor fators-containing supernatants on the induction and the expression of delayed-type hypersensitivity to M. lepraemurium.

Origin of transferred supernatants	Footpad thickness (0.1 mm ± SEM)	
	Induction	Expression
Normal spleen cells	0.45 ± 0.04[a]	0.37 ± 0.04
Infected spleen cells	0.38 ± 0.03	0.20 ± 0.02[c]
Control[b]	0.40 ± 0.04	0.40 ± 0.04

[a] Mean footpad thickness ± standard error of the mean of ten mice per each group.
[b] The control group refers to M.lm-infected mice receiving no transfer of culture supernatants.
[c] Statistically different ($P < 0.001$, as determined by the Student t test) from the value found in recipients of normal culture supernatants.

Partial purification of suppressor factors

On isoelectric focusing (see Fig. 2), the SF that inhibited the response to PHA were found in pH 6.2 to 7.5 fractions. Those suppressing the response to Con A were in the pH 5.1 and 8.4 fractions. Suppressor factors of the response to LPS migrated with the pH 7.5 fraction. Finally, SF of the response to mycobacterial antigens migrated in the pH 7.5 and 4.4 fractions. Interrestingly, the suppressive activity found in the pH 4.4 fraction appeared to be directed against mycobacterial antigens only.

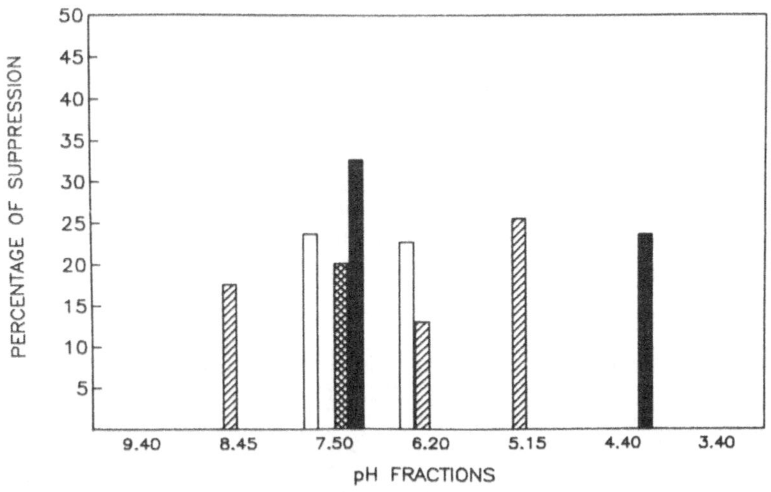

Fig. 2. Isoelectric focusing of splenic culture supernatants from M. lepremurium-infected mice. Open bars represent the inhibition of the response to PHA; left hatched bars, the response to Con A; the right cross-hatched bars, the response to LPS; and the solid bars, the response to mycobacterial antigens.

DISCUSSION

Soluble factors secreted by suppressor cells and able of inhibiting DNA synthesis in spleen cell cultures have been reported by several investigators in mice infected either with a variety of microorganisms (8, 9, 10, 11) or sensitized with non-replicating substances (12, 13). However, very little is known about the mechanisms of production of these SF by suppressor cells in culture. In the present study, spleen cells from M.lm-infected mice were found to produce SF that inhibited the blastogenic responses of normal splenocytes to mycobacterial antigens and to polyclonal mitogens. Interrestingly, these SF were released into the culture supernatant in a cyclic manner; a situation suggesting that, once released, SF were either inactivated or utilized (e.g. via a mechanism of SF-specific membrane receptor) by the cultured spleen cells.

The variations in the time of appearance of suppressive activity in culture supernatants and its distribution on flat bed isoelectric focusing can be interpreted as indicating that several physicochemically distinct SF have been produced. These results would also suggest the release of mycobacterial antigen-specific SF in culture supernatants. Obviously, further experiments would be needed to establish whether specific SF really exist.

Several investigators using unrelated experimental models (11, 13, 14) have shown that antigen-specific SF can be released by first-order suppressor T cells. Once released, these specific factors led to the induction of second-order suppressor T cells which acquired the ability to secrete non-specific SF. Similar mechanisms might be involved in the present system since the "specific" SF, at least in mice infected 9 weeks earlier with M.lm, were detected in the culture supernatants before the nonspecific ones.

In an attempt to isolate the cell population involved in the production of "specific" SF, spleen cells from infected mice were absorbed on mycobacterial antigen-coated petri dishes. In fact, this method led to an enrichment of SF-producing cells but unfortunately, these cells released "specific" and nonspecific SF, as well.

Adoptive transfer experiments have shown that suppressor factors-containing supernatants depressed the expression but not the induction of DTH to M.lm antigens. This situation was not due to the presence of free M.lm bacilli since culture supernatants were filtered through 0.22-μm pore-size membranes. On the other hand, the possibility of a desensitization of recipient mice by soluble M.lm antigens contaminating culture supernatants cannot be completely excluded.

SUMMARY

Suppressor factors (SF) were released into the culture supernatant when spleen cells from M. lepraemurium-infected C57BL/6 mice were incubated at 37°C in the absence of any inducing agents. Some of the SF appeared to be specific in that they inhibited the blastogenic response to mycobacterial antigens by opposition to the others which inhibited the blastogenic responses to PHA, Con A and LPS. All SF seemed to be produced in a cyclic manner. In mice infected 9 weeks earlier, the release of "specific" SF occurred early (4-8 h) during the incubation period whereas, the nonspecific SF were released later on (12-32 h). Adoptive transfers of SF-containing culture supernatants depressed the expression of DTH to M.lm antigens but not its induction.

ACKNOWLEDGMENT

This work was supported by The Order of St. Lazarus of Jerusalem.

REFERENCES

1. **W. E. Bullock, E. M. Carlson, and R. K. Gershon,** The evolution of immunosuppressive cell populations in experimental mycobacterial infection. J. Immunol. 120:1709 (1978).

2. **R. Turcotte,** Suppressor cells in experimental murine leprosy. Int. J. Leprosy 46:358 (1978).

3. **R. Turcotte,** Influence of route of Mycobacterium lepraemurium infection on susceptibility to mouse leprosy and on lymphoblastic transformation. Infect. Immun. 28:660 (1980).

4. **A. Hoffenbach, P. H. Lagrange, and M. A. Bach,** Surface Lyt phenotype of suppressor cells in C57BL/6 mice infected with Mycobacterium lepraemurium. Clin. Exp. Immunol. 54:151 (1983).

5. **S. J. Brett,** T-cell responsiveness in Mycobacterium lepraemurium infections in a "resistant" (CBA) and a "susceptible" (BALB/c) mouse strain. Cell. Immunol. 89:132 (1984).

6. **L. Richard, R. Turcotte, and A. Forget,** Suppressor T cells for delayed-type hypersensitivity in susceptible mice infected with Mycobacterium lepraemurium. Int. J. Leprosy (in press).

7. **L. J. Wysocki, and V. L. Sato,** "Panning" for lymphocytes: A method for cell selection. Proc. Natl Acad. Sci. USA 75:2844 (1978).

8. **R. Turcotte, and S. Lemieux,** Mechanisms of action of Mycobacterium bovis BCG-induced suppressor cells in mitogen-induced blastogenesis. Infect. Immun. 36:263 (1982).

9. **V. Colizzi, J. Ferluga, F. Garreau, M. Malkowski, and G. Asherson**, Suppressor cells induced by BCG release non-specific factors in vitro which inhibit DNA synthesis and interleukin-2 production. Immunology 51:65 (1984).

10. **J. S. Dhaliwal, F. Y. Liew, and F. E. G. Cox,** Specific suppressor T cells for delayed-type hypersensitivity in susceptible mice immunized against cutaneous leishmaniasis. Infect. Immun. 49:417 (1985).

11. **J. Murphy**, Effects of first-order cryptotoccus-specific T-suppressor cells on induction of cells responsible for delayed-type hypersensitivity. Infect. Immun. 48:439 (1985).

12. **G. L. Asherson, and M. Zembala**, T suppressor cells and suppressor factor which act at the efferent stage of the contact sensitivity skin reaction: Their production by mice injected with water-soluble, chemically reactive derivatives of oxazolone and picryl chloride. Immunology 42:1005 (1980).

13. **S. D. Miller, L. D. Butler, and H. N. Claman**, Suppressor T cell circuits in contact sensitivity. 1. Two mechanistically distinct waves of suppressor T cells occur in mice tolerized with syngeneic DNP-modified lymphoid cells. J. Immunol. 129:461 (1982).

14. **M. Taniguchi, and T. Tokuhisa**, Cellular consequences in the suppression of antibody response by the antigen-specific T-cell factor. J. Exp. Med. 151:517 (1980).

IMMUNOREGULATION IN HUMAN TUBERCULOSIS

Jerrold J. Ellner

Division of Infectious Diseases, Department of Medicine, Case Western Reserve University and University Hospitals of Cleveland, Cleveland, OH 44106

INTRODUCTION

Infection of humans with Mycobacterium tuberculosis provides an attractive model for investigating regulation of the immune response for several reasons. First, the causative agent is cultivable on synthetic medium and a cDNA genomic expression library has been prepared. Therefore, purified native and recombinant mycobacterial antigens can be tested directly for immunoregulatory activity. Second, the immune response in healthy subjects with delayed-type hypersensitivity (DTH) to mycobacteria can be contrasted to patients with tuberculosis to elucidate patterns of immunoregulation which are characteristic of disease. Third, although infection with M. tuberculosis or attenuated mycobacteria is an excellent model for DTH in experimental systems, the paradoxic occurrence of anergy in some patients can be explored in the laboratory.

Twenty to 25% of patients with pulmonary tuberculosis, in fact, have negative tuberculin skin tests at the time of diagnosis (1). In some subjects, anergy is nonspecific; in others it is restricted to the response to mycobacterial antigens. Whereas individual studies indicate association of skin test hyporesponsiveness with age, severity of illness, or radiographic manifestations of acute disease, the status of DTH reactivity is not predictable in individual patients. In addition, repeat skin testing of anergic subjects 2-4 weeks after initiation of treatment usually shows conversion to a reactive state. Therefore, lack of response to mycobacterial antigens is not absolute, for example, due to absence of the human equivalent of an immune response gene. Other potential explanations for initially negative tuberculin skin tests (latency to development of DTH, defective chemotaxis, compartmentalization of reactive lymphocytes to tissue sites) seem unlikely on the basis of existing information. This led us to examine the role of active immunosuppression by mycobacterial products and suppressor cells in the anergy present in tuberculous patients.

RESULTS

Nonspecific suppression by mycobacterial polysaccharides and tuberculous plasma

Several observations point to the possible relevance of mycobacterial polysaccharides to suppression of T-cell mediated responses in tuberculosis: skin test nonreactive patients have increased levels of antibody; bacterial polysaccharides typically stimulate a polyclonal B cell response; and mycobacterial polysaccharides elicit antibody production but not DTH. We first confirmed the observation of others that tuberculous plasma was suppressive of PPD-induced blastogenesis in peripheral blood mononuclear cells (PBMC) from healthy tuberculin reactors (2). In contrast to the previous reports, however, suppression was nonspecific, affecting the response to the nonspecific mitogen, phytohemagglutinin, as well as that to PPD (Figure 1).

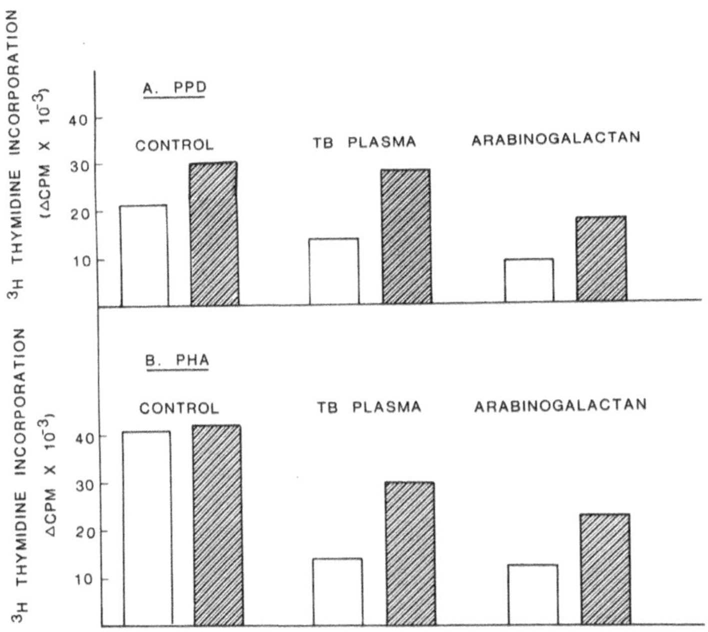

Figure 1. Effect of indomethacin on TB plasma and D-arabinogalactan (AG) suppression of PBMC responses to PPD (panel A) and to PHA (panel B). Data are represented as the mean response in cpm for PBMC cultured without (open bars) or with (hatched bars) 1.0 ug/ml indomethacin. Data are shown for control cell suspensions and for cells cultured with TB plasma or AG. (Reproduced from J. Clin. Invest. 68:153, 1979, by copyright permission of the American Society for Clinical Investigation).

D-arabino-D-galactan, a major cell wall polysaccharide, was purified from M. tuberculosis culture filtrates by affinity chromatography, and also was suppressive of antigen- and mitogen-induced blastogenesis. Suppression by tuberculous plasma and D-arabinogalactan was partly blocked by indomethacin

(Figure 1) and monocyte depletion (not shown). D-arabinogalactan induced four-fold increased production of PGE_2 by human monocytes (2). Prevention of suppression by antibody to mycobacterial polysaccharides and the presence of antibody to polysaccharides in the plasma at a titer of 1:640 (ELISA) suggested that circulating immune complexes containing D-arabinogalactan (or related polysaccharides) were responsible for serosuppression. The mechanism of suppression appears to be monocyte-dependent increased production of immunosuppressive cyclooxygenase products such as PGE_2.

Antigen-specific suppression by circulating monocytes

An effective cell-mediated immune response requires activation of mononuclear phagocytes to destroy the tubercle bacillus. We next investigated the possibility that circulating monocytes activated *in vivo* by exposure to factors derived from *M. tuberculosis*, or products of the host-parasite interaction, might participate in regulatory circuits which suppress T-lymphocyte responses (3). First, patients with tuberculosis were stratified according to level of blastogenic response to tuberculin PPD (Figure 2). Patients lacking significant PPD-induced blastogenesis were similar to those with high responses in terms of age, underlying diseases, extent of pulmonary tuberculosis graded radiographically, and drug treatment regimens. Low responders differed in two ways. First, 6 of 7 had negative intermediate-strength tuberculin skin tests at the time of diagnosis (cf. 1 of 7 high responders; $p<0.01$). Second, a greater proportion of PBMC, prepared by Ficoll-Hypaque sedimentation of heparinized blood, was identified as monocytes by cytochemical criteria (38.6% ± 4.5% non-responders vs. 16.6% ± 3.6% high responders, $p<0.01$). Depletion of adherent cells from PBMC by sequential incubation on plastic surfaces and nylon wool columns increased the response of tuberculin non-responders to PPD by 20.4-fold; the response to streptococcal antigens and PHA was unaffected.

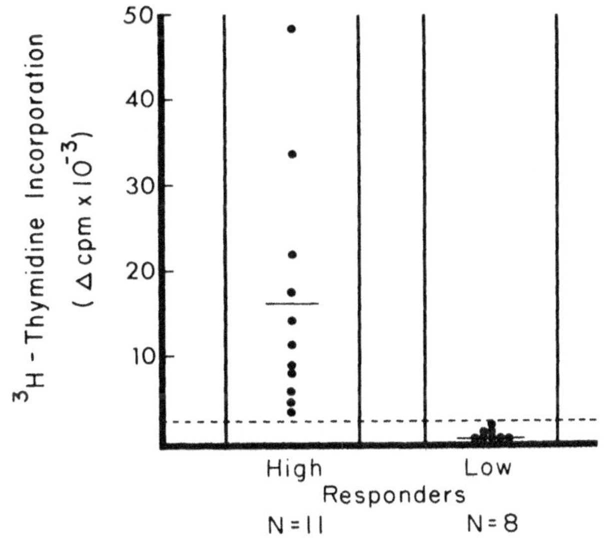

Figure 2. PPD-induced ^3H-thymidine incorporation of PBMC and T cells for representative high and low responder patients. (Reproduced from Ellner JJ, J. Immunol. 121:2573, 1978, copyright by Williams & Wilkins, 1978).

Reconstitution experiments (Figure 3) further established that in addition to their increase in numbers, suppressor adherent cells from patients with tuberculosis were activated to function as antigen-specific suppressor cells. Subsequent studies indicated that the adherent mononuclear cell population with major suppressor cell activity was peroxidase positive, sheep erythrocyte non-rosetting, and reactive with the murine monoclonal antibody OKM1 (4). These characteristics implicate the monocyte as the key suppressor cell.

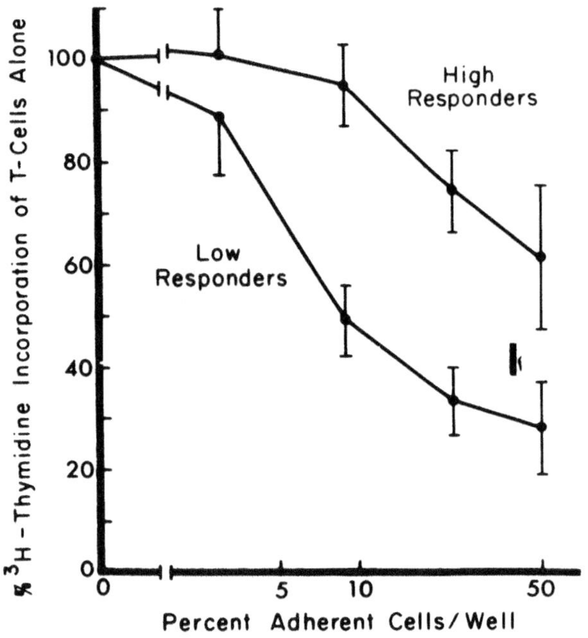

Figure 3. Inhibition of PPD-induced T-cell ^{3}H-TdR by adherent cells. Data are presented as mean ± SEM for six high responders and five low responders. Significant differences between low and high responders were noted at 9%, 23% and 47% adherent cells ($p<0.01$, Student's t test). (Reproduced from Ellner JJ. J. Immunol. 121:2573, 1978, copyright by Williams & Wilkins, 1978).)

Next, we sought to clarify the mechanism and mediators of suppression by monocytes. Surface expression of Class II major histocompatibility complex (MHC) determinants is necessary for immune induction. Monocytes from patients with tuberculosis showed lower levels of reactivity with OKIa1, a mouse monoclonal antibody to the framework of the HLA-DR determinant (5); in addition, their monocytes underwent a burst of synthetic activity during in vitro cultivation. The altered expression of HLA-DR products was associated with suppressor function of the monocytes. It is uncertain whether this represents simply a marker of suppressor cells or is a central feature of the mechanism of suppression.

Recent studies have examined the role of interleukin-1 (IL-1) in suppression by monocytes. Monocytes produce IL-1 when exposed to number of stimuli, including bacterial lipopolysaccharide and PPD (6). Patients with tuberculosis show increased production of IL-1 by monocytes (Figure 4) and an association between suppressor activity and IL-1 production (7). It appears that, in this case, IL-1 may be a mediator of suppression, since crude and recombinant IL-1, in activities resembling those produced by stimulated monocytes, suppressed the response of PBMC from healthy donors to antigens and mitogens and a T-cell line from a tuberculous patient to PPD and interleukin-2 (IL-2) (Wallis RS, Ellner JJ, submitted for publication).

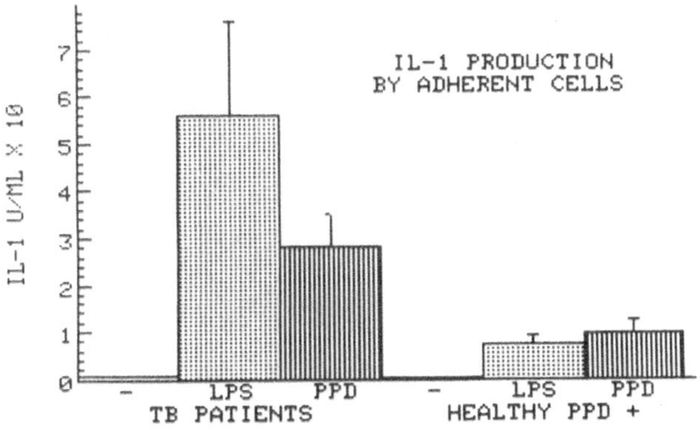

Figure 4. IL-1 activity in supernatants of monocytes cultured for 24 hours with lipopolysaccharide (LPS) or PPD. Data are shown as mean ± SEM, n=7 for each group. (Reproduced from Ellner JJ. J. Lab. Clin. Med. 108:142, 1986, copyright by The C.V. Mosby Company).

Antigen-specific suppression by $Fc_{gamma}R^{+}$lymphocytes

The specificity of suppression by monocytes implies that a lymphocyte specific for tuberculin antigens may be involved in the suppressor cell circuitry. When the traditional helper (OKT4, Leu 4a) and suppressor (OKT8, Leu 2a) subpopulations (and their ratios) were quantified in patients with tuberculosis by reactivity with monoclonal antibodies and indirect immunofluorescence, they were not differentiable from control subjects (Kleinhenz ME, Ellner JJ, submitted for publication). In contrast, nonadherent cells identified by rosetting with IgG sensitized ox erythrocytes as $Fc_{gamma}R^{+}$ were increased in patients (42 ± 4% compared to 28 ± 3% healthy subjects). As contrasted to controls, cells from patients also showed direct responsiveness to tuberculin PPD. Depletion experiments indicated that $Fc_{gamma}R^+$ cells functioned as antigen-specific suppressor cells in some patients. In fact, subjects hyporesponsive to PPD could be divided into two groups: a minority showed depressed responses which were reconstituted to normal levels by depletion of monocytes; in the remainder, monocyte depletion had no effect, whereas PPD-induced blastogenesis was boosted, although not to normal levels, by depletion of $Fc_{gamma}R^+$ lymphocytes. The data indicate parallel suppressor circuits involving $Fc_{gamma}R^+$ cells or monocytes. The dual mechanisms resemble observations in leprosy (10). On the other hand, monocyte-mediated suppression of tuberculin responses is not effected through $Fc_{gamma}R^+$ or Leu 2a lymphocytes (data not shown).

Regulation of metabolism of interleukin-2

The fit of IL-2 in its receptor leads to clonal expansion of activated T-lymphocytes. We examined IL-2 production and the generation of IL-2 receptors in patients with tuberculosis (8). PPD-stimulated production of IL-2 by T-cells correlated with blastogenesis and was decreased in tuberculosis (Figure 5).

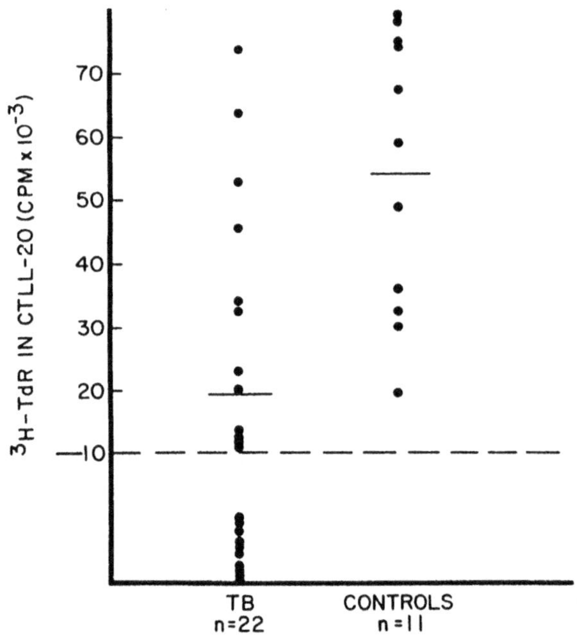

Figure 5. IL-2 activity in supernatants of PPD-stimulated T-cell cultures for patients with tuberculosis (TB) and controls, - - -, Mean IL-2 activity of controls -2 SD. This line separates patients with tuberculosis into normal producers of IL-2 (above line) and low producers of IL-2 (below line). (Reproduced from Toossi Z, et al. J. Exp. Med. 163:1162, 1986, by copyright permission of The Rockefeller University Press).

When patients were divided into normal and low producers of IL-2 by T-cells, modulatory effects of adherent cells only were observed in normal producers (Figure 6). This suggests that in patients with low PPD-induced blastogenesis, IL-2 production may be low, but suppressor adherent cells block blastogenesis at another step in activation. In this regard, surface expression of the IL-2 receptor also was evaluated. PPD-induced anti-TAC reactivity (anti-TAC is a murine monoclonal antibody which reacts with the human IL-2 receptor) was 31.9 ± 8.0% in 3 healthy donors and 5.4 ± 2.9% in 4 tuberculous patients. It is not yet clear whether adherent cells modulate expression of IL-2 receptors in tuberculosis.

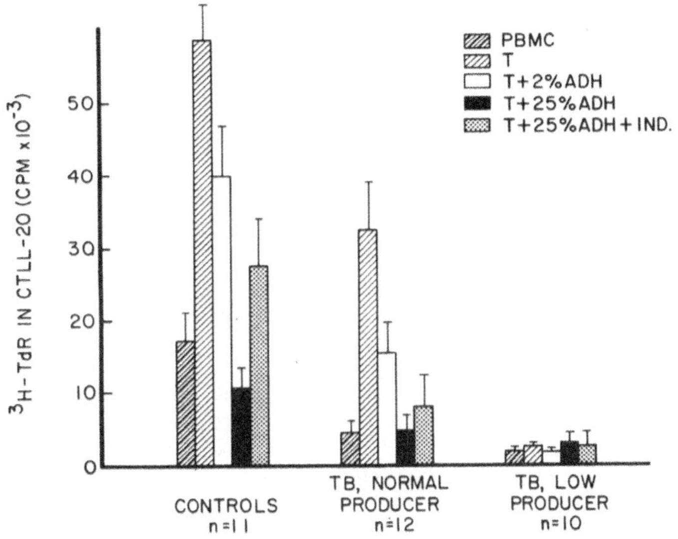

Figure 6. PPD-induced IL-2 activity in cultures of PBMC, T-cells (T), T cells + 2% adherent cells (ADH), T cells + 25% ADH, and T cells + 25% ADH in the presence of 1 ug/ml indomethacin. Each bar represents mean ± SEM. (Reproduced from Toossi Z, et al. J. Exp. Med. 163:1162, 1986, by copyright permission of The Rockefeller University Press).

DISCUSSION

Our findings on the immune response in tuberculosis pose three main questions:

1. Is disturbed immunoregulation cause or effect of tuberculosis?

Skin test anergy and *in vitro* hyporesponsiveness are transient states, reverting during therapy of tuberculosis. Nonetheless, the existence of HLA-associations with tuberculosis suggests that host factors influence the course of *M. tuberculosis* infection. We speculate that HLA-DR phenotype determines the level and patterns of regulation of the immune response following exposure to tuberculosis. This hypothesis must be tested in family studies which examine linkage of HLA-phenotype with tuberculin reactivity and occurrence of disease.

2. What is the basis for antigen-specificity of suppression by monocytes in tuberculosis?

Antigen-specificity of suppression may reside in the antigen, or its processing, or in obligatory interactions with T-lymphocytes. PPD is a direct stimulus for IL-1 production (6). Given the data supporting a suppressive role for IL-1 in tuberculosis, the apparent specificity of suppression could reflect stimulus-specific preferential induction of IL-1 release. This, in turn, would imply that some mycobacterial antigens or epitopes might be phlogistic and immunosuppressive, whereas others could activate cellular immune responses. Cytophilic antibody on monocytes directed against mycobacteria also might lead to differential binding, uptake and processing of tuberculin antigens which could be manifest as specificity of suppression. The main alternative to direct effects of antigen is that specificity is due to obligatory interactions of monocytes with antigen-specific lymphocytes. Based on available data, leading contenders for cellular interlocutor are adherent $Fc_{gamma}R^{+}$ lymphocytes (large granular lymphocytes) and nonadherent $OKT4^{+}$ $Leu\ 8^{+}$ cells (suppressor-inducer subset).

3. What are the molecular mediators of suppression by adherent cells?

The data implicating IL-1 in suppression have been presented. In balance, existing evidence is indirect. The lack of consistent spontaneous elaboration of suppressor factors during *in vitro* cultivation of monocytes increases the complexity of directly establishing the suppressive role of IL-1 in tuberculosis. It seems possible that other macromolecular factors, some of which may be novel, participate in suppression by mononuclear phagocytes. For example, we have studied a factor produced by the human macrophage-like cell line U937 (9); this factor interferes with blastogenesis mainly through the exquisite sensitivity of IL-2 receptor expression to its action. Such a factor possesses features of an antagonist of IL-1 and could be important in immune homeostasis as well as pathophysiologic states.

Although each infectious disease may well have a unique pattern of immunoregulation, available data indicate at least some common mechanisms. Dual regulatory circuits involving T-cells and adherent mononuclear cells occur, for example, in leprosy (10), filariasis (11) and schistosomiasis (12). It may well be that a wide variety of infectious agents induce activation of mononuclear phagocytes, and perhaps large granular lymphocytes, to suppress the immune response through common pathways.

ACKNOWLEDGEMENTS

I wish to acknowledge the participation and insights provided by my colleagues: Thomas M. Daniel, Hiroshi Fujiwara, Bernice Z. Schacter, Philip J. Spagnuolo, Zahra Toossi, David J. Tweardy, and Kay Edmonds.

REFERENCES

1. Rooney, J.J. Jr., J.A. Crocco, S. Kramer, and H.A. Lyons. 1976. Further observations on tuberculin reactions in tuberculosis. Am. J. Med. 60:517.
2. Kleinhenz, M.E., J.J. Ellner, P.J. Spagnuolo, and T.M. Daniel. 1981. Suppression of lymphocyte responses by tuberculous plasma and mycobacterial arabinogalactan: monocyte-dependence and indomethacin reversibility. J. Clin. Invest. 68:153.
3. Ellner, J.J. Suppressor adherent cells in human tuberculosis. 1978. J. Immunol. 121:2573.
4. Kleinhenz, M.E., and J.J. Ellner. 1985. Immunoregulatory adherent cells in human tuberculosis: radiation-sensitive antigen-specific suppression by monocytes. J. Infect. Dis. 152:171.
5. Tweardy, D.J., B.Z. Schacter, and J.J. Ellner. 1984. Association of altered dynamics of monocyte surface expression of human leukocyte antigen DR with immunosuppression in tuberculosis. J. Infect. Dis. 149:31.
6. Wallis, R.S., H. Fujiwara, and J.J. Ellner. 1986. Direct stimulation of monocyte release of interleukin-1 by mycobacterial protein antigens. J. Immunol. 136:193.
7. Fujiwara, H., M.E. Kleinhenz, R.S. Wallis, and J.J. Ellner. 1986. Increased interleukin-1 production and monocyte suppressor cell activity associated with human tuberculosis. Am. Rev. Respir. Dis. 133:73.
8. Toossi, Z., M.E. Kleinhenz, and J.J. Ellner. 1986. Defective interleukin-2 production and responsiveness in human pulmonary tuberculosis. J. Exp. Med. 163:1162.
9. Fujiwara, H., and J.J. Ellner. 1986. Spontaneous production of a suppressor factor by the human macrophage-like cell line U937. I. Suppression of interleukin-1, interleukin-2 and mitogen-induced blastogenesis in mouse thymocytes. J. Immunol. 136:181.
10. Bloom, B.R., and V. Mehra. 1984. Immunological unresponsiveness in leprosy. Immunol. Rev. 80:5.
11. Piessens, W.F., F. Partono, S.L. Hoffman, S. Ratiwayanto, P.W. Piessens, J.R. Palmieri, I. Koiman, D.T. Dennis, and W.P. Carney. 1982. Antigen-specific suppressor T-lymphocytes in human lymphatic filariasis. N. Engl. J. Med. 307:144.
12. Olds, G.R., A. El Kholy, and J.J. Ellner. 1983. Two distinctive patterns of monocyte immunoregulatory and effector functions in heavy human infections with *Schistosoma mansoni*. J. Immunol. 131:954.

MACROPHAGE ACTIVATION IN THE ACQUIRED IMMUNODEFICIENCY SYNDROME

Henry W. Murray

Division of Infectious Diseases, Cornell University Medical College, New York, NY

In view of the clear documentation that T-cell function in the acquired immunodefiency syndrome (AIDS) is grossly impaired, the striking susceptibility of AIDS patients to infections caused by intracellular micro-organisms is not only not surprising but is predictable. Indeed, if one draws up a list of the pathogens against which successful host defense is thought to require an intact cell-mediated immune response (1) and compares this to a list of the pathogens which regularly infect patients with AIDS (2) (Table 1), the two lists are virtually superimposable. In addition, many of the AIDS pathogens are known to be intracellular organisms which, although capable of causing quite different clinical manifestations, share the common feature of being able to enter and replicate within unstimulated macrophages (1). In the presence of a normal, effective T cell-dependent immune response, however, presumed to be largely mediated by antigen-triggered lymphokine secretion with resultant macrophage activation, these same intracellular pathogens are killed or their growth is inhibited. Thus, the particular spectrum of opportunistic micro-organisms which consistently infect AIDS patients, the frequent failure of these patients to respond to appropriate antimicrobial therapy, their propensity for relapse despite adequate treatment, and the eventual uniformly fatal outcome of these infections all serve to graphically indicate that the process of macrophage activation in patients with AIDS is either profoundly disordered or more likely, has not taken place at all (3). Histopathologically, these clinical observations are expressed by the absence of granuloma formation, little or no inflammatory cell infiltrates, and overwhelming numbers of micro-organisms in wide-spread and numerous foci of tissue infection.

With the concept of T cell-dependent macrophage activation in mind, the studies reviewed here have been directed at four inter-related questions concerning the immunopathogenesis of opportunistic infections in AIDS: (a) Are AIDS patients' T cells capable of generating macrophage-activating lymphokines? (b) Are AIDS patients' mononuclear phagocytes intrinsically defective in antimicrobial activity? (c) Can AIDS patients' macrophages express the activated state once provided with exogenous activating lymphokines? and (d) Can treatment with such lymphokines activate the AIDS mononuclear phagocyte in vivo?

Table 1. Opportunistic Pathogens in AIDS (2)

Pneumocystis carinii
Toxoplasma gondii
Cryptosporidium
Isospora belli
Cytomegalovirus
Herpes simplex virus
Candida albicans
Histoplasma capsulatum
Cryptococcus neoformans
Salmonella sp.
Mycobacterium avium-intracellulare

LYMPHOKINE-GENERATING CAPACITY OF AIDS T CELLS

Crude Lymphokines

In response to stimulation with either non-specific mitogens or specific microbial antigens, peripheral blood mononuclear cells (PBMC) from healthy individuals readily secrete soluble T cell products (lymphokines) which in vitro activate both human monocyte-derived and tissue-derived (alveolar) macrophages. Lymphokine-induced effects can be measured by two linked expressions of the activated state - augmented oxidative metabolism (e.g. H_2O_2 release) and enhanced antimicrobial activity against intracellular pathogens (5-9). In the absence of lymphokine stimulation, these macrophages are normally quiescent in vitro and generate little H_2O_2 and support microbial replication. In our initial study of AIDS patients with opportunistic infections, we tested AIDS PBMC for the ability to generate these crude macrophage-activating lymphokines (3). We found several patients whose cells could produce active lymphokines in response to mitogen (concanavalin A); no patient, however, responded to specific antigen with the production of effective activating lymphokines (Table 2) (3). This T cell deficit also correlated closely with lymphocyte proliferative activity; responses to mitogen were highly variable (absent to near-normal), while antigen-induced proliferation was typically absent (3).

Gamma Interferon

Since gamma interferon (IFN-γ) has been recently shown to be a key macrophage-activating component of crude T cell-derived lymphokines (5-7,9-14), we also examined the capacity of PBMC from AIDS patients with opportunistic infections to specifically generate this T cell product. As shown in Table 3, cells from one-third of our initially-studied patients secreted normal IFN-γ levels (≥300 U/ml) in response to mitogen (concanavalin A). In response to previously encountered and clinically-relevant microbial antigens (e.g. Toxoplasma gondii and Candida albicans), however, 13 of 14 tested patients failed to secrete any detectable IFN-γ (<10 U/ml); the one responder produced a barely measurable level (20 U/ml) (3). We have now extended this analysis to a total of 52 AIDS patients with opportunistic infections, and using specific toxoplasma and cytomegalovirus (CMV) antigens, have found that the failure to produce any antigen-stimulated IFN-γ is typical of these patients (Table 4). Thus, we consider absent antigen-induced IFN-γ production to be the functional immunophenotype of AIDS patients whose immune deficit has progressed sufficiently to render them subject to opportunistic infections. We have also identified this specific defect in patients with

Table 2. Failure of AIDS Peripheral Blood Mononuclear Cells to Generate Crude Macrophage-Activating Lymphokines (3)

Normal Macrophages Stimulated With:[a]	Antimicrobial Activity		Oxidative Activity
	% Toxoplasmas Killed	% Inhibition of C. psittaci Replication	Fold Increase in H_2O_2 Release
(A) Medium alone	4±2	0	-[b]
(B) Con A-lymphokines from:			
Controls	38±5	84±3	5.9±1.4
AIDS patients	9±4	21±7	1.5±0.3
(C) Antigen-lymphokines from:			
Controls	52±3	85±2	5.0±0.7
AIDS patients	2±1	5±3	1.0±0.2

[a]Monocyte-derived macrophages from healthy controls were treated for 72 hours before infection or assay with medium alone or 10 per cent mitogen-induced or antigen-induced lymphokines generated from cultures of mononuclear cells from controls or patients with AIDS. Lymphokines induced by antigen (toxoplasma antigen) were from subjects with positive serum Sabin-Feldman dye tests (3).

[b]Control macrophages treated with medium alone released 104±33 nmol of hydrogen peroxide (H_2O_2) per milligram of protein in 90 minutes.

the prodromal AIDS-related complex (ARC), and have shown that impaired secretion of antigen-stimulated IFN-γ is an accurate predictor of who is at high risk for progressing to full-blown AIDS and developing opportunistic infections (16). Since almost one-third of our AIDS patients secreted normal levels of IFN-γ in response to non-specific mitogen stimulation (Table 4) (3, 15, 16), it is clearly preferable and we believe more accurate to test T cell function in patients with AIDS or ARC using only specific antigens. In our laboratory, we routinely utilize (a) T. gondii lysate antigen for patients with positive serum Sabin-Feldman dye tests, (b) C. albicans sonicate antigen for those with oral candidiasis or the few patients with positive candida skin tests, (c) cytomegalovirus (CMV) antigen if the serum complement fixation titer is ≥1:8, or (d) tetanus toxoid for those previously immunized (3, 15-17).

It is also worth pointing out that although most of our AIDS patients have been quite lymphopenic with markedly decreased numbers of peripheral blood T4+ cells (Table 4) and that this quantitative abnormality alone may largely explain the failure to proliferate or produce IFN-γ in response to soluble antigen, we have observed several patients with fully-established AIDS (opportunistic infections) who have normal absolute numbers of circulating T4+ cells. Nevertheless, these patients' PBMC also failed to secrete IFN-γ in response to specific antigen. We presume this observation reflects cytopathic (but non-cytolytic) effects induced by HTLV-III/LAV (human immunodeficiency virus (HIV)) infection. In addition, we have also found that the production of IFN-γ stimulated by T. gondii and CMV antigen is strictly T4+ cell-dependent (18). Thus, given HIV's tropism for and capacity to destroy T4+ cells, defective antigen-induced IFN-γ secretion does not appear surprising.

Table 3. Production of IFN-γ by Mononuclear Cells From AIDS Patients With Opportunistic Infections (3)

Patients	IFN-γ Production (U/ml)		
	Con A	*T. gondii* Antigen	*C. albicans* Antigen
Healthy Controls			
Range	300-6000	300-3000	100-300
Mean±SEM	1884±194	1108±93	200±41
AIDS Patients			
No. 1	40	-[a]	<10
2	20	-	-[a]
3	350	-	<10
4	150	<10	-
5	400	<10	-
6	20	<10	-
7	60	<10	<10
8	120	<10	-
9	1000	20	<10
10	<10	-	<10
11	300	<10	-
12	20	<10	-
13	<10	<10	-
14	10	<10	-
15	10	<10	-
16	2000	-	-

[a]Not applicable since either the serum Sabin-Feldman dye test was negative or there was no evidence of mucosal candidiasis.

Interleukin 2

Since interleukin 2 (IL-2), another lymphokine implicated in a variety of cellular immune reactions, is readily produced by normal T cells in response to mitogen and antigen (17), we also measured the IL-2 activity in the supernatants of the AIDS patients' PBMC cultures. Although IL-2 by itself does not directly activate macrophages (10), our interest in IL-2 generation stemmed from prior observations indicating that the presence of IL-2 plays an important role in the capacity of T cells to produce IFN-γ (18,19). As shown in Table 5, PBMC from only one of 32 (3%) AIDS patients with opportunistic infections or Kaposi's sarcoma secreted normal levels of IL-2 in response to a specific antigen, and 21 (66%) failed to produce any detectable IL-2 (17). Thus, deficient antigen-induced IL-2 production also appears to be typical of patients with or at high risk for developing opportunistic infections. If IL-2 is indeed required for T cell production of IFN-γ (17-19), these results suggest that impaired IFN-γ secretion may largely reflect or in fact be due to absent antigen-stimulated IL-2 generation. Antigen-induced IL-2 production is also T4+ cell-dependent (18).

Table 4. IFN-γ Production and T4+ Cell Number in 52 AIDS Patients With Opportunistic Infections (OI) (15)

	Healthy Control	AIDS + OI
A. IFN-γ Production		
Mitogen[a]		
Mean ± SEM (U/ml)	1401±160	269±128
% Normal (≥200 U/ml)	100	27
% Undetectable (<10 U/ml)	0	24
Antigen[b]		
Mean ± SEM (U/ml)	843±106	13±3
% Normal (≥100 U/ml)	100	1
% Undetectable (<10 U/ml)	0	78
B. T4+ Cells		
Mean ± SEM (per mm^3)	853±53	63±9
% Normal (≥328/mm^3)	100	0
% <33/mm^3	0	28

[a]Mitogen (Con A).
[b]Antigens (*T. gondii* or cytomegalovirus (CMV) for seropositive patients).

Table 5. Interleukin 2 Production by AIDS Mononuclear Cells in Response to Specific Microbial Antigen (14)[a]

	IFN-γ Production		
Patients	Normal[b]	Abnormal but detectable	Undetectable[c]
Total Group (n=32)	1/32 (3%)	10/32 (31%)	21/32 (66%)
Opportunistic infections (n=21)	0/21 (0%)	6/21 (29%)	15/21 (71%)
Kaposi's sarcoma (n=11)	1/11 (9%)	4/11 (36%)	6/11 (55%)

[a]Antigens included *T. gondii*, tetanus toxoid, cytomegalovirus, *C. albicans*, and *H. simplex* virus (14).
[b]Normal IL-2 production in response to these antigens (14): *T. gondii*, 33.9±2.7 U/ml (14-45); tetanus toxoid, 11.9±1.8 U/ml (2.2-20), cytomegalovirus, 3.6±0.5 U/ml (2.0-4.8); *C. albicans*, 20.2±4.2 U/ml (5.3-40); and *H. simplex* virus, 9.9±1.7 U/ml (2.8-19).
[c]<0.1 U/ml of IL-2 (14).

AIDS MONOCYTE AND MACROPHAGE FUNCTION

Monocytes

The second question we asked was whether AIDS mononuclear phagocytes might also be defective in antimicrobial effector cell function. In these studies, we tested AIDS monocytes for their ability to (a) stain for myeloperoxidase, (b) generate and release H_2O_2 (a key antimicrobial oxygen intermediate), (c) respond to both inert (zymosan) and viable (*T. gondii*) phagocytized targets with oxidative burst activity, and (d) to kill or inhibit *T. gondii* and *Chlamydia psittaci*. These latter two intracellular pathogens were selected for use in order to test the effectiveness of both the oxygen-dependent and oxygen-independent mechanisms of the AIDS monocyte. Activity against *T. gondii* is primarily oxygen-dependent (11), while oxygen-independent mechanisms are sufficient to inhibit *C. psittaci* replication (20,21). As shown in Table 6, fresh monocytes from AIDS patients with opportunistic infections were indistinguishable from monocytes from healthy controls with regard to both oxidative and in vitro antimicrobial activities (3), indicating that AIDS peripheral blood mononuclear phagocytes showed neither intrinsic nor acquired defects in effector cell function.

Macrophages

Given that AIDS monocytes appeared to behave in a normal fashion, we proceeded to test AIDS macrophages for the capacity to respond to lymphokines, and once stimulated, to express the activated state by displaying enhanced oxidative and antimicrobial activity. In these experiments, AIDS monocyte-derived macrophages were cultivated with crude lymphokines prepared from cells from healthy donors. As shown in Table 6, once properly stimulated, macrophages from AIDS patients with opportunistic infections readily generated increased levels of H_2O_2 and exerted normal levels of enhanced intracellular activity against both *T. gondii* and *C. psittaci* (3). As in our experiments with AIDS monocytes, these in vitro observations also suggested that AIDS macrophages had no defect in either the ability to respond to exogenous lymphokines with activation or once activated to exert effective antimicrobial activity. To extend this analysis from the peripheral blood-derived macrophage to the tissue macrophage, we also studied alveolar macrophages from 11 AIDS patients undergoing diagnostic broncho-alveolar lavage (9). After 72 hours in culture, unstimulated alveolar macrophages from all individuals examined (three healthy volunteers, 12 non-AIDS patients, 11 AIDS patients) released comparably low levels of H_2O_2 and readily supported the intracellular replication of both *T. gondii* and *C. psittaci* (Table 7). Cells cultivated with crude (normal) lymphokines during this 72 hour period, however, displayed the activated phenotype in that they produced two- to three-fold more H_2O_2 and exerted both antitoxoplasma and antichlamydial activity (Table 7). Once similarly activated, AIDS alveolar macrophages behaved identically to cells from the controls (9). It is also worth pointing out that AIDS alveolar macrophages were fully capable of being activated despite being obtained from an in vivo environment in which both pulmonary Kaposi's sarcoma and opportunistic infections had developed (9).

RESPONSES OF AIDS MACROPHAGES TO IFN-γ IN VITRO

Since treatment with IFN-γ is one of the immunotherapeutic avenues now being tried in AIDS patients (see below), we also utilized the preceding models to determine the in vitro responsiveness of AIDS monocytes and macrophages to this particularly key activating lymphokine (5-7,9-14). As shown in Tables 6 and 7, AIDS peripheral blood- and tissue-derived (alveolar) macrophages readily responded to treatment with 300 U/ml of both partially-purified and recombinant (r) IFN-γ, and attained levels of activation

Table 6. Activities of AIDS Peripheral Blood Monocytes and Monocyte-Derived Macrophages (3)

	Oxidative Activity		Antimicrobial Activity	
	H_2O_2 Release (nmol/mg/90 min)	Fold Increase in H_2O_2 Release	% Toxoplasmas Killed at 4 hr	% Inhibition of C. psittaci at 20 hr
Monocytes[a]				
Control	939±61	-	38±7	86±3
AIDS	877±55	-	40±5	81±3
Macrophages stimulated with[b]				
Medium alone				
Control	115±26	-	2±1	0
Normal lymphokines				
Control	-	4.6±0.6	43±4	88±3
AIDS	-	5.6±0.4	39±3	89±3
IFN-γ				
Control	-	5.8±0.5	41±3	89±4
AIDS		6.2±0.7	37±4	90±3

[a]Monocytes were cultivated one day before infection or assay.
[b]Monocytes were first cultivated for >7 days, then treated for 72 hours with medium alone, 10 percent active (normal) lymphokines, or 300 U or partially purified or recombinant gamma interferon per milliliter.

Table 7. Responsiveness of AIDS Tissue (Alveolar) Macrophages to Activating Lymphokines and Recombinant IFN-γ (9)

Source and Treatment of Alveolar Macrophages	Oxidative Activity	Antimicrobial Activity	
	Fold Increase in H_2O_2 Release	Fold Increase in Toxoplasmas/100 Cells	% Inhibition of C. psittaci Replication
Healthy Controls			
Medium Alone	-	7.7	0
Lymphokine	2.5	2.7	74
IFN-γ	3.1	2.4	67
AIDS Patients			
Medium Alone	-	7.4	0
Lymphokines	2.2	2.4	71
IFN-γ	2.5	1.8	78

identical to that displayed by in vitro-activated macrophages from healthy controls (3,9). In separate studies, we found that AIDS monocytes also responded to pulses of rIFN-γ with normal levels of enhanced oxidative and antimicrobial activity (22). Fresh monocytes treated with 300 U/ml for 24 hours and then cultivated in medium alone remained fully activated for up to 5-7 days (not shown) (22).

RESPONSE OF AIDS MONONUCLEAR PHAGOCYTES TO rIFN-γ IN VIVO

To determine if IFN-γ could also activate the AIDS mononuclear phagocyte in vivo, we examined monocytes from AIDS patients before and after a 24-hour intravenous infusion of either 30 or 500 μg/M^2 of rIFN-γ (22). The rationale for this phase 1 trial stemmed not only from the preceding in vitro results, but also from accumulated data which has indicated that IFN-γ can directly activate macrophages both in vitro and in vivo: (a) more than a dozen different intra- and extracellular pathogens are susceptible to the IFN-γ-activated macrophage in vitro (reviewed in 14), (b) parenterally-administered rIFN-γ can activate the tissue macrophage in animals (12) and the blood monocyte in patients with cancer (23) and lepromatous leprosy (24), and (c) that rIFN-γ can act therapeutically in both experimental models of systemic intracellular infections (25-28) and in patients with leprosy (24). Our studies also confirmed that rIFN-γ can activate the blood monocyte in AIDS patients (22). In comparison to pre-infusion levels of activity, monocytes obtained after a 24-hour infusion of rIFN-γ (30 to 500 μg/M^2) remained activated in vitro for up to 5 days and showed 3.2- to 5.9-fold increases in H_2O_2 release and 49 to 68% increases in the capacity to inhibit _T. gondii_ replication (not shown) (22).

CONCLUSION

From the preceding in vitro and in vivo studies, it seems reasonable to conclude that both the peripheral blood monocyte and the tissue macrophage in AIDS patients with opportunistic infections show neither intrinsic abnormalities in intracellular antimicrobial activity nor any defect in the capacity to achieve the activated state once properly provided with effective T cell-derived activating signals. It is clear, however, that the AIDS T cell defect extends to the failure to secrete antigen-induced macrophage-activating lymphokines, in particular IFN-γ, thus, rendering macrophages persistently susceptible to and entirely unable to contain newly-acquired or reactivated infections caused by intracellular pathogens. In all likelihood, the failure to generate IFN-γ in patients with fully-established AIDS largely reflects an absolute deficiency of T4+ helper cells; in some patients, however, qualitative defects in T4+ cell function and/or perhaps abnormalities more proximal to T4+ cell activation (e.g. accessory cell function) may also be involved. Irrespective of the mechanism responsible for absent secretion of T cell lymphokines, it is clear that macrophage activation is grossly impaired or entirely fails to occur in AIDS and that this acquired immunodeficiency is persistent, progressive, and ultimately accompanied by a uniformly fatal outcome once expressed clinically by the development of an opportunistic infection. Given this background, attempts to therapeutically or prophylactically induce macrophage activation in vivo by administering agents such as IFN-γ clearly are appropriate from both a clinical as well as a scientific standpoint.

REFERENCES

1. McLeod, R., E.J. Wing, J.S. Remington. 1984. Lymphocytes and macrophages in cell-mediated immunity. In Mandell, G.L., R.G. Douglas, Jr., J.E. Bennett, eds. Principles and Practice of Infectious Diseases. New York: John Wiley, p. 72-93.
2. Fauci, A.S. 1985. The acquired immunodeficiency syndrome: an update. Ann. Intern. Med. 102:800-813.
3. Murray, H.W., B.Y. Rubin, H. Masur, and R.B. Roberts. 1984. Impaired production of lymphokines and immune (gamma) interferon in the acquired immunodeficiency syndrome. N. Engl. J. Med. 310:883-889.
4. Seligmann, M., L. Chess, J.L. Fahey, A.S. Fauci, P.J. Lachman, J. Age-Stehr, N. Jacob, A.J. Pinching, F.S. Rosen, T.J. Spira, and J. Wybran. 1984. AIDS - an immunologic re-evaluation. N. Engl. J. Med. 311:1286-1292.
5. Nathan, C.F., H.W. Murray, M.E. Wiebe, and B.Y. Rubin. 1983. Identification of interferon-γ as the lymphokine that activates human macrophage oxidative metabolites and antimicrobial activity. J. Exp. Med. 158:670-689.
6. Murray, H.W., D.M. Cartelli. 1983. Killing of intracellular *Leishmania donovani* by human mononuclear phagocytes: evidence for oxygen-dependent and independent leishmanicidal activity. J. Clin. Invest. 72:32.
7. Rothermel, C.D., B.Y. Rubin, and H.W. Murray. 1983. γ-interferon is the factor in lymphokine that activates human macrophages to inhibit intracellular *Chlamydia psittaci* replication. J. Immunol. 131:2542-2544.
8. Nash, T.W., D.M. Libby, M.A. Horwitz. 1984. Interaction between the Legionnaire's disease bacterium (*Legionella pneumophila*) and human alveolar macrophages. J. Clin. Invest. 74:771-782.
9. Murray, H.W., R.A. Gellene, D.M. Libby, C.D. Rothermel, B.Y. Rubin. 1985. Activation of tissue macrophages from AIDS patients: in vitro response of AIDS alveolar macrophages to lymphokines and gamma interferon. J. Immunol. 135:2374.
10. Nathan, C.F., T.J. Pendergast, M.E. Weibe, E.R. Stanley, E. Platzer, H.G. Remold, K. Welte, B.Y. Rubin, H.W. Murray. 1984. Activation of human macrophages. Comparison of other cytokines with interferon-γ. J. Exp. Med. 160:600-605.
11. Murray, H.W., B.Y. Rubin, S.M. Carriero, A.T. Denn, A.M. Harris, E.A. Jaffe. 1985. Human mononuclear phagocyte antiprotozoal mechanisms: oxygen-dependent versus oxygen-independent activity against intracellular *Toxoplasma gondii*. J. Immunol. 134:1982.
12. Murray, H.W., G.L. Spitalny, C.F. Nathan. 1985. Activation of mouse peritoneal macrophages in vitro and in vivo by gamma interferon. J. Immunol. 134:1619.
13. Murray, H.W., B.Y. Rubin, C.D. Rothermel. 1983. Killing of intracellular *Leishmania donovani* by lymphokine-stimulated human mononuclear phagocytes: evidence that interferon-γ is the activating lymphokine. J. Clin. Invest. 72:1506-1510.
14. Nathan, C.F. Interferon-gamma and macrophage activation in cell-mediated immunity. In Mechanisms of Host Resistance to Infectious Agents, Tumors, and Allografts, R.M. Steinman and R.J. North, eds. The Rockefeller University Press, New York, 1986, pp. 165-184.
15. Murray, H.W., D. Scavuzzo, B.Y. Rubin, R.B. Roberts. $T4^+$ cell production of gamma interferon and the clinical spectrum of patients at risk for and with AIDS (submitted).
16. Murray, H.W., J.K. Hillman, B.Y. Rubin, C.D. Kelly, L.M. Tyler, D.M. Donnelly, S.M. Carriero, R.B. Roberts. 1985. Patients at risk for AIDS-related opportunistic infections: clinical manifestations and impaired gamma interferon production. N. Engl. J. Med. 313:1504.

17. Murray, H.W., K. Welte, J.L. Jacobs, B.Y. Rubin, R. Mertelsmann, R.B. Roberts. 1985. Production of and in vitro response to interleukin 2 in the acquired immunodeficiency syndrome. J. Clin. Invest. 76:1959.

18. Kelly, C.D., K. Welte, H.W. Murray. Antigen-stimulated human gamma interferon production: differential dependence on interleukin 2 and its receptor (submitted).

19. Vilcek, J.D., Henriksen-Destefano, D. Siegel, A. Klion, R.J. Robb, J. Le. 1985. Regulation of IFN-γ induction in human peripheral blood cells by exogenous and endogenously produced interleukin 2. J. Immunol. 135:1851.

20. Murray, H.W., G.I. Byrne, C. Rothermel. 1985. Lymphokine enhances oxygen-independent activity against intracellular pathogens. J. Exp. Med. 158:234.

21. Rothermel, C.D., B.Y. Rubin, E.A. Jaffee, H.W. Murray. 1986. Oxygen-independent inhibition of intracellular Chlamydia psittaci growth by human monocytes and gamma interferon-activated macrophages. J. Immunol. 137:689.

22.Murray, H.W., D. Scavuzzo, J.L. Jacobs, M.H. Kaplan, D.M. Libby, R.B. Roberts. In vitro and in vivo activation of human mononuclear phagocytes by gamma interferon: Studies with normal and AIDS monocytes (submitted).

23. Nathan, C.F., C.R. Horowitz, J. de al Harpe, S. Vadham-Raj, S. Sherwin, H. Oettgen, S. Krown. 1985. Administration of recombinant interferon-γ to cancer patients enhances monocyte secretion of hydrogen peroxide. Proc. Natl. Acad. Sci. USA 82:8686-8690.

24. Nathan, C.F., G. Kalpan, W.R. Lewis, A. Nusrat, M.D. Witmer, S.A. Sherwin, C.K. Job, C.R. Howowitz, R.M. Steinman, Z.A. Cohn. 1986. Local and systemic effects of low doses of recombinant interferon-γ after intradermal injection in patients with lepromatous leprosy. N. Engl. J. Med. 315:6-15.

25. McCabe, R.E., B.J. Luft, J.S. Remington. 1984. Effect of murine interferon-γ on murine toxoplasmosis. J. Infect. Dis. 150:961-962.

26. Kiderlen, A.F., S.H.E. Kaufmann, M.-L. Lohmann-Matthes. 1984. Protection of mice against the intracellular bacterium Listeria monocytogenes by recombinant immune interferon. Eur. J. Immunol. 14:964-970.

27. Edward, C.K. III, H.B. Hedegaard, A. Zlotnik, T.R. Gangadharam, R.B. Johnston, Jr., M.J. Pabst. 1986. Chronic infection due to Mycobacterium intracellulare in mice: association with macrophage release of prostaglandin E2 and reversal by injection of indomethacin, muramyl dipeptide, and interferon-γ. J. Immunol. 136:1820.

28. Murray, H.W., J. Stern. K. Welte, B.Y. Rubin, S.M. Carriero, C.F. Nathan. Experimental visceral leishmaniasis: production of interleukin 2 and gamma interferon, tissue immune reaction, and response to treatment with interleukin 2 and gamma interferon (submitted).

DECREASED MITOGENIC RESPONSE OF MURINE SPLEEN CELLS FOLLOWING INTRAPERITONEAL INJECTION OF SEROVAR-SPECIFIC GLYCOPEPTIDOLIPID ANTIGENS FROM THE MYCOBACTERIUM AVIUM COMPLEX

Lucilla C. Hooper and William W. Barrow

Department of Microbiology and Immunology, Texas College of Osteopathic Medicine, Fort Worth, Texas 76107

INTRODUCTION

Mycobacteria in the Mycobacterium avium complex have recently become clinically important opportunistic pathogens with a demonstrated ability to cause severe disseminated infections in patients suffering from AIDS (6,7,9,13). Although there are a variety of other nontuberculous mycobacteria that can infect humans, it appears that only certain serovars of the MAC are the most common to be associated with individuals who have AIDS (14). It has been suggested that the increased number of MAC infections in AIDS patients may be due to an immunologic defect which selectively favors these mycobacteria over other nontuberculous mycobacteria (14).

Although members of the MAC are similar to other mycobacteria regarding their ability to survive in host macrophages as intracellular parasites, the one feature that helps to differentiate them is a group of C-mycosidic polar glycopeptidolipid antigens (GPL) (3) which have been identified as major constituents of the superficial L_1 layer (1,16). The GPL components are serovar specific antigens which are used in the serologic (15) and thin-layer chromatographic (TLC) (4) identification of members of the MAC and because of their superficial location, may be important in cellular immunity.

In an effort to generate cell mediated immune reactions in mice, we observed that the GPL antigens from serovar 20 have the ability to suppress the response of murine splenic lymphocytes to the T-cell mitogens, concanavalin A (ConA) and phytohemagglutinin (PHA). This suppression was found to take place up to three weeks following an intraperitoneal injection of from 10 to 200 µg of the purified GPL antigens and was dependent upon a group of nonadherent Thy 1.2^+ cells.

Although we were unable to generate cell mediated immune responses to the GPL antigens of serovar 20, it was determined that the GPL components cause a low level non-specific inflammatory response when injected intraperitoneally (i.p.) and are apparently nontoxic. These findings imply that the GPL antigens may be the sensitins(s) that Collins suggested as an explanation for the apparent predilection of certain MAC serovars for persons suffering from AIDS (5).

MATERIALS AND METHODS

Antigen Extraction and Purification

The GPL antigens were extracted from lyophilized Mycobacterium intracellulare serovar 20 with chloroform-methanol (2:1) and purified by means of column chromatography using silicic acid Celite and DEAE cellulose in succession (1,16). Antigens were routinely stored at -20°C in chloroform. Prior to use, an appropriate amount was transferred to a sterile glass vial and dried under a stream of nitrogen. Dried antigen preparations were then suspended in sterile saline by sonication.

Immunization of Mice

Female C57BL/6 mice were immunized with GPL-MBSA suspended in a water-in-oil emulsion containing incomplete Freund adjuvant as described in an earlier report (2,16). Each mouse received 0.1 ml of emulsion by subcutaneous injection on the dorsal side on day 0 and 7. Mice received either 250 μg of the GPL-MBSA complex or 250 μg of MBSA suspended in 0.1 ml of a water-in-oil emulsion containing Freund's incomplete (FIC) or complete adjuvant (FCA), respectively.

Elicitation of Peritoneal Macrophages by GPL Antigens

Three weeks following the final immunization, immunized and non-immunized mice were challenged by an i.p. injection of 200 μg GPL antigens suspended in 0.1 ml saline. At 1, 2, 3 and 4 days postchallenge, mice were sacrificed by cervical dislocation and cells removed by irrigation of peritoneal cavity with 2.0 ml of ice-cold NCTC medium 109 (Difco Laboratories, Detroit, MI.) containing 5 U of heparin per ml of solution. Collected cells were counted and viability evaluated by trypan blue exclusion to be always >97%. Differential peritoneal cell counts were determined and macrophages estimated cytochemically on smears stained for nonspecific esterase (10).

Cell volumes were adjusted to 2.0×10^6 cells/ml and added in triplicate to either eight-chamber tissue culture slides or twenty-four well tissue culture plates. Cultures were allowed to incubate for 2 h at 37°C, after which nonadherent cells were removed by washing monolayers with Medium 109. Monolayers in chamber slides were assessed for those cells which had spread and also possessed one or more of the following morphological features: ruffled membrane, increased vacuolation and increased granulation. Percentages were determined on quadruplicate counts of 100 adherent cells, and mean and standard deviation computed.

Adherent cell monolayers in multi-well plates were lysed with 0.05% Triton X-100 in phosphate buffered saline (PBS), and levels of 5'-nucleotidase (5'-ND) were assessed by the Arkesteijn enzyme kinetic method using a commercial kit (Sigma Chemical Co., St. Louis, MO.). Protein was determined by the method of Lowry (11). Levels of 5'-ND were also determined on peritoneal macrophages that had been elicited 3 days previously with either 30 μg lipopolysaccharide (LPS, Salmonella typhimurium, Sigma) or 1.0 ml thioglycollate (BBL, Cockeysville, MD.).

Lymphocyte Blastogenesis

After appropriate time intervals following injection of GPL antigens, mice were killed by cervical dislocation and spleens aseptically removed. A single-cell suspension was layered over Histopaque separation gradient medium (Sigma) and centrifuged at 250 x g for 30 min. The buffy layer was aspirated and washed 2-3 times in RPMI-1640 medium containing L-glutamine (2 mM) and penicillin and streptomycin (100 units/ml) (RPMI), then suspended in RPMI containing 10% heat inactivated fetal bovine serum (RPMI-complete) (12). Cells were adjusted to 2 x 10^6 cells/ml and added to a 96 well microtiter plate at a concentration of 2 x 10^5 or 4 x 10^5 cells/well, in triplicate. Mitogens were added to each well at concentrations previously determined to give maximum response. Concanvalin A (Sigma) was added at a concentration of 3 µg/well and PHA (Sigma or Wellcome Res. Lab, Beckenham, England) at a concentration of 0.2 µg/well. Plates were incubated at 37°C, 5% CO_2, for 72 hr, with the last 6 hr consisting of a pulse with 1 µCi ^3H-(methyl)-thymidine/well. Following pulse, the cells were harvested onto glass filter paper and thymidine uptake determined by counting filters in Beta Gel (WestChem, San Diego, CA.). Response to mitogens was determined for each group and suppression determined by comparing the response of each GPL-treated group to the response of the untreated (control) group. Samples were assayed in triplicate and the net cpm (ncpm) determined by subtracting the mean cpm of the untreated (control) cultures from the mean cpm of the mitogen-treated cultures. Percent change (or suppression) was determined by the following formula (12):

$$\% \text{ Change} = 1 - \frac{\text{ncpm GPL treated animals}}{\text{ncpm untreated animals}} \times 100$$

Statistical analysis was conducted by using an unpaired student t-test to compare the mean cpm of the untreated vs. the treated animal.

In some experiments, spleen cells were treated with 1:20 anti-Thy-1.2 monoclonal antibody (Accurate Chemical and Scientific Corp., New York) at 4°C for 1 h. followed by Lo-Tox-M rabbit complement (Accurate Chem.) at 37°C for 1 h. In other experiments, spleen cells were incubated on plastic for 2 h at 37°C to remove adherent cells.

RESULTS

Changes in Peritoneal Cell Populations Following GPL Challenge

Response to i.p. injection of 200 µg GPL antigens was monitored in three groups of C57BL/6 mice by observing the percent distribution of lymphocytes, monocytes, and polymorphonuclear leukocytes (PMN). Non-immunized had no treatment prior to injection of antigens, Sham had previously been immunized with FIA emulsion, and Immune had been immunized with 250 µg GPL-MBSA suspended in FIA. Percent distribution of cell types throughout 4 days postchallenge is given in Table 1.

Intraperitoneal injection of GPL antigens resulted in an increase in the percentage of PMNs in the peritoneal cavity of all three groups of mice followed by a return towards normal values (Table 1). In all three groups, the increase in PMNs at day 1 was significant (P<0.02) when compared to values obtained following injection of sterile saline in which case the PMNs increased to only 3% throughout 4 days. In contrast, the levels of lymphocytes and monocytes remained similar in the Sham and Immune groups following GPL challenge, suggesting that no apparent cell mediated immune (CMI) response had taken place. This assumption is further substantiated by the fact that these mice also failed to respond to footpad challenge with GPL antigens (data not reported). An i.p. injection of 1.0 ml of thioglycollate resulted in an increase in total cells from 2.1 x 10^6 cells/ml to 14.5 x 10^6 cells/ml at 24 hr and 10.0 x 10^6 cells/ml at three days of which 50% and 16% were PMNs, respectively.

Table 1. Numbers and differential peritoneal cell counts of mice injected with 200 μg GPL antigens. Values represent the mean and standard deviation of two separate experiments involving groups of three mice each.

Treatment	Day	Total cells/ml (10^6)	Cell Type (%) Lymph	Mono	PMN
Nonimmunized	0	3.6 ± 1.2	40 ± 15	56 ± 13	3.6 ± 4
	1	4.5 ± 0.1	18 ± 13	59 ± 1.4	24 ± 15
	2	5.4 ± 1.0	29 ± 2.6	59 ± 3.8	13 ± 2.6
	3	5.9 ± 0.1	35 ± 19	51 ± 11	15 ± 8.5
	4	6.6 ± 1.3	44 ± 4.9	47 ± 5.2	9 ± 1.0
Sham	0	4.2 ± 0.5	53 ± 4.0	43 ± 2.5	2 ± 1.0
	1	3.0 ± 0.2	59 ± 2.1	31 ± 1.4	8.5 ± 0.7
	2	3.4 ± 2.0	61 ± 1.4	31 ± 2.1	7 ± 0
	3	6.6 ± 3.2	57 ± 3.5	32 ± 9.9	9 ± 4.2
	4	5.6 ± 0.8	58 ± 7.6	28 ± 7.5	12 ± 1.5
Immune	0	4.2 ± 0.5	53 ± 4.0	43 ± 2.5	2 ± 1.0
	1	3.8 ± 0.4	55 ± 8.5	26 ± 16	18 ± 9.2
	2	4.5 ± 0.6	56 ± 2.8	29 ± 7.0	14 ± 5.7
	3	5.3 ± 1.0	60 ± 13	35 ± 11	5 ± 1.4
	4	5.0 ± 1.2	59 ± 4.7	34 ± 8.2	7 ± 3.5

Influence of GPL Challenge on Macrophage Spreading

Intraperitoneal injection of GPL antigens resulted in an increase in the number of adherent cells which spread rapidly on glass (Table 2). The increases in the number of those cells which spread rapidly were significant ($P<0.05$) when compared to the Control group (no immunization/ saline challenge). One observation that persisted throughout this study was the distinct morphology of macrophages removed from mice which had been injected i.p. with GPL antigens; they appeared more vacuolated and ruffled than those of the control group (Figures 1 A-C).

Table 2. Effect of GPL challenge on peritoneal macrophage spreading. Values represent the mean and standard deviation of two separate experiments involving groups of three mice each.

	Percentage of cells spread at two hours			
Days postchallenge	Control [a]	Nonimmune [b]	Sham [b]	Immune [b]
1	3±2	43±4	59±8	34±4
2	13±5	54±14	56±5	55±6
3	15±7	51±7	38±4	50±4
4	16±4	45±5	43±4	53±4

[a] Challenged with sterile saline
[b] Challenged with 200 μg GPL suspended in sterile saline

5'Nucleotidase Levels in Adherent Peritoneal Cells Following Challenge with GPL Antigens.

An i.p. injection of GPL antigens resulted in a significant decrease in the level of 5'-ND detected in peritoneal macrophages obtained three days following injection (Table 3, Groups B, C, and D). This response was similar to that observed with thioglycollate (Table 3, Group E) but not as great as that observed when LPS was injected i.p. (Table 3, Group F). In preliminary experiments, injection of 50 μg LPS caused death within 72 h, therefore the LPS dose was decreased to 30 μg and even so, the mice became noticeably lethargic and toxic in appearance. For all experiments involving injection of GPL antigens, no adverse reactions were observed in mice, even though some mice received up to 200 μg GPL i.p. No decrease in 5'-ND was observed in mice which received an i.p. injection of sterile saline (Table 3, Group A).

Response of Immune Murine Spleen Cells to in vitro Challenge with Homologous Antigens

C57BL/6 mice which had been immunized with either MBSA or GPL-MBSA were sacrificed at three weeks following the second injection and their spleen cells removed and challenged in vitro against homologus antigens. Mice which had been immunized with MBSA or GPL-MBSA responded to in vitro challenge with MBSA (Table 4, Groups 1-4), whereas mice which had been immunized with GPL-MBSA did not produce a significant response when challenged with GPL (Table 4, Groups 2-4).

Response of Murine Spleen Cells to Mitogens

In one set of experiments involving immunization with GPL-MBSA, mice were injected i.p. with 200 μg purified GPL antigens three weeks following immunization. Three days following i.p. injection of GPL, spleen cells were removed and challenged in vitro with MBSA and GPL and also with the mitogens ConA and PHA. Again there was a significant response to MBSA but not to GPL (Table 4, Group 4) and in addition it was observed that there was a significant reduction in the response of the spleen cells to ConA and PHA (Table 5). A significant reduction in the response to ConA and PHA was also observed in spleen cells removed from nonimmunized mice which had received an i.p. injection of 200 μg GPL antigens (Table 5).

Table 3. Effect of GPL challenge on 5'-nucleotidase activity in peritoneal macrophages

		5'-Nucleotidase Activity		
Group	Challenge	Day 0	Day 3	P value
A (nonimmunized)	saline	52 ± 11	55 ± 2	NS
B (sham)	GPL	58 ± 11	10 ± 1	0.01
C (immunized)	GPL	37 ± 8	20 ± 0	0.01
D (nonimmunized)	GPL		14 ± 5	0.01
E (nonimmunized)	thioglycollate		10 ± 3	0.01
F (nonimmunized)	LPS		ND	0.01

Immunized C57BL/6 mice were injected with 250 μg GPL-MBSA suspended in FIA emulsion and sham mice received only FIA emulsion. Mice were challenged i.p. with either saline (Group A), 200 μg GPL antigens (Groups B-D), 1.0 ml thioglycollate (Group E), or 30 μg LPS (Group F). Adherent cells were obtained from peritoneal exudates either immediately before challenge (Day 0) or three days postchallenge (Day 3) and assayed for 5'-ND and protein. Values are expressed as nmole AMP hydrolyzed/min/mg protein and represent mean and SD determined from 3 experiments involving groups of three mice each. Significance was determined by using an unpaired student t test. Experimental values were compared with those obtained for Group A (nonimmunized) at time zero. ND = nondetectable.

In an additional set of experiments (Table 6), nonimmunized mice were injected i.p. with 200 μg GPL antigens and their spleen cells challenged in vitro one or three weeks later with ConA and PHA. In groups which received the injection one week prior to spleen cell assay there was a significant decrease in the response to PHA in 3 out of 5 groups. In the two groups in which ConA was tested, no significant decrease was observed at one week. At three weeks following the i.p. injection of GPL antigens, all 3 groups demonstrated a significant decrease in the response to PHA but only one group demonstrated a significant decrease in response to ConA.

To determine the range of activity for the GPL antigens, mice were injected i.p. with varying amounts of the antigens and their spleen cells tested for responsiveness to mitogens three weeks following injection. It was observed that optimum concentration to produce significant suppression to mitogen stimulation was between 10 and 500 μg of the GPL antigens (Table 7).

Although spleen cells from GPL treated mice had a significant suppression in their response to mitogens, this suppression was not maintained when those cells were mixed with equal numbers of normal spleen cells (Table 8, Experiment 1). However, when GPL treated spleen cells were exposed to anti-Thy 1.2 and complement and then mixed in equal numbers with normal spleen cells, there was a reversal in the suppression (Table 8, Experiment 1) indicating that Thy 1.2^+ cells were responsible for the suppression.

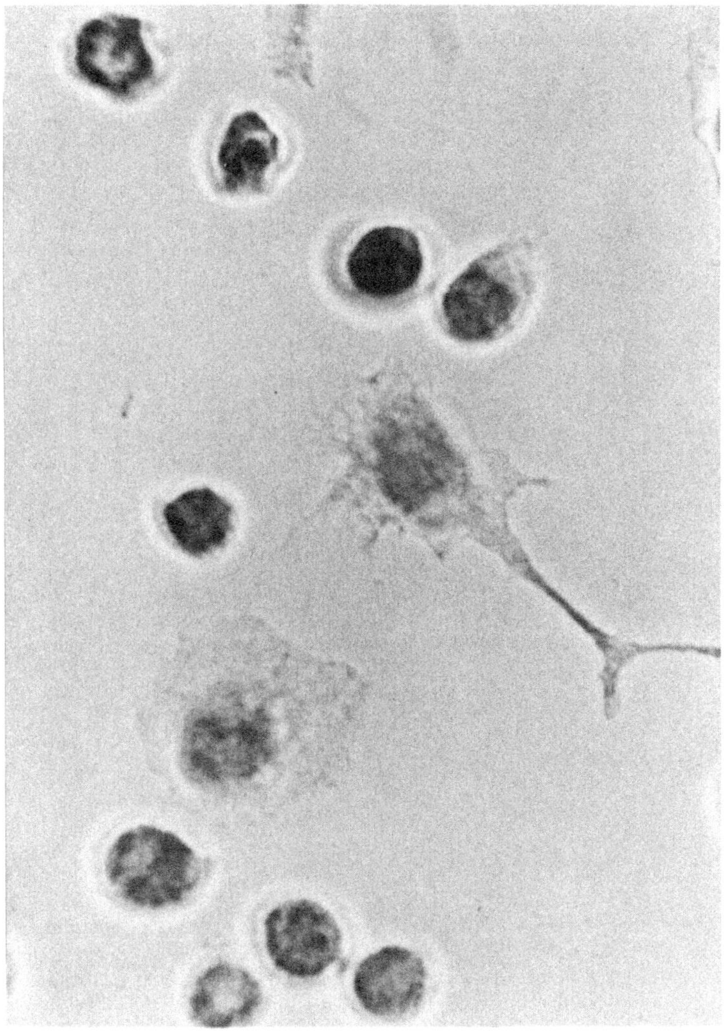

Figure 1A

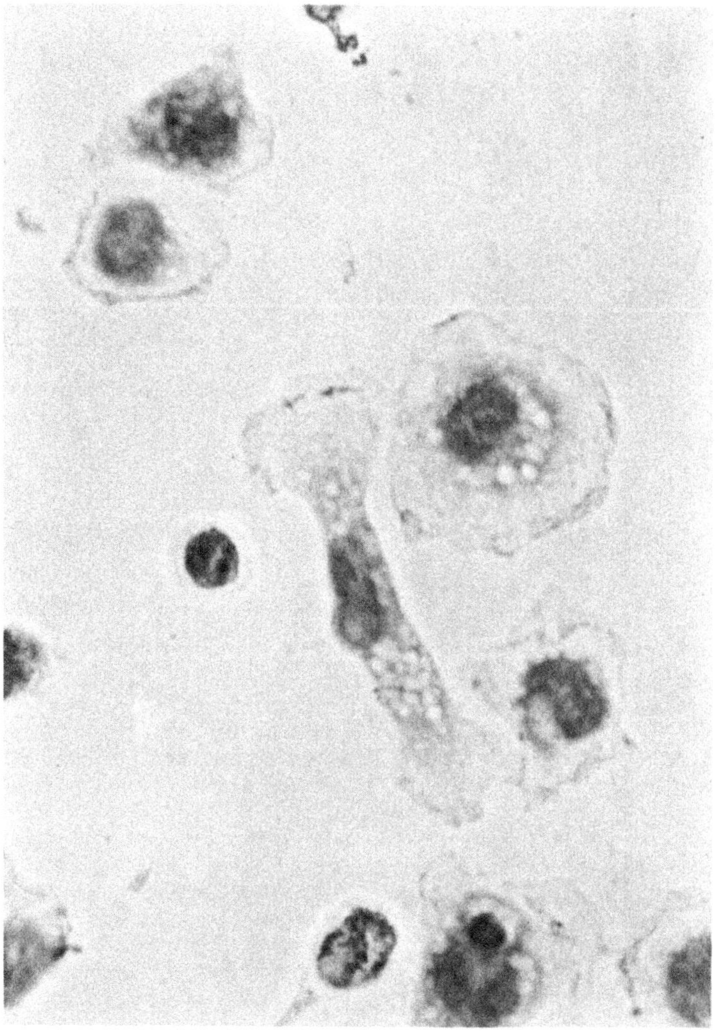

Figure 1B

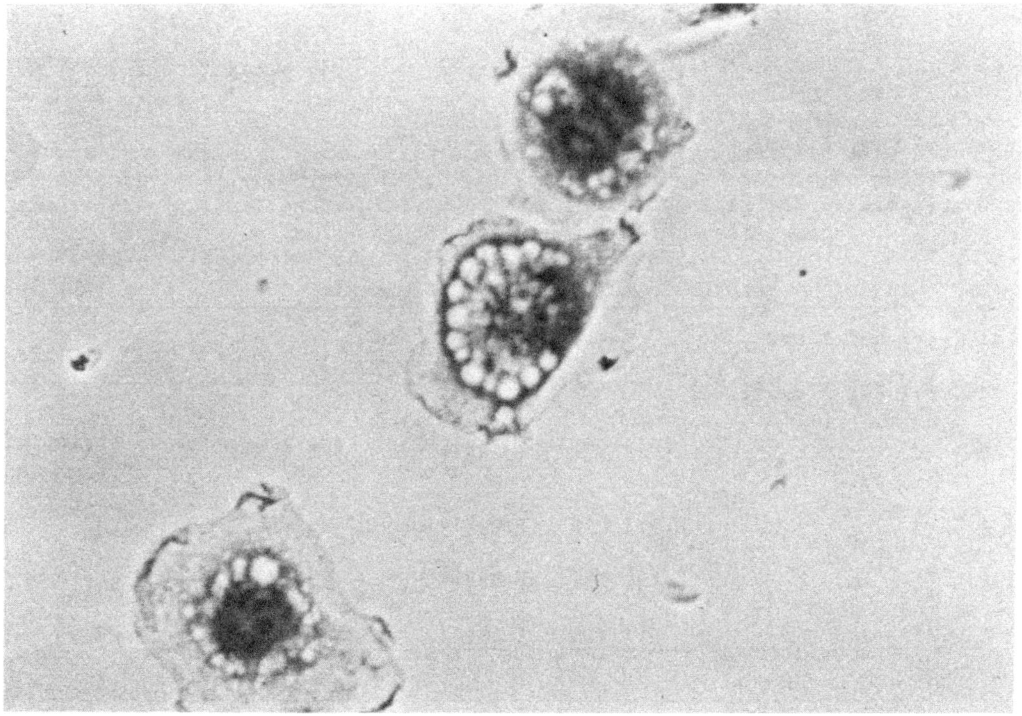

Figure 1C

Figure 1. Morphology of GPL elicited adherent peritoneal cells. Fields represent adherent cell populations removed 48 h following i.p. injection of 200μg GPL antigens and allowed to adhere for 2 h: (A) nonimmunized, saline challenge; (B) sham immunized; (C) GPL-MBSA immunized.

Table 4. Blastogenic response of immune murine spleen cells to homologous antigens. Numbers represent the mean and standard deviation of counts per minute obtained from three separate experiments involving three mice in each group. Cultures contained 2 x 10^5 cells/well.

Group	Donor of Spleen Cells	^{3}H-Thymidine Uptake by Cells Cultivated: Alone	with MBSA (μg)	with GPL (μg)	% Change
1	MBSA-immunized	444 ± 3.5	1,438 ± 581 (1)		+ 2,159
			4,864 ± 2,150 (5)		+ 12,000
			5,566 ± 860 (10)		+ 18,873
2	GPL-MBSA immunized	1,329 ± 976	3,972 ± 4,009 (10)		+ 8,426
				1,068 ± 822 (1)	- 943
				693 ± 460 (5)	- 3,632
3	GPL-MBSA immunized	13,704 ± 2,617	28,012 ± 21,893 (10)		+ 38,569
				13,322 ± 1360 (1)	- 257
				10,862 ± 3053 (5)	-3,484
4	GPL-MBSA immunized	899 ± 320	1,958 ± 1,216 (10)		+ 21,080
				818 ± 458	- 143

Table 5. Mitogen response of spleen cells from mice previously immunized with GPL-MBSA and subsequently challenged with GPL, intraperitoneally. Numbers represent the mean and standard deviation from triplicate cultures obtained from two different groups containing three mice each. Cultures contained 2×10^5 cells/well.

Donor Spleen Cells	^3H-Thymidine Uptake by Cells Cultivated				
	Alone	with PHA	Suppression (%)	with ConA	Suppression (%)
Non-immunized	654 ± 64	$3,161 \pm 465$	-	$116,473 \pm 3,889$	-
Non-immunized[a]	281 ± 86	$1,604 \pm 272$	48	$53,032 \pm 11,044$	55
Immunized[a]	1108 ± 484	$1,051 \pm 310$	102	$37,905 \pm 11,014$	68

[a] These mice received an i.p. injection of sterile saline containing 200 μg GPL antigens 3 days prior to mitogen assay.

Table 6. Mitogen response of spleen cells from mice previously injected, i.p. with 200 μg GPL. Numbers represent the mean and standard deviation of triplicate cultures from groups containing three mice each. Cultures contained 2 x 10^5 cells/well.

Donor Spleen Cells	Time[a] (wk)	^{3}H-Thymidine Uptake by Cells Cultivated: Alone	with PHA (cpm x 10^{-3})	% Suppression (P value)	with ConA (cpm x 10^{-3})	% Suppression
Normal[b]	--	327 ± 118	35.1 ± 5.9	-	48.3 ± 11	-
GPL[c]	1	631 ± 77	26.8 ± 6.4	25 (NS)	41.5 ± 9.0	6 (NS)
	1	361 ± 110	14.1 ± 2.1	60 (.001)	43.3 ± 8.0	2 (NS)
	1	223 ± 13	11.0 ± 1.7	69 (.001)	ND	
	1	182 ± 23	28.4 ± 1.4	20 (NS)	ND	
	1	226 ± 36	15.1 ± 2.5	57 (.002)	ND	
Normal[b]	3	280 ± 116	39.2 ± 8.0	-	13.3 ± 2.4	-
GPL[c]	3	166 ± 20	12.2 ± 2.1	69 (.02)	11.0 ± 2.6	17 (NS)
	3	215 ± 85	10.1 ± 1.2	74 (.02)	6.6 ± 2.0	51 (.02)
	3	245 ± 57	19.4 ± 3.2	50 (.02)	10.4 ± 1.6	22 (NS)

a Time elapsed between antigen injection and mitogen assay.
b Received i.p. injection of sterile saline.
c Received i.p. injection of sterile saline containing 200 μg GPL.

Table 7. Mitogen response of spleen cells from mice previously injected, i.p. with varying amounts of GPL. Numbers represent the mean and standard deviation from triplicate cultures from groups containing three mice each. Cultures contained 2 x 10^5 cells/ well.

Amount GPL (ug)[a]	^{3}H-Thymidine Uptake by cells Cultivated: Alone (cpm)	with PHA (cpm x 10^{-3})	% Suppression (P value)	with ConA (cpm x 10^{-3})	% Suppression (P value)
0	113 ± 21	10.6 ± 0.6	-	27.7 ± 7	-
10	81 ± 8	6.6 ± 0.3	38 (.001)	21.0 ± 2.2	24 (NS)
50	88 ± 17	7.9 ± .03	25 (.002)	6.5 ± 1.8	77 (.007)
100	117 ± 22	7.4 ± 1.8	30 (.04)	7.5 ± 0.4	73 (.008)
500	180 ± 23	15.5 ± 1.3	-46	21.7 ± 2.0	22 (NS)

[a] Mice were injected with indicated amounts of GPL suspended in sterile saline.

When spleen cells from GPL treated mice were enriched for nonadherent cells and mixed with normal spleen cells in a 1:3 ratio (normal:GPL treated), a suppression in the response to PHA was observed (Table 8, Experiment 2) that was significantly greater (P=0.001) than when normal nonadherent cells were mixed with normal cells in a 1:3 ratio (Table 8, Experiment 2). A significant difference in suppression was not observed when an adherent cell population from GPL treated mice was mixed with normal spleen cells (Table 8, Experiment 2). In addition, cell mixing with normal and GPL treated nonadherent cells (1:3) resulted in a significant suppression in the response to PHA and Con A. These results suggest that nonadherent cells are a major contributing factor to the suppression observed in GPL treated mice.

DISCUSSION

From the results of our investigation it is apparent that the GPL antigens of serovar 20 are relatively nontoxic and capable of producing a nonspecific inflammatory response. In addition, injection of these mycobacterial antigens by an intraperitoneal route results in significant reduction in the response of splenic lymphocytes to the T-cell mitogens, ConA and PHA. Cell mixing experiments indicate that the GPL-induced suppression is low level and appears to be dependent upon a group of nonadherent cells which are Thy-1.2$^+$.

Previous studies in our laboratory have revealed that the GPL antigens are inert to macrophage degradation (8); therefore it is possible that during a chronic MAC infection, substantial amounts of these antigens would accumulate and persist in lymphoid tissue thus causing impairment of the immune system. These findings suggest that the GPL antigens of the MAC may be at least one factor which could predispose infected patients to subsequent reinfection or inactivation of a previous MAC

Table 8. Mitogen response of spleen cells from mice previously injected i.p. with GPL antigens. Numbers represent mean and standard deviation from triplicate cultures containing 4×10^5 cells/well.

Experiment 1	^{3}H-Thymidine Uptake by Cells Cultivated				
Donor Spleen Cells	Alone	with PHA (cpm x 10^{-3})	% Suppression (P value)	with ConA (cpm x 10^{-3})	% Suppression (P value)
Normal[a]	535 $\pm$ 122	41.4 $\pm$ 1.9	-	45.5 $\pm$ 2.6	-
GPL[b]	218 $\pm$ 18	19.3 $\pm$ 1.3	53 (<0.001)	32.6 $\pm$ 5.9	28 (0.03)
Normal + GPL	312 $\pm$ 124	40.6 $\pm$ 6.8	2 (NS)	54.6 $\pm$ 3.7	-20
Normal + GPL (anti-Thy)[c]	404 $\pm$ 137	46.2 $\pm$ 8.7	-12	53.0 $\pm$ 0.7	-17
Normal (anti-Thy)	555 $\pm$ 51	0.3 $\pm$ 0.05	99	1.1 $\pm$ 0.3	98
GPL (anti-Thy)	323 $\pm$ 122	0.5 $\pm$ 0.2	99	1.1 $\pm$ 0.04	98

Table 8. (Continued)

Donor Spleen Cells	^{3}H-Thymidine Uptake by Cells Cultivated: Alone	with PHA (cpm x 10^{-3})	% Suppression (P value)	with ConA (cpm x 10^{-3})	% Suppression (P value)
Experiment 2					
Normal	705 ± 161	60.5 ± 8.3	-	133.2 ± 1.6	-
GPL[b]	1257 ± 10	53.8 ± 17.6	11 (NS)	146.5 ± 28.6	-10
Normal + Normal (NA)[d]	5353 ±1171	51.9 ± 4.9	14 } (0.01)	82.2 ± 21.3	38 } (NS)
Normal + GPL (NA)	2578 ± 193	24.7 ± 4.5	59	95.1 ± 18.6	29
Normal + Normal (Ad)[e]	4147 ±1043	24.3 ± 2.4	60 } (NS)	35.3 ± 6.5	74 } (NS)
Normal + GPL (Ad)	2340 ± 444	19.6 ± 0.9	68	15.9 ± 5.8	88
Normal (NA) + GPL (NA)	273 ± 90	16.7 ± 3.5	72 (0.001)	46.4 ± 6.9	65 (<0.001)

a Normal received i.p. infection of sterile saline three weeks prior to assay.
b GPL received i.p. injection of sterile saline containing 200 μg GPL three weeks prior to assay.
c Spleen cells treated with anti-Thy 1.2 and complement
d NA = nonadherent spleen cells
e Ad = adherent spleen cells

infection, providing their T-cell defense system became defective (i.e. as the result of an infection with HTLV-III). Because of their lack of toxicity, their limited inflammatory capabilities, inertness to macrophage degradation and ability to suppress mitogenic responses of splenic lymphocytes, the GPL antigens may be the common link that explains the selective ability of certain MAC serovars to infect persons suffering from AIDS. A similar scenario has recently been proposed by Collins (5).

ACKNOWLEDGEMENT

This work was supported by Grant AI-21946 from NIAID.

REFERENCES

1. Barrow, W. W., Ullom, B. P., and Brennan, P. J. 1980. Peptidoglycolipid nature of the superficial cell wall sheath of smooth-colony-forming mycobacteria. J. Bacteriol. 144:814-822.

2. Barrow, W. W., and Brennan, P. J. 1982. Immunogenicity of type-specific C-mycoside glycopeptidolipids of mycobacteria. Infect. Immun. 36:678-684.

3. Brennan, P. J., and Goren, M. B. 1979. Structural studies on the type-specific antigens and lipids of the *Mycobacterium avium-Mycobacterium intracellulare-Mycobacterium scrofulaceum* serocomplex. J. Biol. Chem. 254:4205-4211.

4. Brennan, P. J., Souhrada, M., Ullom, B., McClatchy, J. K., and Goren, M. B. 1978. Identification of atypical mycobacteria by thin-layer chromatography of their surface antigens. J. Clin. Microbiol. 8:374-379.

5. Collins, F. M. 1986. *Mycobacterium avium*-complex infections and development of the Acquired Immunodeficiency Syndrome: Casual opportunist or causal co-factor? Int. J. Lepr. 54:458-474.

6. Fainstein, V., Bolivar, R., Mavligit, G., Rios, A., Luna, M. 1982. Disseminated infection due to *Mycobacterium avium-intracellulare* in a homosexual man with Kaposi's sarcoma. J. Infect. Dis. 145:586.

7. Greene, J. B., Sidhu, G. S., Lewin, S., Levine, J., Masur, H., Simberkiff, M. S., Nicholas, P., Good, R. C., Zolla-Pazner, S. B., Pollock, A. A., Tapper, M. L. and Holzman, R. S. 1982. *Mycobacterium avium-intracellulare*: a cause of disseminated life-threatening infection in homosexuals and drug abusers, Ann. Intern. Med. 97:539-546.

8. Hooper, L. C., Johnson, M. M., Khera, V. R., and Barrow, W. W. 1986. Macrophage uptake and retention of radiolabeled glycopeptidolipid antigens associated with the L_1 layer of *Mycobacterium intracellulare* serovar 20. Infect. Immun. 54:133-141.

9. Kiehn, T. E., Edwards, F. F., Brannon, P., Tsang, A. Y., Maio, M., Gold, J. W. M., Whimbey, E., Wong, B., McClatchy, J. K. and Armstrong, D. 1985. Infections caused by Mycobacterium avium complex in immunocompromised patients: Diagnosis by blood culture and fecal examination, antimicrobial susceptibility tests, and morphological and seroagglutination characteristics. J. Clin. Microbiol. 21:168-173.

10. Li, C. Y., Lam, K. W., and Yam, L. T. 1973. Esterases in human leukocytes. J. Histochem. Cytochem. 21:1-12.

11. Lowery, O., Rosebrough, N. J., Farr, A. L., and Randall, R. J. 1951. Protein measurement with folin phenol reagent. J. Biol. Chem., 193:265-275.

12. Luster, M. I., Dean, J. H., and Moore, J. A. 1982. Evaluation of immune functions in toxicology, In: "Principles and Methods of Toxicology," Hayes, A. W., ed., New York, pp. 561-586.

13. Macher, A. M., Kovacs, J. A., Gill, V., Roberts, G. D., Ames, J., Park, C. H., Straus, S., Lane, H. C., Pararillo, J. E., Fauci, A. S. and Masur, H. 1983. Bacteremia due to Mycobacterium avium-intracellulare in the acquired immunodeficiency syndrome. Ann. Intern. Med. 99:782-785.

14. Masur, H. 1982. Mycobacterium avium-intracellulare: Another scourge for individuals with the Acquired Immunodeficiency Syndrome. J.A.M.A. 248:3013.

15. Schaefer, W. B. 1965. Serologic identification and classification of the atypical mycobacteria by their agglutination. Am. Rev. Respir. Dis. 92:85-93.

16. Tereletsky, M. J., and Barrow, W. W. 1983. Postphagocytic detection of glycopeptidolipids associated with the superficial L_1 layer of Mycobacterium intracellulare, Infect. Immun. 41:1312-1321.

LEGIONELLA PNEUMOPHILA IMMUNITY AND IMMUNOMODULATION: NATURE AND MECHANISMS

Herman Friedman, Thomas W. Klein, Raymond Widen, Catherine Newton, D. Kay Blanchard and Yoshima Yamamoto

Department of Medical Microbiology and Immunology, University of South Florida College of Medicine, Tampa, FL 33612

Legionella pneumophila is considered the etiologic agent of legionellosis and may cause severe respiratory infection in susceptible individuals, including man and guinea pigs (1-8). These organisms are fastidious opportunistic pathogens which are ubiquitously found in nature but only occasionally causes disease in man under normal circumstances. Guinea pigs are extremely susceptible to these bacteria and are widely used as an animal model for legionellosis. In contrast, rodents such as mice and rats are highly resistant to infection by these bacteria (7,8,10,11). Mice are difficult to infect with strains of *Legionella* highly virulent for guinea pigs. In several situations, it has been observed that *Legionella* may infect immunocompromised individuals, although no particular immunological lesion has been associated with acquisition of the disease (12-14). Indeed, in the first recognized outbreak of legionellosis, i.e., the upper respiratory infection in Pennsylvania State Legionnaires attending a convention in Philadelphia, specific immunologic depression was not observed although individuals who developed the disease drank more liquor, smoked more cigarettes and generally had less sleep than those companions who did not contact the disease.

Recently, legionellosis has been associated mainly with individuals who have either an immunodeficiency or are immunocompromised due to drugs used for transplants or because of other co-existing infections such as that associated with AIDS (13,14). Several studies have been concerned with the immune responsiveness to *Legionella* organisms in man, including the possible role of serum antibodies versus cellular immunity (15,16). Despite the ubiquitousness of this organism in the environment and the general rarity of fatal infection in recent years, attempts have been made in a number of laboratories to develop animal models for this disease. *L. pneumophila* was originally isolated by intraperitoneal (i.p.) injection of guinea pigs with biopsy and autopsy material from patients. The sensitivity of guinea pigs to infection has made it a prime candidate for successful and potentially valid animal models. Although the natural route of infection of man is thought to be by the aeorsol route, the lung pathology of guinea pigs inoculated i.p. does not differ significantly from that observed in animals receiving organisms intranasally or by the aeorsol route. The histology of lungs of such infected animals is similar to that seen in legionellois patients (17-19). Both aeorsol and intracheal (i.t.)

routes of infection of guinea pigs has been shown to produce fatal disease accompanied by at least some of the following signs of true infection: weight loss, fever, pneumonia, bacterial multiplication *in vivo* and specific antibody responses as well as delayed skin hypersensitivity.

Mice and rats are relatively resistant to *Legionella* infection by either the i.p. route or even the aerosol route. For example, studies in rats using i.p. infection with mucin coated organisms reportedly resulted in death within 24 hrs after inoculation of a large inoculum (7,8). Lung pathology was not consistent with human disease and death appeared due to toxicity. Also, mice generally sucuumbed within 24 hrs due to a toxic-like syndrome after inoculation of relatively large numbers of organisms (11). Similarly, mice have been used for infection with smaller numbers of *Legionella* when they are rendered immunologically immunocompromised by immunosuppressive drugs such as cyclophosphamide or when innately immunocompromised because of the lack of a thymus, i.e., athymic mice. Recent studies in this laboratory have shown that the i.t. infection route of mice also results in disease, and one strain of mice showed moderately heightened susceptibility to smaller numbers of *Legionella* as compared to other strains, suggesting a genetic predisposition.

Legionella Antigens - There is now much information concerning the ecological niche of various species of *Legionella*, the ubiquitousness of these organisms, as well as their physiology and biochemistry. However, little is known about the role of immunity to resistance to infection. In this regard, there have a number of studies attempting to determine the antigenic determinants of these bacteria in relationship to protective immunity. Studies have shown that both man and experimental animals readily produce antibodies as well as develop cellular immunity when either injected with vaccines prepared from whole bacteria or after infection with these organisms (20-26). Furthermore, it is now known that the outer membrane protein rich antigens from these bacteria are strong immunogens, as is purified flagella and LPS components of these bacteria (27-32). Early studies showed that immunization of guinea pigs with killed bacteria in complete Freund's adjuvant (CFA) or with antigenic faction, such as the outer membrane proteins, resulted in resistance of these animals when challenged at a later time with viable *Legionella* which are normally lethal. Similar results have been obtained with mice, i.e., immunity has been induced by either whole bacterial cells in adjuvant or by serogroup specific antigen preparations. In most cases challenge infection of vaccinated animals was performed by the i.p. route, which is obviously not considered a natural route of infection. Attempts have been made to protect guinea pigs from challenge infection by aeorsol exposure; i.p. injection of killed bacteria or purified fractions thereof induced less protection against such aeorsol challenge. In other studies, however, aeorsol infection with sublethal doses of these bacteria has induced resistance to aeorsol infection at a later time with otherwise lethal numbers of bacteria. Specific protection has been achieved with crude as well as purified antigens and low levels of cross serogroup protection has been observed. In studies with guinea pigs resistance has been achieved with lipid-protein-carbohydrate complexes considered rich in lipopolysaccharide (LPS). This component has been purified and isolated from several *Legionella* strains and protection has been shown to be both serogroup as well as cross serogroup specific. Protection has also been achieved in mice using vaccines prepared from killed organisms.

Protection against lethality associated with infection of mice with large numbers of bacteria presumably resulted from anti-toxic effects. Checkerboard type protection studies with preparations from homologous serogroup antigens, i.e., serotype specific, gave better protection against infection but, in agreement with previous studies with guinea pigs, some cross serogroup protection was observed. Thus, despite a number of early reports that serum antibody may possibly protect guinea pigs or mice from lethality due to *L. pneumophila*, there has been no convincing evidence that this occurs with syngeneic sera or with models of death due to infections as opposed to toxicity.

Humoral Antibody to Legionella - Patients who recover from *Legionella* develop antibody detected by a variety of assays including microhemagglutination against whole *Legionella* vaccines. Other tests have been developed including complement fixation and immunoflourescent assays which readily show appearance of serum antibodies, both of the IgG and IgM classes, following infection (11,16, 25,26). Vaccination of experimental animals such as guinea pigs or mice results in rapid appearance of specific serum antibodies (33-36). However, there have been no reports indicating that such antibody *in vitro* has lytic capacity against viable bacteria even in the presence of complement. Thus it seems plausible that antibody induced against *Legionella* may not be protective. Some studies have shown that passive immunization of experimental animals such as guinea pigs or mice with antiserum may protect against serogroup specific *Legionella*. In earlier studies, Hedlund et al. found that AKR mice could be protected against death but not illness with goat antiserum raised to formalized bacteria (9). Rolstad and Berdal, using a rat model in the which the LD_{50} was $6x10^8$ organisms, reported passive protection with murine immune serum (10). In both cases animals became ill within 4-6 hrs and died within 24 hrs when injected with the large inoculum of *Legionella*, suggesting that toxic death, possibly due to endotoxin, occurred and protection may be a possible model for endotoxin immunity but not against active infection. Studies in this laboratory have failed to show that immune serum antibody can protect guinea pigs from acute infection although spleen cells from immune but not nonimmune donor guinea pigs could transfer resistance to challenge infection with *Legionella* (Table 1). Adherent,

Table 1. Survival of recipient guinea pigs challenged with viable *Legionella* after transfer of spleen cells or serum from normal or immune donors

Recipient treatment		Survival (survivors/total)	Percent survivors
none (medium control)		5/17	29
spleen cells			
non-immune	$1x10^7$ cells	2/5	40
	$5x10^7$	1/8	12
immune	$1x10^7$	7/10	70
	$5x10^7$	14/16	88
	serum[b]	3/8	38

[a] Groups of normal strain 2 guinea pigs infected i.p. with either medium (Hanks' balanced saline) or spleen cells from normal or *Legionella* immune ($2x10^5$ bacteria 4 weeks earlier) spleen cells or serum. Recipients challenged 24 h later with lethal numbers of *Legionella* i.p. and death determined 3-6 days later.

[b] One ml serum with anti-*Legionella* microagglutinin titer of 1:1280 injected i.p.

not nonadherent cells, were responsible for the adoptive protection (Table 2). In these experiments it was found that spleen cells from infected guinea pigs of the same inbred strains could initiate protection in naive recipients after active immunization. However such resistance was due to cell populations rich in macrohages, not lymphocytes. Adoptive transfer of resistance occurred also with elicited peritoneal cells or adherent spleen cell populations (Table 2).

Delayed Hypersensitivity Reactions - There have been no reported studies concerning the development of delayed cutaneous hypersensitivity in man to *Legionella* following infection as occurs in many other infections. However, there have been a number of studies showing that animals, either infected with living *Legionella* or injected with a vaccine in adjuvant, develop delayed skin hypersensitivity. For example, Wong et al. reported that immunized guinea pigs readily develop cutaneous hypersensitivity when challenged with serogroups specific antigen intradermally several weeks afterward (37). Studies in this laboratory showed that guinea pigs infected with sublethal numbers of *Legionella*, either virulent or avirulent, evince cutaneous hypersensitivity evident by skin inoculation tests with either sonicates or purified antigens from the bacteria (Table 3). Following active infection or challenge immunization of guinea pigs maximum cutaneous hypersensitivity occurred 4-5 weeks after initial exposure to the bacteria or 2-3 wks after a booster immunization (38). Guinea pigs infected with smaller numbers of virulent organisms developed more intense delayed hypersensitivity reaction than those injected with less virulent organisms, suggesting that the degree of virulence of the bacteria was directly related to development of delayed cutaneous hypersensitivity reactions.

In vitro correlates of delayed hypersensitivity have also been readily observed, both in man and experimental animals. For example, it was reported that peripheral blood monocytes from patients after recovery from *Legionella* infection showed marked blastogenesis *in vitro* when stimulated with sonicates of these bacteria (39,40). A stimulation index of 20-30 or greater occurred in the lymphocyte blastogenic assay as measured by thymidine uptake when peripheral blood cells from legionellosis patients were stimulated *in vitro* with the bacteria. However, a significant stimulation index occurred, albeit less than observed with individuals who had no evidence of clinical infection with these organisms, indicating a sensitivity to *Legionella* in "nor-

Table 2. Survival of guinea pigs challenged with *Legionella* after transfer of different cell population from *Legionella* immune donor guinea pigs

Recipient treatment[a]	Survival (survivor/treatment)	Percent survival
none (medium control)	0/3	0
spleen cells unfractionated	3/3	100
nonadherent cells	0/3	0
peritoneal exudate cells	3/3	100

[a] Groups of normal guinea pigs given eigher $10x10^7$ spleen cells from donor guinea pigs, G-10 and nylon wool passed nonadherent splenocytes or thiolycollate induced peritoneal exudate cells; cell recipients challenged 24 hrs later by i.p. inoculation of *Legionella*.

mal" individuals. In this laboratory using the blastogenic assay with lymphoid cells from either guinea pigs or mice direct correlation was evident between responsiveness of lymphoid cells with the degree of sensitization as a function time of previous sensitization by either infection or immunization (Table 3). A good correlation of lymphocyte blastogenic reactions with skin hypersensitivity responses was evident. Furthermore, spleen cells from normal nonsensitized guinea pigs showed no significant blastogenic reaction to Legionella antigen, either whole killed vaccine, sonicates thereof or purified antigens (41-43). However, within several weeks after sublethal infection or immunization of guinea pigs a marked blastogenic response occurred when spleen cells were stimulated with Legionella antigen but not with antigens from other bacteria such as E. coli.

Macrophage migration inhibition factor (MIF) tests also showed development of sensitization of guinea pigs following either infection or immunization (Table 3). No evidence of positive reactions occurred with spleen cells from nonsensitized normal guinea pigs. Within 2-3 weeks after either sublethal infection or immunization both direct and indirect MIF assays showed development of delayed hypersensitivity reactions (44). Spleen cells from sensitized guinea pigs, but not from normal guinea pigs, failed to migrate normally in vitro when incubated with Legionella sonicates but not with sonicates from other bacteria. In the indirect assay, cell free supernatants from spleen cells from Legionella sensitized guinea pigs following exposure to Legionella antigens in vitro markedly inhibited in vitro migration of indicator lymphoid cells from either normal guinea pigs or mice, showing that MIF activity was induced (44). Such activity occurred only with supernatants from spleen cells from sensitized but not normal guinea pigs following stimulation in vitro with Legionella antigens but not with antigens from other bacteria.

Results of studies with spleen cells from mice exposed to sublethal numbers of viable Legionella or immunized with whole Legionella vaccine in adjuvant or sonicates thereof were similar to those with guinea pigs cells. However, a major difference was observed. Similar

Table 3. Comparative reactivity of guinea pigs after sensitization by i.p. infection with L. pneumophila

Time in weeks after sensitization[a]	Cellular Hypersensitivity		
	skin reaction[b]	MIF production[c]	blastogenesis[d]
none (normal	0	0	0
1-2	0	0	0
3-4	3^+	2^+	3^+
5-6	4^+	4^+	4^+
8-10	4^+	4^+	4^+

[a] Groups of guinea pigs infected i.p. with 2×10^6 L. pneumophila at indicated time before testing.

[b] Cutaneous skin hypersensivity reactions 48 h. after i.d. injection with 10 ug Legionella sonicate; 0 = no reaction; 2^+ = 8-10 mm reaction; 4^+ = 12 mm or greater reaction.

[c] Migration inhibition reactivity; 2^+ = 20-30% inhibition; 4^+ = 40% or greater inhibition of migration.

[d] Spleen cell blastogenesis with 10 ug Legionella sonicate; 0 = SI of 1 or less; 3^+ = SI of 3-5; 4^+ = SI of 5 or more.

to the situation with man, spleen cells from normal nonsensitized mice evinced a consistent reactivity to Legionella antigen in vitro as shown by the thymidine uptake reaction (45-47). A stimulation index of 8-10 was evident for spleen cells from normal mice treated in vitro with Legionella antigens for 48 hrs (Table 4). Following sensitization of mice by either infection with sublethal numbers of bacteria or injection of Legionella vaccine in adjuvant spleen cells showed marked responsiveness to homologous Legionella antigen by the blastogenic reaction. A stimulation index of 40-50 or more was evident in many instances when spleen cells were obtained from mice 3-4 weeks after sensitization (Table 4). Furthermore, a striking difference was noted between responses of spleen cells from sensitized animals versus those from normal animals. Maximum responses of spleen cells stimulated with Legionella antigen in vitro using cells from normal animals occurred on day +3 of cultures. By day 5 after the initiation of cultures the spleen cells were much less active in thymidine uptake. In contrast, spleen cells from mice sensitized 3-4 weeks or more earlier by injection with live Legionella or Legionella vaccine in adjuvant gave a peak response still on day +3 after in vitro sensitization but on day 5 thymidine uptake was still markedly elevated, suggesting that this may reflect a "booster" or an anamnestic type reaction relative to the reaction of spleen cells from nonsensitized mice (47). Thus the kinetics of responses indicated a difference between normal mice versus those which had been previously exposed to Legionella. The peak blastogenic responsiveness of spleen cells from sensitized mice was approximately 4 wks after exposure to the bacteria.

In other studies on the kinetics of the blastogenic responses, it was found that early after infection with sublethal numbers of bacteria or injection of killed bacterium there was a finite but marked depression of early blastogenic responsiveness. This was most evident 3-5 days after exposure of the animals to Legionella. Whereas spleen cells from normal mice resulted in a SI of approximately 10 following optimal in vitro stimulation with Legionella, spleen cells from Legionella injected mice generally showed an SI of less than 2-4 during the first 2-5 days after exposure to the organism. Such hyporesponsiveness was not only specific for the Legionella antigen but also occurred with other nonspecific stimulators, including E. coli LPS, considered a B

Table 4. Effect of infection of mice with L. pneumophila on responsiveness of spleen cells in vitro to Legionella sonicate

Time after sensitization (days)[a]	Splenic blastogenesis[b]	
	cpm ± S.E.	S.I.
None (normal control)	10,310±458	8.6±1.3
5-10	12,420±590	9.5±1.2
15-20	18,960±1,400	18.6±2.5
25-30	68,530±3700	34.5±4.6
35-40	86,450±7810	49.6±3.2
45-60	80,690±6530	45.5±4.6
70-90	75,360±4350	41.6±3.5

[a] Groups of DBA/2 mice injected i.p. with $1x10^7$ viable Legionella at indicated time before testing.

[b] Average blastogenic response of $5x10^6$ spleen cells for 3-4 mice per group stimulated for 48 hr in vitro with 10 ug L. pneumophila sonicate.

cell stimulator, as well as the plant mitogens Con A and PHA, considered T cell mitogens. Maximum depression of these nonspecific responses paralleled depression of the response to Legionella antigen. Thus early after either sublethal infection or immunization of mice with Legionella there was not only a specific suppression of responsiveness to Legionella antigen but also a nonspecific suppression to other stimuli. The significance of such suppressions to possible mechanisms of Legionella infectivity is not clear.

Since the strains of mice studied are relatively resistant to Legionella infection, and generally 10^8 or more bacteria are needed to induce lethality and this generally occurs within 24 hrs due to a toxic reaction, the relevance of suppression with such mice is not clear. However, recent studies with A/J mice showed that at least this one strain of mouse is more susceptible to Legionella and their peritoneal macrophages, unlike those from other mouse strains, appear similar to those from guinea pigs and even peripheral blood monocytes of man in that they are susceptible rather than resistant to infection in vitro with Legionella.

Mediators of cellular immunity are also readily induced by Legionella antigens (48,49). As indicated above, MIF activity was apparent in spleen cells from guinea pigs after sensitization with Legionella. In the mouse model interleukin 1 and interleukin 2 were readily induced by Legionella antigens (Table 5). Furthermore, interferon and tumor necrosis factor (TNF) were also readily induced by these bacteria and their antigens (Table 5). Spleen cells from Legionella sensitized mice, but not normal mice, when treated with Legionella antigen resulted in formation of lymphokine which caused proliferation of CTLL/2 cells requiring exogenous IL 2 for proliferation.

Interferon was readily induced in spleen cell cultures from both normal and Legionella sensitized mice following stimulation with antigen from these bacteria in vitro. Most of the interferon induced was of the gamma type as shown by characterization studies showing acid

Table 5. Induction of soluble mediators of immunity by Legionella preparations

Mouse group[a]	Stimulator[b]	Mediator[c]			
		IL-1	IL-2	IFN	TNF
none	none	0	0	0	0
	Legionella vaccine	3+	0	2+	4+
	LPS	3+	0	3+	4+
Legionella immune	none	0	0	0	0
	Legionella vaccine	4+	4+	4+	4+
	LPS	4+	4+	4+	4+

[a] Spleen cells ($5x10^6$) from Legionella immune mice stimulated in vitro with indicated Legionella antigen.

[b] Legionella (10^6 killed bacteria) or LPS (10 ug) added to spleen cells from normal DBA/2 mice or mice immunized 25-35 days earlier with 10^7 Legionella in CFA.

[c] Indicated lymphokine determined by biologic assay in cell free supernatants from $5x10^6$ spleen cells form normal or immunized mice stimulated for 24 hrs with indicated Legionella antigens.

lability and neutralization with monoclonal antibody to interferon. The gamma interferon induced by Legionella antigen was IL 2 dependent since only target spleen cells pretreated with IL 2 produced IFN upon stimulation with Legionella antigen. Furthermore, TNF was readily induced by Legionella antigens in vitro as well as in vivo. Following i.t. infection of normal mice with viable Legionella TNF was found in the lung lavage fluids shortly following the appearance of interferon. In addition, treatment of mice with dextran sulfate prior to infection with viable Legionella decreased considerably the amount of TNF produced. This is consistent with the observation that macrophages are the source of this factor. Treatment of mice with rTNF and also rIFN resulted in increased survival of animals challenged with viable Legionella via i.t. inoculation. Thus it appears that lymphokines, including TNF, may be important in resistance to these bacteria.

Interaction of Legionella with Phagocytes

Studies concerning the histology of lung tissue of patients who succumb to legionellosis have shown that alveolar macrophages are filled with replicating Legionella. It is now apparent that these bacteria have a predilection for macrophages and that phagocytosis readily occurs with these bacteria. Horwitz and Silverstein first showed that peripheral blood monocytes from normal and convalescent individuals readily phagocytize Legionella in vitro (50). Cultures of human monocytes from peripheral blood together with as few as one organism per 100 mononuclear cells resulted in rapid intracellular growth of the bacteria with peak growth four days after initiation of culture. Bacteria were rapidly phagocytized by peripheral blood monocytes from individuals with no evidence of prior exposure to Legionella. However, phagocytosis by mononuclear cells occurred most efficiently in the presence of both antibody and complement. Horwitz and Silverstein reported that human antibody plus complement promoted association of the bacteria with monocytes in cultures and may mediate a modest amount of bacterial killing by these cells (50-52). However, a majority of the bacteria survive despite antibody and complement and proceed to replicate intracellularly. Morever, blood mononuclear cells incubated with Concanavalin A or supernatants of such cultures inhibited intracellular multiplication of Legionella. Such activated monocytes not only contained fewer bacteria but also exerted bacterostatic control over those which were interiorized.

Recently Horwitz showed that interferon addition to monocytes resulted in inhibition of growth of Legionella but did not cause the killing of the bacteria. Furthermore, monocytes from patients recovered from legionellosis readily inhibited growth of the organism in vitro. Studies by Kishimoto et al. showed that Legionella could infect alveolar cells of monkeys at a ratio of bacteria to cells of 100 (53). Intracellular replication was evident within 3 hrs and extensive within 24 hrs. Electron micrographic studies showed that macrophages were packed with bacterial cells. Although only a small percentage of Legionella were phagocytized, those that were grew quite well. The uptake of Legionella by rat alveolar and mouse peritoneal macrophages has also been studied. Radiolabelled organisms were interiorized in the presence of immune serum and this was serogroup specific. The specificity of the immune serum was demonstrated by removal of opsonic activity upon absorption with purified homologous Legionella antigen but not with heterologous antigen. Kishimoto also reported on the interaction of L. pneumophila with guinea pig peritoneal macrophages in vitro (54). Normal macrophages required immune serum to phagocytize the bacteria, either virulent or avirulent, but macrophages from previously infected animals were much more phagocytic. Virulent organisms multiplied intracellularly while avirulent bacteria did not.

Studies in this laborabory have confirmed that macrophages from normal guinea pigs readily ingest Legionella and that the bacteria grow well in these cells (Table 6). In contrast, when peritoneal macrophages are obtained from Legionella immune guinea pigs, inhibition of ingestion and growth of the bacteria occurs. Furthermore, when Concanavalin A stimulated macrophage cell free supernatants are added to macrophages from normal guinea pigs, inhibition of growth occurs and this depends upon the dose of the supernatant used (Table 7). This suggests that lymphokines related to cellular immunity induce resistance of guinea pig macrophages to Legionella replication.

In contrast to the situation with macrophages from guinea pigs, peritoneal macrophages from mice are highly resistant to Legionella growth (Table 6). The marked difference in phagocytic activity of macrophages from guinea pigs vs mice in comparison to phagocytosis of Listeria or staphylococci is noteworthy, indicating the distinct difference in regards to phagocytosis of Legionella by guinea pig vs mouse cells. However, macrophages from guinea pigs and mice generally respond similarly to zymosan or other phagocytosis inducers in terms of their biochemistry. Recently, it has been found that peritoneal macrophages from the A/J strain of mouse, but not from other mouse strains tested such as BALB/c, C_3H/HeJ, C_3/HeN, DBA/2, etc., are susceptible to growth of Legionella in vitro. Macrophages from normal A/J mice permit replication of Legionella similar to macrophages from guinea pigs. There was no apparent difference in the ability of macrophages from A/J mice vs those from other mouse strains to phagocytise other bacteria. Furthermore, cell free culture supernatants rich in lymphokines from several mouse strains were capable of activating macrophages from A/J mice to resist Legionella growth in vitro. In

Table 6. Comparative growth in vitro of L. pneumophila in peritoneal exudate macrophages from normal guinea pigs or mice

Ratio of Legionella to macrophages[a]		Legionella growth (PFU $\log_{10}$/ml) on day[b]				
		0	+1	+2	+3	+5
guinea pigs	2:1	5.4±0.3	6.5±0.4	6.4±6.5	7.1±0.2	--
	0.2:1	4.2±0.2	5.5±0.3	6.4±0.8	6.9±0.3	--
	0.02:1	3.3±0.3	4.9±0.4	6.2±0.3	6.6±0.3	--
	0.002:1	2.7±0.2	4.1±0.3	5.9±0.6	6.5±0.7	--
mouse	65:1	6.2±0.3	5.9±0.3	4.8±0.2	5.4±0.5	5.0±0.2
	6.5:1	5.1±0.4	4.8±0.3	4.6±0.3	4.6±0.4	4.2±0.3
	0.6:1	4.1±0.2	3.6±0.3	--	2.2±0.5	2.2±0.4
	0.06:1	3.3±0.2	2.0±0.5	--	1.0	1.0
	0.006:1	2.3±0.3	1.3±0.5	--	1.0	1.0

[a] Indicated ratio of viable Legionella cultured with macrophages from either normal guinea pigs or DBA/2 mice for 3-5 days in vitro; phagocytosis for 30 min at 37°C, cells then washed with Hanks' balanced salt solution and cells recultured in RPMI 1640 medium with 15% fetal calf serum and incubated for indicated additional time before determining CFU 1 ratio.

[b] Average CFU $\log_{10}$/ml ± SD for at least 3 separate macrophage cultures per variable for each day of culture.

addition, macrophages from A/J mice immunized with Legionella become highly resistant to growth of the bacteria in vitro similar to macrophages from other mouse strains or macrophages from sensitized but not normal guinea pigs. Recombinant DNA derived interferon, when added to cultures of macrophages from A/J mice, rendered these cells much more resistant to replication of Legionella, suggesting that interferon may be important in resistance mechanisms. This activity was associated with gamma but not alpha/beta interferon.

DISCUSSION AND CONCLUSIONS

L. pneumophila is a ubiquitous intracellular opportunistic pathogen which has a predilection for rapid growth in macrophages, at least from susceptible animals such as guinea pigs and, more recently, A/J mice, as well as human which show susceptibility to infection by these bacteria. Legionella have been shown to replicate in cultures of macrophages not only from the lung but also from the peritoneum and spleen. Electron microscopy studies have shown that these bacteria are associated with phagosomal vesicles in human and guinea pig monocytes and macrophages. Histological studies of human and animal tissue, as well as in vitro experiments using phagocytes or cell lines, suggest that these bacteria are facultative intracellular pathogens which grow best in macrophages. The multiplication of Legionella in human monocytes as well as in macrophages from guinea pigs and mice appears to be inhibited by lymphokines, especially interferon. Such studies focus attention on immunity as a mechanism not only for resistance to these organisms but also to growth of the bacteria in the situation of compromised intracellular immunity. It remains to be determined, however, whether T cells or their products are the mechanism of activation of monocytes or macrophages with enhanced bacterostatic activity or whether T cells can actually mediate immunity, at least in animal model systems.

Table 7. Effect of cell free Con A induced supernatants from normal guinea pigs spleen cells on growth of Legionella treated guinea pig macrophages

Treatment of macrophage culture[a]	CFU per day in culture[b]			
	0	+1	2	+5
None (medium control)	3.2±0.4	4.1±0.5	5.4±0.6	6.4±0.5
Con A supernatants 1.0 ug	--	3.6±0.4	3.9±0.2	2.1±0.2
4.0 ug	--	3.5±0.2	3.1±0.1	1.0
16.0 ug	--	3.3±0.2	3.1±0.2	1.0

[a] Cultures of peritoneal macrophages from normal guinea pigs pretreated for 24 hrs at 37°C with 30% cell free culture supernatants from $5x10^6$ spleen cells from normal guinea pigs after stimulation in vitro with indicated concentration of Con A for 24 hr. Control supernatants from spleen cell cultures treated with medium alone (other controls consisted of medium from untreated cells or Con A only were negative).

[b] Average CFU log_{10}/ml lysate of treated guines pig macrophages incubated at ratio of 10^5 Legionella per 10^6 macrophages for 15 min., washed and then recultured for 1-5 days with medium before determining bacterial CFU per ml lysate.

Mitogenesis of peripheral blood leukocytes from patients stimulated with *Legionella* antigen appears to show that lymphocytes do respond to these bacteria and that T cells are involved. Nevertheless, definitive studies concerning specific involvement of T cells or other cells of the immune system in immunity or resistance to these bacteria is still lacking. There has been considerable work to date suggesting that antibody may be related to *Legionella* infection. However, the observation that antibody is present in individuals prior to clinical infection with *Legionella* and the increased titers of antibody after infection probably indicates a lack of association with protective immunity. The findings by Horwitz and Silverstein, as well as by others, that antibody and complement are not lytic for these organisms, at least *in vitro*, and that antibody may promote phagocytosis of the bacteria by monocytes and/or macrophages *in vitro* but does not inhibit the replication of the bacteria in these cells cast further doubt on the role of antibody in protection against *Legionella*.

The possibility that antibody may serve as a "blocking" factor and protect the bacteria from destruction by macrophage or T lymphocytes and/or other cells of the T cell lineage such as NK or cytolytic cells has not been examined in detail, but the possibility of such a "negative" effect of antibody on host immunity against *Legionella* has not been eliminated.

The susceptibility of guinea pigs versus rodents such as rats and mice to infection with *Legionella* organisms, including those which are considered highly virulent for guinea pigs and man, suggests some genetic basis for resistance versus susceptibility. Although mice are generally susceptible to infection by *Listeria* and their monocytes replicate these bacteria, there appears to be no correlation with resistance vs susceptibility to *Listeria* in regards to *Legionella*. Whatever the genetic mechanism involved in susceptibility to *Listeria* vs *Legionella* this is apparently not a general phenomenon.

Purification of antigens from *Legionella* has resulted in different antigenic components which appear to induce different levels of protection. These different components may also activate different cell types including antibody-producing B lymphocytes and their progeny, macrophages or T cells. How such antigens, including LPS rich fractions, suppress immune responses, especially cell mediated responses, at least early after exposure, is not yet clear. Nevertheless, it appears that antigenic components of *Legionella* may induce antibody within a short period of time, whereas cell mediated immunity is a much later event. Progression of disease may be due either to a "blocking" effect of antibody on induction of cellular immunity to *Legionella* or to the fact that the *Legionella* antigens may induce a temporary but still significant depression of cellular immunity, at least early after infection. Various studies have shown that bacterial antigens, including LPS-rich components as well as whole bacteria and their components, may induce anergy. This can occur with *Legionella*, at least in the mouse model system. Thus future studies to examine in more detail the nature of the mechanism of immunosuppression vs immunomodulation induced by *Legionella* and its components are warranted.

SUMMARY

L. pneumophila is a faculative intracellular opportunistic pathogen ubiquitously present in the environment. Much is now known concerning the ecological niche of this organism as well as many other characteristics of these bacteria, including physiology and biochemistry. However, much less is known about immune mechanisms responsible for host resistance vs susceptibility. Not only outer membrane protein rich fractions but also LPS-rich components are potent immunogens, both in experimental animals such as susceptible guinea pigs and more resistant rodent species like rats and mice. Immunity to these organisms can be readily observed by a variety of serologic techniques. Antibody titers increase rapidly after exposure of individuals to these bacteria either by infection or immunization. However, such antibody does not appear to play an important role in host resistance. Serum antibody plus complement is not lytic for the bacteria in vitro. Furthermore, antibody appears to promote the phagocytosis of the bacteria by monocytes and/or macrophages in culture but such phagocytosis does not result in killing of the bacteria, merely an enhanced uptake and subsequent replication of the organisms. Studies on cellular immunity have focused attention on the role of T lymphocytes, monocytes and macrophages. In addition, cutaneous hypersensitivity is readily induced by infection or immunization of experimental animals with Legionella or antigenic components. In vitro correlates of hypersensitivity is also readily evident after infection or immunization. Although lymphoid cells from guinea pigs only show evidence of responsivenss to Legionella antigens by the lymphocyte blastogenic reaction after animals have been sensitized, peripheral blood monocytes from man as well as splenocytes from mice show evidence of responsiveness to Legionella even before known infection or sensitization. However, higher blastogenic responses become evident after sensitization or infection. In addition, interleukins, such as interleukin 1 and 2, as well as interferon and tumor necrotizing factor, appear in response to Legionella antigens and seem to play a role in resistance mechansisms. Cellular replication of Legionella in monocytes from man as well as macrophages from susceptible animals seems related to susceptibility or resistance to these organisms. Further analyses of the nature and mechanism of humoral vs cellular immune responses to Legionella antigens will provide valuable information about immunity and resistance to these intracellular pathogens in susceptible individuals.

REFERENCES

1. Fraser, D.W., T.R. Tsai, W. Orenstein, W.E. Parkin, H.J.Beecham, P.G. Sharrar, J. Harris, G.F. Mallison, S.M. Martin, J.E. McDade, C.C. Shepart, P.S. Brachman, and The Field Investigation Team. 1977. Legionnaires' disease. Description of an epidemic of pneumonia. N. Engl. J. Med. 297:1198.
2. Meyer, R.P. and S.M. Finegold. 1980. Legionnaires' disease. Ann. Rev. Med. 31:219.
3. Fraser, D.W., C. Bopp, I.K. Wachsmuth, J.C. Feeley, and T. Tsai. 1978. Antibiotic treatment of guinea pigs infected with agent of Legionnaires' disease. Lancet. 1:175.
4. Chandler, F.W., J.E. McDade, M.D. Hicklin, J.A. Blackmon, B.M. Thomason, and E.P. Ewing. 1979. Pathologic findings in guinea pigs inoculated intraperitoneally with the Legionnaires' disease bacterium. Ann. Inter. Med. 90:671.
5. Berendt, R.F., H.W. Young, R.G. allen, and G.L. Knutsen. 1980. Dose-response of guinea pigs experimentally infected with aerosols of Legionella pneumophila J. Infect. Dis. 141:186.
6. Katz, S.M., and S. Hashemi. 1982. Electron microscopic examination of the inflammatory response to Legionella pneumophila in guinea pigs. Lab. Invest. 46:24.
7. Winn, W.C., Jr., G.S. Davis, D.W. Gump, J.E. Craighead, and H.N. Beaty. 1982. Legionnaires' pneumonia after intratracheal inoculation of guinea pigs and rats. Lab. Invest. 47:568.

8. Davis, G.S., W.C. Winn, Jr., D.W. Gump, J.E. Craighead and H.N. Beaty. 1982. Legionnaires' pneumonia after aerosols exposure of guinea pigs and rats. Am. Rev. Respir. Dis. 126:1050.
9. Hedlund, K.W., V.G. McGann, D.S. Copeland, S.F. Little and R.G. Allen. 1979. Immunological protection against the Legionnaires' disease bacterium in the AKR/J mouse. Ann. Intern. Med. 90:676-679.
10. Rolstadt, B. and P.B. Berdal. 1981. Immune defenses against Legionella pneumophila in rats. Inf. and Immun. 32:805-812.
11. Eisenstein, T.K. and H. Friedman. 1985. Immunity to Legionella in Legionellosis. 2nd ed., p.159-169, CRC Press, Boca Raton, Florida.
12. Saravolatz, L.D., K.H. Burch, E. Fisher, T. Madhavan, D. Kiani, T. Neblett and E.L. Quinn. 1979. The compromised host and Legionnaires' disease. Ann. Intern. Med. 90:533.
13. Cutz, E., P.S. Thorner, P. Rao, S. Toma, R. Gold and E.W. Gelfand. 1982. Desseminated Legionella pneumophila infection in an infant with severe combined immunodeficiency.
14. Saravolatz, L.D., K.H. Burch, E. Fisher, T. Madhavan, D. Kiani, T. Neblett and E.L. Quinn. 1979. The compromised host and Legionnaires' disease. Ann. of Inter. Med. 90:533-537.
15. Arko, R.J., K.H. Wong and J. Feeley. 1979. Immunologic factors affecting the in vivo and in vitro survival of the Legionnaires' disease bacterium. Ann. Inter. Med. 90:630-683.
16. Friedman, A.P. and S.M. Katz. 1981. The prevalence of serum antibodies to Legionella pneumophila in patients with chronic pulmonary disease. Am. Rev. Respir. Dis. 123:238-239.
17. Davis, G.S., W.C. Winn and H.N. Beaty. 1981. Legionnaires' disease: Infections caused by Legionella pneumophila and Legionella-like organisms. Clin. Chest. Med. 2:145-66.
18. Winn, W.C.,Jr. and R.L. Myerowitz. 1981. The pathology of the Legionella pneumonias. A review of 74 cases and the literature. Human Pathol. 12:401-422.
19. Winn, W. 1984. Pathology and pathogenesis of Legionella infections. In: Legionella, (C.Thornsberry, A. Ballows, J.C. Feeley and W. Jakubowski, eds.). p. 115-122. Amer. Soc. Microbiol. Press, Washington, D.C.
20. Berendt, R.F., H.W. Young, R.G. Allen et al. 1980. Dose response of guinea pigs experimentally infected with aerosols of Legionella pneumophila. J. Infect. Dis. 141:186-192.
21. Broome, C.V., W.B. Cherry, W.C. Winn,Jr. and B.R. MacPherson. 1979. Rapid diagnosis of Legionnaires' disease by direct immunofluorescent staining. Ann. Inter. Med. 90:1-4.
22. Edson, D.C., H.E. Stiefel, B.B. Wentworth and D.D. Wilson. 1979. Prevalence of antibodies to Legionnaires' disease. A seroepidemiologic survey of Michigan residents using the hemagglutination test. Ann. Inter. Med. 90:691-694.
23. Holliday, M.G. 1980. The diagnosis of Legionnaires' diesease by counterimmunoelectrophoresis. J. Clin. Pathol. 33:1174-1181.
24. Horwitz, M.A. 1982. Demonstration of cell-mediated immunity in Legionnaires' disease. Clin. Res. 30:369A.
25. Wilkinson, H.W., B.J. Fikes and D.D. Cruce. 1979. Indirect immunofluorescence test for serodiagnosis of Leginnaires disease: evidence for serogroup diversity of Legionnaires' disease bacterial antigens and for multiple specificity of human antibodies. J. Clin. Microbiol. 9:379-383.
26. Wilkinson, H.W., A.L. Reingold, B.J. Brake, D.L. McGiboney, G.W. Gorman and C.V. Broome. 1983. Reactivity of serum from patients with suspected legionellosis against 29 immunofluorescence assay. J. Infect. Dis. 147:23-31.

27. Elliot, J.A., W. Johnson and C.M. Helms. 1981. Ultrastructural localization and protective activity of high-molecular-weight antigen isolated from Legionella pneumophila. Infec. Immun. 31:822-824.
28. Johnson, W., J.A. Elliott, C.M. Helms and E.D. Renner. 1979. A high molecular weight antigen in Legionnaires' disease bacterium: isolation and partial characterization. Ann. In. Med. 90:638-641.
29. Elliott, J.A. and W. Johnson. 1981. Immunological and biochemical relationships among flagella isolated from Legionella pneumophila serogroups 1, 2, and 3. Inf. and Immun. 33:602-609.
30. Friedman, H., R. Widen, T. Klein and W. Johnson. 198 . Legionella pneumophila-induced immunostimulation and blastogenesis of normal mouse spleen cells in vitro. Proc. Soc. Exp. Biol. Med. 174:212-216.
31. Friedman, H., R. Widen, T. Klein and W. Johnson. 1984. Immunostimulation by Legionella pneumophila antigen preparations in vivo and in vitro. Infec. Immun. 43:347-352.
32. Friedman, H., C. Newton, K.D. Blanchard, T.W. Klein, R. Widen and K.H. Wong. 1986. Immunogenicity and adjuvanticity of lipopolysaccharide from Legionella pneumophila. Proc. Soc. Exp. Biol. Med. (in press).
33. Vogel, F.R., T.W. Klein, S. Specter, M. Hitchings and H. Friedman. 1981. Detection of antibodies for Legionella pneumophila in immune guinea pig serum by solid phase immunofluorescence. J. Clin. Microbiol. 13:726-729.
34. Friedman, H., R. Widen and T. Klein. 1983. Cellular immunity to Legionella antigen. Clin. Immunol. Newsletter, 4:92-96.
35. Friedman, H., T. Klein and R. Widen. 1983. Cellular and humoral immunity to Legionella pneumophila. In: Infect. Colloquium 1: p.99-111. C. Krasemann, ed. W. deGruytes Press, Amsterdam, The Netherlands.
36. Friedman, H., R. Widen, and T. Klein. 1983. Immunodiagnostic assays for legionellosis. Lab. Mgmt. 21:19-24.
37. Wong, K.H., P.R.B. McMaster, J.C. Feeley, R.J. Arko, W.O. Schalla and F.W. Chandler. 1980. Detection of hypersensitivity to Legionella pneumophila in guinea pigs by skin test. Cur. Microbiol. 4:105-110.
38. Klein, T., H. Friedman and R. Widen. 1984. The relative potency of virulent vs avirulent Legionella pneumophila for the induction of cell-mediated immunity. Infec. Immun. (in press).
39. Plouffe, J.F. and I.M. Bair. 1981. Lymphocyte transformation to Legionella pneumophila. J. Clin. Lab. Immunol. 5:149-152.
40. Plouffe, J.F. and I.M. Baird. 1982. Lymphocyte blastogenic responses to L. pneumophila in acute legionellosis. J. Clin. Lab. Immunol. 7:43-44.
41. Friedman, H., T. Klein and R. Widen. 1984. Immunity to Legionella pneumophila. In: Legionella, p. 145-152. J.C. Feeley, C. Thornsbery, A. Balows and W. Jakubowski. eds. Amer. Soc. Microbiol. Washington, D.C.
42. T. Klein, R. Widen, K. Cabrian, L. Searles and H. Friedman. 1984. Development of cellular immunity in guinea pigs exposed to Legionella pneumophila. In: Legionella, p.178-180. J.C. Feeley, C. Thornsberry, A. Balows and W. Jakubowski, eds. Amer. Soc. Microbiol., Washington, D.C.
43. Widen, R., I. Lee, T. Klein and H. Friedman. 1983. Blastogenic responsiveness of spleen cells from guinea pigs sensitized to Legionella pneumophila antigen. Proc. Soc. Exp. Biol. Med.,143:547-544.
44. Friedman, H., R. Widen, I. Lee and T. Klein. 1983. Cellular immunity to Legionella pneumophila in guinea pigs assessed by direct and indirect migration inhibition reactions in vitro. Infec. Immun. 41:1132-1137.

45. Friedman, H., R. Widen, T. Klein, L. Searles and K. Cabrian. 1984. Legionella pneumophila-induced blastogenesis of murine lymphoid cells in vitro. Infect. Immun. 43:314-319.
46. Friedman, H., C. Newton, A. Friedman, R. Widen, T. Klein. 1986. Blastogenic responsiveness of spleen cells from Legionella pneumphila-infected mice immunosuppressed with cyclophosphamide. Current Microbiol. 14:35-39.
47. H. Friedman, R.Widen, C. Newton and T. Klein. 1986. Distinctive cytokinetics of blastogenic responses by spleen cells from Legionella pneumophila sensitized mice. Current Microbiol. (in press).
48. Widen, R., C. Newton, T.W. Klein, and H. Friedman. 1985. Interleukin induction by Legionellia pneumophila antigens. Proc. Am. Soc. Mibriol. Ann. Mtg. p.82.
49. Blanchard, D.K., T.W. Klein, H. Friedman and W.E. Stewart II. 1985. Kinetics and characterization of interferon induction by murine spleen cells stimulated with Legionella pneumophila antigen. Infec. Immun. 49:719-723.
50. Horwitz, M.A. and S.C. Silverstein. 1981. Interaction of the Legionnaires' disease bacterium (Legionella pneumophila) with human phagocytes. I. J. Exp. Med. 153:386-397.
51. Horwitz, M.A. and S. C. Silverstein. 1981. Interaction of the Legionnaires' disease bacterium (Legionella pneumophila) with human phagocytes. II. J. Exp. Med. 153:398-406.
52. Horwitz, M.A. 1984. Interactions between Legionella pneumophila and human mononuclear phagocytes. p. 159-166. In: Legionella C. Thornsberry, A. Balows, J.C. Feeley and W. Jakubowski, eds. Amer. Soc. Microbiol. Press. Washington, D.C.
53. Kishimoto, R.A., M.D. Kastello, J.D. White, F.G. Shirey, V.G. McGann, E.W. Larson and K.W. Hedlund. 1979. In vitro interaction between normal cynomolgus monkey alveolar macrophages and Legionnaires' disease bacteria. Infec. Immun. 25:761-763.
54. Kishimoto, R.A., J.D. White, F.G. Shirey, V.G. McGann, R.F. Berendt, E.W. Larson and K.W. Hedlund. 1981. In vitro response of guinea pig peritoneal macrophages to Legionella pneumophila. Inf. and Immun. 31:1209-1213.

IMMUNOMODULATION AND *CHLAMYDIA*: IMMUNOSUPPRESSION AND THE PROTECTIVE IMMUNE RESPONSE TO *C. PSITTACI* IN MICE

Gerald I. Byrne, Lynne E. Guagliardi, Robin E. Huebner and Donna M. Paulnock

Department of Medical Microbiology
University of Wisconsin Medical School
1300 University Avenue
Madison, WI 53706

INTRODUCTION

The main point of this presentation will be to describe the immunosuppressive events that accompany acquired protective immunity to *Chlamydia psittaci* in the mouse. As a prelude to the presentation and discussion of the experimental data, it is important to understand some aspects of the biology of chlamydiae, the diseases that these organisms cause and what is already known concerning immune responses to chlamydiae.

A. Biology of Chlamydia

Chlamydia comprise a genus of procaryotes that are obligate intracellular microbes. These organisms replicate only within the confines of a membrane-bound vesicle in the cytoplasm of susceptible eucaryotic host cells. In addition to their obligate intracellular requirements, chlamydiae also undergo a unique cycle of cellular differentiation that involves the orderly alternation of two distinct developmental forms. One form is termed the elementary body (EB), and the other is called the reticulate body (RB), and the process of cellular differentiation in chlamydiae is called the developmental cycle. EB and RB can be distinguished from each other morphologically and functionally (Table 1). EB are small (0.2 µm diameter) rigid cells, suited for transitory existence between host cells. They are metabolically inert, but are adapted for attachment and uptake into susceptible host cells. The uptake process is mediated by adhesins on the EB surface that initiate attachment to host cell surface glycoproteins. It is significant that once uptake has been completed, the chlamydiae-containing endocytic vesicle does not fuse with host cell lysosomes. Thus, chlamydiae are not subjected to the battery of degradative enzymes that normally results from the phagocytic process.

Once uptake has been completed, differentiation of EB to RB occurs. This process may take several hours to complete, and it is not known how it is triggered, although reduction of disulfide-linked surface proteins is thought to be involved. Once RB have been formed, the replicative phase of chlamydial development begins. RB replicate by binary fission, and multiple rounds of replication occur within the cytoplasmic vesicle (inclusion). This process can continue for one, two, or even three days, depending on the specific chlamydial strain and host cell involved. Eventually an intracellular chlamydial microcolony is formed. The numbers of chlamydiae can increase from a single infectious EB per host cell to a thousand or more per intracellular inclusion. At a point when the chlamydial inclusion nearly fills the entire cytoplasmic space of the infected host cell, a second round of chlamydial differentiation begins. At this time, each metabolically active RB differentiates back to an infectious EB. It is at this point in the developmental cycle that infectious progeny can be detected. Soon after RB to EB differentiation has been completed, host cell lysis occurs and a new population of EB is released. The cycle of intracellular chlamydial development as described here is idealized to the version seen under carefully controlled laboratory conditions in cell culture systems. There is, however, good evidence that a substantively similar set of events occurs during actual chlamydial infections. In the natural setting, chlamydiae infect either mucosal epithelial cells or mononuclear phagocytes depending on the chlamydial strain and the type of infection.

B. Diseases caused by Chlamydia

Diseases caused by Chlamydia have been described in human populations since the beginning of recorded history. Accurate descriptions of trachoma, a potentially blinding, chronic chlamydial infection of the conjunctiva are found in early Chinese and Egyptian writings. Major cities in the Mideast, such as Bagdad, Damascus, and Babylon were constructed with streets called straights and these led to the cities of the blind. These cities within cities, with their high-walled straight-avenue entrance roads, were necessary to provide space for the thousands of people who were blinded each year due to trachoma. But trachoma is not just a disease of antiquity. Even today, trachoma remains the premier cause of preventable blindness in the world.

TABLE 1. Distinguishing characteristics of chlamydial developmental forms [a]

Characteristic	Elementary Body (EB)	Reticulate Body (RB)
size	200-400 nm	600-1,000 nm
rigid cell wall	+	-
RNA to DNA ratio	less than 1	3-4
infective	+	-
induce endocytosis	+	-
inhibit lysosome fusion	+	-
directly toxic to host cells (in large numbers)	+	-
metabolic activity	-	+
cell division	-	+

[a] Adapted from Moulder[1]

Trachoma, although clearly a significant world-wide health problem, is not a direct threat for people who live in industrialized countries; but other human chlamydial diseases are epidemic in the developed world. Genital chlamydial infections currently exhibit the highest incidence of sexually transmitted diseases in both Europe and the United States. Chlamydial urethritis in men occurs approximately twice as frequently as gonorrhea and chlamydial cervicitis in women is at least as common as gonococcal cervicitis. The major complications associated with chlamydial genital infections are similar to those seen with gonococcal genital infections. Spread by direct extension from the cervix to the uterus and fallopian tubes can lead to tubal damage and female infertility. Chlamydial salpingitis (inflammation of the fallopian tube) is more insidious than gonococcal pelvic inflammatory disease, but can be even more sinister in nature. Often no symptoms initially manifest, but tubal damage none-the-less occurs and therefore infertility problems can arise without the infected individual or the clinician being aware of any on-going infectious process. An additional major complication of chlamydial genital infections is the risk of the neonate acquiring *Chlamydia* from an infected mother at parturition. Most frequently ocular (conjuncivitis) and pulmonary (pneumonitis) diseases result in the neonate, but other manifestations of systemic chlamydial infection such as myocarditis are possible.

Other, less frequently encountered chlamydial diseases also affect humans. A second sexually transmitted disease called lymphogranuloma venereum is caused by a distinct biovar of *C. trachomatis*. This disease differs from other chlamydial genital infections in that there is an initial lesion at the site of infection and lymph node involvement is prominent. Arthritis seen as part of the triad of diseases (arthritis, urethritis and conjunctivitis) and termed Reiters syndrome can have a chlamydial etiology. In addition to diseases caused by *C. trachomatis*, the other species of *Chlamydia*, *C. psittaci*, also can cause disease in humans. Ornithosis, a systemic disease acquired via the respiratory route by inhalation of infected material

TABLE 2. Spectrum of Chlamydial infections

Agent	Disease	Complications
C. psittaci		
many avian strains	ornithosis	endocarditis life-threatening if not treated
TWAR strain	Interstitial (atypical) pneumonia	increased susceptibility to other pulmonary diseases
C. trachomatis		
A, B, Ba, C serovars	trachoma	blindness with repeated infections
L_1, L_2, L_3 serovars	lymphogranuloma venereum (LGV)	sterility reported
D, E, F, G, H, I, J K serovars	urethritis cervicitis	epididymitis, proctitis endometritis, salpingitis (PID)
	neonatal conjunctivitis pneumonitis	Failure to thrive

from various avian reservoirs, is a serious, but fortunately infrequent, zoonotic disease. Human to human transmission of an apparently unique C. psittaci biovar (TWAR) has been implicated as a cause of interstitial (atypical) pnemonia. If the rather limited serologic studies that have thus far been reported concerning TWAR are more broadly confirmed[2,3], it may be that C. psittaci is responsible for a significant number of atypical pneumonias. The salient features of human chlamydial diseases are summarized in Table 2.

More detailed accounts of Chlamydia and chlamydial diseases may be found in a variety of recent reviews, compendia and published symposia. Several of these are listed in the reference section[4-10].

C. Immune Responses to Chlamydia

Given the importance of chlamydial diseases, it is surprising that little is understood concerning the immune response to the chlamydiae. This is in part due to the difficulty in establishing relevant animal models, but also because relevant immune responses may be subtle and overlooked in the face of dramatic but irrelevant responses. In addition, multiple serovars are recognized for C. trachomatis, and although C. psittaci has not been systematically serotyped, probably multiple serovars exist for the latter species also. Thus, if protective immunity is associated with recovery from any chlamydial infection, it may be serovar or even sub-serovar specific so that reinfections with distinct serovars are possible.

A variety of immune responses are augmented during active chlamydial infection, but there is no compelling evidence to suggest that long-lived protection from reinfection is a component of responses resulting from naturally occurring chlamydial diseases. On the contrary, demonstrable immune responses to chlamydiae are frequently associated with adverse effects. For example, tissue damage associated with chronic ocular chlamydial infections exhibits a strong immunopathologic component[11]. Similarly, tubal damage that may accompany either frank or sub-clinical chlamydial salpingitis is more a result of the host's response to the presence of chlamydiae than to direct effects of the multiplication of organisms or the production of toxic products at the infected site.

Despite the apparent lack of protective immunity during natural chlamydial infections, it is possible to demonstrate protective immunity under certain experimental circumstances. Evidence is also accumulating to indicate that responses directed against specific polypeptide components of the chlamydial outer envelope may be requisite for protective immunity, at least for some chlamydial infectons[12].

II. MURINE MODEL OF PROTECTIVE IMMUNITY OF CHLAMYDIA PSITTACI

When considering any animal model of chlamydial infections, it is important to know if the experimental model is applicable to actual chlamydial diseases. The murine model described here is not intended to mimic modes of transmission of chlamydiae and damage that results at the site of actual chlamydial infection (i.e. mucosal surfaces or the lung). Our model was developed to determine it if is possible to establish protective immunity against an easily demonstrable chlamydial disease. In this respect it serves as a model for all chlamydial infections. Variations of the basic system probably can be developed to evaluate strain differences and compare protection against challenge at a variety of sites. This, however, was not our initial intent.

A. Immunization of Mice and Protection from Lethal Challenge

During the past several years a murine model for protective immunity to chlamydiae has been developed and studied. The system involves first immunizing inbred mice (several strains have been used) intramuscularly (IM) with a very low dose (about 10^2) of viable C. psittaci, strain 6BC. Beginning at 1 week post immunization, animals acquire the capacity to survive an otherwise lethal high dose (10^6 viable EB) intraperitoneal (IP) challenge with the homologous strain. We have not examined if these animals survive challenge to other C. psittaci strains or to C. trachomatis. Immunization with 6BC does not, however, protect against challenge by the unrelated bacterium, Listeria monocytogenes.

The nature of the cellular infiltrate to IP challenge also has been investigated. When mock-immunized animals are challenged and the cellular exudate examined at various times after challenge, a slow influx of polymorphonuclear leukocytes (PMN) is observed over the course of 3 or 4 days until the animals die from the challenge dose. Mononuclear phagocytes recovered from mock-immunized animals are filled with developing chlamydiae. Histologic observations indicate that the chlamydiae become systemic, causing lesions in other organs. In contrast, the post-challenge inflammatory exudate recovered from immunized animals exhibits different cellular influx kinetics and the population of cells recruited into the peritoneal cavity is distinct from the normal inflammatory exudate population. In the immune animal, a PMN response occurs rapidly (by 4 hours) and is cleared rapidly, often by 8-12 hours and always by 24 hours. Chlamydial inclusions are not observed in mononuclear phagocytes and when these cells are plated and infected in vitro with C. psittaci, they do not support growth. This is similar to, but not analogous with, in vitro activation of mononuclear phagocytes by gamma interferon. Thus, the initial response of immunized animals to the homologous chlamydial strain is markedly different than the response that occurs in unimmunized animals. These aspects of early events in the immune response to chlamydiae are summarized in Table 3.

TABLE 3. Early responses to intraperitoneal chlamydial infection in immunized and unimmunized mice

Parameter	Response in Unimmunized	Response in Immunized
Survive IP infection	No	Yes
Resist challenge by L. Monocytogenes	No	No
Splenomegaly	No	Marked
PMN influx	Slow	Rapid
Mononuclear Phagocytes	Support chlamydial growth in vivo and in vitro	Do not support chlamydial growth in vivo or in vitro
Gross Pathology	Systemic infection uncontrolled	Systemic infection resolved with cellular response

B. Measurement of Immune Responses by Immunized Mice

To confirm that protected animals responded in ways other than the development of a heightened inflammatory exudate to IP chlamydial challenge, splenocytes from immunized animals were tested for their proliferative responses to chlamydial antigens. As a control for these experiments, responses to the mitogen concanavalin A (Con A) also were tested. It was found that once animals acquired protective immunity, suppression of lymphocyte proliferative responses also occurred. A similar finding had been noted by Lammert and Wyrick[13]. These authors ascribed the observed suppression to the presence of suppressive components of the chlamydial cell or products directly elaborated by the chlamydiae. In contrast to the earlier report, we found that the development of suppression was clearly associated with a cellular component and linked to the development of protective immunity. Transfer of suppression was effected when spleen cells from immune animals were irradiated and added to normal splenocytes. The degree of suppression was dependent on the ratio of irradiated immune cells to normal cells. It was significant that the development of immunosuppression accompanied the onset of protective immunity. The observed suppression was transient. Responses that were suppressed 10 days after immunization returned to normal by 30 days post immunization. Protection from IP challenge is not a transient phenomenon. Once rendered immune, mice maintain their ability to survive IP challenge for 100 days or longer. A specific suppressive sub-population has not as yet been identified, but hints regarding the characteristics of these cells are beginning to emerge. Suppression was abolished when spleen cells from immune animals were treated with L-leucyl leucine methyl ester. This compound has demonstrable toxicity for cells after it enters the lysosome compartment[14]. Initially it was thought to be specific for mononuclear phagocytes, but it is now believed that other pinocytically active cells, such as cytotoxic T cells also are affected by it[15].

In addition to suppression of blastogenic responses, evidence for *in vivo* suppression also was observed. Animals immunized against chlamydiae were injected IP with sheep red blood cells (SRBC). When antibody secreting cells were quantitated by a plaque assay against SRBC, the number of splenic plaque forming cells was dramatically reduced as compared to plaque forming cells recovered from mock-immunized, SRBC-injected, mice.

Thus, the immunosuppression was not restricted to either the humoral or cellular arm of the immune response, and was a general rather than an antigen-specific phenomenon. To gain some insight concerning the immune mechanisms that prevailed in immunosuppressed mice, experiments were carried out to determine if spleen cells from immunized animals secreted lymphokines. Previous work had provided data to show the induction of lymphokines contributed to the intracellular control of chlamydial growth *in vitro*[16], and that gamma interferon was the effector lymphokine in spleen cell preparations[17]. It was of interest, therefore, to determine if spleen cells from immunosuppressed mice could be induced to produce lymphokines that were active in the control of chlamydial replication. It was found that spleen cells from immune mice that suppressed lymphocyte proliferative responses, produced antichlamydial lymphokines by mitogen induction. Thus, the soluble mediator compartment of the immune response remained intact in these otherwise

TABLE 4. Immune Responses of C3H Mice before and after Immunization Against C. psittaci

Parameter	Pre-immune Response	Response 10 d Post-Immunization	Response 30 d Post-Immunization
Con A blastogenesis	+	-	+
LPS blastogenesis	+	-	+
antigen blastogenesis	-	-	+
inhibit control Con A proliferation	-	+	-
inhibit control LPS proliferation	-	+	-
PFCs to SRBC	+	-	Not done
lymphokine production	+	+ +	Not done

+ means intact response, - means suppressed response, + + means augmented response.

suppressed animals. Data related to the measurement of immune responses in immunized mice are summarized in Table 4.

III. DISCUSSION AND CONCLUSIONS

Immunosuppression is a key element in the pathogenesis for a number of human pathogens. Suppressive events are well described for viral[18,19] bacterial[20-25], protozoan[26-28], and trematode[29] infections. Clearly, deciphering the complex of disease and suppressive events in AIDS[18] has resulted in renewed interest in pathogen-mediated suppression of immunity[22,24,28]. Immunosuppression generally falls into two broad catagories. Either the suppression is restricted to the infectious agent that caused depressed immunity[28-30] (antigen specific suppression) or it is manifest as a general suppression of responsiveness[21-23]. Systems also have been described where components elaborated by or directly associated with the pathogen are suppressive[31-33]. In addition, suppression has been associated with the induction of a suppressor cell. Suppressor lymphocytes, suppressive mononuclear phagocytes[20,23,27], and interactions between subpopulations of different cell types resulting in suppression[34] all have been described.

Despite the diversity of observed suppressor mechanisms for various pathogens, a common feature between most pathogen-associated immunosuppressive events is that induction of suppression correlates with increased pathogen virulence and thus is perceived as a fitness trait that contributes to the pathogenesis of disease. The system that has been described here for the induction of immunosuppression by C. psittaci in the mouse contrasts with the notion of suppression as a contributing factor to pathogenesis of the disease process. We found that measurements of immunosuppression accompanied the development of protective immunity. We have not as yet resolved if suppressive and protective aspects of the immune response are causally related or whether they are simultaneous independent events occurring in response to a live chlamydial inoculum. Results of this study suggest that great care should be given to the interpretation of in vitro immunosuppression resulting from an ongoing infectious process. In this context, it is important to note what the overall status of the infected individual is before relating immunosuppression to impaired *in vivo* protective immunity.

IV. SUMMARY

Mice immunized intramuscularly with a low dose, viable inoculum of *C. psittaci* survived an otherwise lethal intraperitoneal challenge with the homologous chlamydial strain. Immunized animals were not protected from intraperitoneal challenge by the unrelated pathogen, *Listeria monocytogenes*. Spleen cells from animals that exhibited protective immunity were suppressed in their proliferative responses to mitogens or chlamydial antigen in an *in vitro* blastogenic assay. This suppression was transferrable to normal spleen cells by adding irradiated cells from immunized animals to normal cell populations. The degree of normal cell blastogenic suppression was dependent on the ratio of irradiated immune to normal cells present in the assay medium. Suppression of humoral responses was demonstrated *in vivo*. Immunized animals were incapable of producing antibody secreting cells to sheep red blood cells after an intraperitoneal inoculation of SRBC. Unimmunized animals produced a significant number of plaque forming cells as measured by a direct plaque forming cell assay. Lymphokine activity was not impaired in spleen cells from mice that exhibited other manifestations of suppression. Taken together, these data provide evidence to indicate that the induction of suppression may not correlate with increased pathogenesis, but rather be closely associated with protective immunity. Data also provide circumstantial evidence to indicate that lymphokine induction may be important in the development of protective immunity to *C. psittaci* in the mouse.

V. ACKNOWLEDGMENTS

This work was supported by grant number Al-19782 from the National Institutes of Health. We thank Sherideen Stoll for her help in preparing the manuscript.

VI. REFERENCES

1. J.W. Moulder, A model for studying the biology of parasitism, *Chlamydia psittaci*, and mouse fibroblasts (L cells), *BioScience* *58*:875 (1969).
2. P. Saikku, S.-P. Wang, M. Kleemola, E. Brander, E. Rusaneu, and J.T. Grayston, An epidemic of mild pneumonia to an unusual strain of *Chlamydia psittaci*, *J. Infect. Dis.* *151*:832 (1985).
3. J.T. Grayston, C.-C. Kuo, S.-P. Wang, and J. Altman., A new *Chlamydia psittaci* strain, TWAR, isolated in acute respiratory tract infections, *N. Engl. J. Med.* *315*:161 (1986).
4. J. Schachter, and H.D. Caldwell, Chlamydiae, *Ann. Rev. Microbiol.* *34*:285 (1980).
5. P.-A. Mardh, K.K. Holmes, J.D. Oriel, P. Piot, and J. Schachter (ed.), "Chlamydial Infections," Proceedings of the 5th International Symposium on Human Chlamydial Infections, Elsevier Biomedical Press, New York (1982).
6. S. Darouger (ed.), Chlamydial Disease, *in*: "British Medical Bulletin," Churchill Livingstone Inc., New York (1983).

7. J.W. Moulder, Looking at Chlamydiae without looking at their hosts, ASM News 50:353 (1984).
8. S. Ladany, and I. Sarov, Recent advances in Chlamydia trachomatis, Eur. J. Epidemiol. 1:235 (1985).
9. D. Oriel, G. Ridgway, J. Schachter, D. Taylor-Robinson, and M. Ward (ed.), "Chlamydial infections," Proceedings of the 6th International Symposium on Human Chlamydial Infections, Cambridge University Press, New York (1986).
10. P. Reeve, (ed.), "Chlamydial Infections," Springer-Verlag, Heidelberg (1987).
11. J. Schachter, Immunity, in: "Chlamydial Infections," P. Reeve (ed.), Springer-Verlag, Heidelburg (1987).
12. R.C. Brunham, I. MacLean, J. McDowell, R. Peeling, K. Persson, and S. Osser, Chlamydia trachomatis antigen specific serum antibodies among women who did and did not develop acute salpingitis following therapeutic abortion, in: "Chlamydial Infections," Oriel et. al. (ed.), Cambridge University Press, New York (1986).
13. J.K. Lammert, and P.B. Wyrick, Modulation of the host immune response as a result of Chlamydia psittaci infection, Infect. Immun. 35:537 (1982).
14. D.L. Thiele, M. Kurosaka, and P.E. Lipsky, Phenotype of the accessory cell necessary for mitogen-stimulated T and B cell responses in human peripheral blood: delineation by its sensitivity to the lysosomotropic agent L-Leucine methyl ester, J. Immunol. 131:2282 (1983).
15. D.L. Thiele, P.E. Lipsky, The immunosuppressive activity of L-Leucyl-L-Leucine methyl ester: selective ablation of cytotoxin lymphocytes and monocytes, J Immunol. 136:1038 (1986).
16. G.I. Byrne, and C.L. Faubion, Lymphokine-mediated microbistatic mechanisms restrict Chlamydia psittaci growth in macrophages, J Immunol. 128:469-474.
17. G.I. Byrne, and D.A. Krueger, Lymphokine-mediated inhibition of Chlamydia replication in mouse fibroblasts is neutralized by anti-gamma interferon immunoglobulin, Infect. Immun. 42:1152 (1983).
18. I.J. Selikoff, A.S. Teirstein, and S.Z. Hirschman (ed.), "Acquired Immune Deficiency Syndrome," Ann. NY Acad. Sci. 437 (1984).
19. C.G. Orosz, N.E. Zinn, R.G. Olsen, and L.E. Mathes, Retrovirus mediated immunosuppression II. Felv-uv alters in vitro murine T lymphocyte behavior by reversibly impairing lymphokine secretion, J. Immunol. 135:583 (1985).
20. H. Kirchner, H.T. Holden, and R.B. Herberman, Splenic suppressor macrophages induced in mice by injection of Corynebacterium parvum, J Immunol. 120:1709 (1978).
21. W.E. Bullock, E.M. Carlson, and R.K. Gershon, The evolution of immunosuppressive cell populations in experimental mycobacterial infection, J. Immunol. 120:1709 (1978).
22. F.M. Collins, and S.R. Watson, Suppressor T cells in BCG-infected mice, Infect. Immun. 25:491-496 (1979).
23. T.R. Jerrells, Immunosuppression associated with the development of chronic infections with Rickettsia tsutsugamushi adherent suppressor cell activity and macrophage activation, Infect. Immun. 50:175 (1985).
24. R.L. Modlin, V. Mehrs, L. Wong, Y. Fugimiya, W.-C. Chang, D.A. Horwitz, B.R. Bloom, T.H. Rea, and P.K. Pattengale, Suppressor T lymphocyte from lepromatous leprosy skin lesions, J. Immunol. 137:2831 (1986).

25. R. Turcotte, D. LeGault, Mechanisms underlying the depressed production of interleukin-2 in spleen and lymph node cell cultures of mice infected with Mycobacterium bovis BCG, Infect. Immun. 51:826 (1986).
26. S.R. Wellhausen, and J.M. Mansfield, Characteristics of the splenic suppressor cell-target cell interactions in experimental African trypanosomiasis, Cell Immunol. 54:414 (1980).
27. E.A. Peterson, F.A. Neva, C.N. Oster, and H.B. Diaz, Specific inhibition of lymphocytes-proliferation responses by adherent suppressor cells in diffuse cutaneous leishmaniosis, N. Engl. J. Med. 306:387 (1982).
28. A.D. Nickol, and P.F. Bonventre, Visceral leishmaniosis in congenic mice of susceptible and resistant phenotypes: T-lymphocyte-mediated immunosuppression, Infect. Immun. 50:169 (1985).
29. C.W. Todd, R.W. Goodgame, and D.G. Colley, Immune responses during human schistosomiosis mansoni. V. Suppression of schistosome antigen-specific lymphocyte blastogenesis by adherent/phagocyte cells, J. Immunol. 122:1440 (1979).
30. A. Haregewoin, T. Godal, A.S. Mustafa, A. Belehu, and T. Yemaneberhan, T-cell conditioned media reverse T-cell unresponsiveness in lepromatous leprosy, Nature 303:342 (1983).
31. U. Persson, Lipopolysaccharide-induced suppression of the primary immune response to a thymus-dependent antigen, J. Immunol. 118:789 (1977).
32. P.S. Holt, and M.L. Misfeldt, Alteration of murine immune response by Pseudomonas aeruginosa exotoxin A, Infect. Immun. 45:227 (1984).
33. V. Mehra, P.J. Brennan, E. Rada, J. Convit, and B.R. Bloom, Lymphocyte suppression in leprosy induced by unique M. leprae glycolipid, Nature 308:194 (1984).
34. J.D. Stobo, Immunosuppression in man: suppression by macrophages can be mediated by interactions with regulatory T cells, J. Immunol. 119:918 (1977).

PARADOXES OF IMMUNITY AND IMMUNOSUPPRESSION IN SALMONELLA INFECTION

Toby K. Eisenstein, Niloofer Dalal, Loran Killar,
Joo-Chiang Lee, and Rosana Schafer

Department of Microbiology and Immunology
Temple University School of Medicine
Philadelphia, Pa.

INTRODUCTION

There is continuing interest in mechanisms of immunity to systemic Salmonella infection, as concepts regarding the relative contributions of humoral and cellular immunity to host defense against these organisms form the theoretical basis for development of improved vaccines against typhoid fever (1,2). (Experimentally, investigations are carried out using a mouse model of systemic infection with Salmonella typhimurium, as S. typhi is not virulent for mice.) Although the current typhoid vaccine, consisting of acetone-killed cells, has been shown to be protective in humans (3), it has an undesirable level of toxicity (1). Recent efforts have focused on live, attenuated strains of S. typhi which can be given orally, as an alternative vaccine strategy. A galE mutant, Ty21a, has been shown to have efficacy in a field trial in Egypt (4), although results have been less promising in field trials in Chile (5). One drawback of the Ty21a strain is that the exact nature of the genetic lesions which confer loss of virulence are not known (6). Stocker and colleagues have developed a series of mutants in various species of Salmonella which are blocked in aromatic synthesis due to transposon-mediated gene deletions or inversions (7,8). Based on high levels of protection induced in mouse models of typhoid fever using these aroA$^-$ strains of S. typhimurium, Stocker has developed attenuated S. typhi with similar types of lesions for potential use in humans against typhoid fever (9). In addition, there is also considerable interest in using these aro$^-$ strains as vectors for cloned genes of other organisms such as E. coli enterotoxins (10,11).

Our laboratory has carried out extensive investigations into the mechanisms of protection induced by one of the aroA$^-$ strains, designated SL3235. We have shown that this strain induces very high levels of protection against challenge with virulent Salmonella (12), but that protection is accompanied by a profound immunosuppression of splenic mitogenic responses (13), and of the in vivo and in vitro plaque-forming cell (PFC) responses to sheep red blood cells (SRBC). The paradox of protection in the face of parameters of immunosuppression will be considered from a theoretical and practical standpoint.

MATERIALS AND METHODS

Mice. C3HeB/FeJ and C3H/HeJ mice were purchased from Jackson Laboratories. C3H/HeNCrlBR mice were obtained from Charles River Breeding Laboratories. The characteristics of the mouse strains are shown in Table 1.

Table 1. Characteristics of Mouse Strains

Strain	LPS Responsiveness	Salmonella Susceptibility	Macrophage Activation[a]
C3H/HeJ	Defective	Hypersusceptible $LD_{50} < 7$ cells	Defective
C3HeB/FeJ	Normal	Hypersusceptible $LD_{50} < 2$ cells	Normal
C3H/HeNCrlBR	Normal	Resistant $LD_{50} = 10^3$	Normal

[a]See ref. 25.

Organisms. S. typhimurium, SL3235, is a smooth (0;4,12), attenuated strain, blocked in synthesis of aromatic compounds by a lesion in the aroA gene (7). The LD_{50} of this strain is greater than 10^7 cells by the ip route. The virulent strain is W118-2, which has an LD_{50} of less than 10 cells ip (14).

Mitogenicity assay. Responses to Con A and LPS were assayed in 96-well plates with 8×10^5 spleen cells in 200 µl of RPMI 1640 per well with 20 µl of mitogen or medium added. All variables were tested in triplicate and results expressed as mean counts per minute (12,15).

Macrophage enrichment. Macrophages were purified from spleens by fibronectin adherence using flasks coated with gelatin and human plasma according to the method of Freundlich and Avdalovic (16,17).

Macrophage depletion. Macrophages were depleted from spleen cell suspensions by two rounds of plastic adherence and passage over Sephadex G-10 as described by Ly and Mishell (18).

Plaque-forming cell assays. In vivo plaque-forming cells (PFCs) were enumerated by the Cunningham slide modification of the Jerne plaque technique carried out on dissociated spleen cells (19). In vitro generation of PFCs was carried out using Mishell-Dutton cultures (20). All variables were tested in triplicate.

Macrophage-mediated tumor cytotoxicity assay. P815 mastocytoma cells, labeled with ^{51}Cr, were incubated in 96-well plates for 16 hr with unelicited peritoneal macrophages from normal or immune mice, at various effector to target ratios ranging from 12.1:1 to 100:1. Chromium release in quadruplicate cultures was quantitated as % specific ^{51}Cr release = [(experimental release - spontaneous release)/(total releasable counts - spontaneous release)] 100.

RESULTS

Protection with SL3235. The high levels of protection engendered by live SL3235 in all three mouse strains are shown in Table 2. In contrast, acetone-killed cells were not protective in the Salmonella-hypersusceptible C3H/HeJ and C3HeB/FeJ mice, but could protect the more resistant C3H/HeNCrlBR strain (21). Acetone-killed cells did result in significant prolongation of median time to death in the hypersusceptible strains (21). The live SL3235 also induced transient cross-protection against *Listeria monocytogenes* that was strong at 21 days, waning at 28 days, and not detectable 12 weeks post-immunization (Table 3). In contrast, the protection against virulent *Salmonella* challenge was still strong 7 months post-immunization (Table 3). The loss of cross-protection to *Listeria* waned with elimination of the SL3235 from the spleen (Fig. 1).

Spleen cell transfers. To ascertain whether the high level of protection induced by SL3235 was mediated by T-cells, spleen cell transfers from SL3235-immunized C3H/HeJ mice into naive HeJ recipients were carried out. Unfractionated spleen cell suspensions taken 1 week after SL3235 administration were able to transfer protection, with 5/6 mice surviving a challenge dose of 40 cells. However, similar unfractionated suspensions taken from donors 2, 3, 4 or 12 weeks post-immunization, did not confer protection at comparable or lower challenge doses, even though the donors were highly immune (no survivors, data not shown). Fractionation of 1-week immune spleen cells showed that removal of plastic adherent cells decreased ability to transfer protection, and nylon wool nonadherent cells, which were enriched for T-cells, were nonprotective (Table 4). However, a population of fibronectin-adherent cells from 1-week spleen cells was found to transfer protection (Table 5). The protective cells represent a macrophage-enriched population (70% as judged by latex bead ingestion). Thus, macrophage-enriched, but not T-cell-enriched immune cells were able to transfer Salmonella immunity to C3H/HeJ mice.

Macrophage-mediated tumor cytotoxicity. The results presented above provided evidence for macrophage activation as an important effector mechanism for the immunity induced by live SL3235. To further test the extent of macrophage activation, peritoneal cells of SL3235-immunized mice were assayed for activation as judged by tumoricidal capacity. Seven to 10 days post-SL3235 inoculation, activated macrophages cytotoxic for P815 mastocytoma cells were found (Fig. 2). Acetone-killed cells could activate C3HeB/FeJ macrophages to be fully cytotoxic, but could only prime cells of C3H/HeJ mice to respond to LPS or γ-interferon in vitro before exhibiting cytotoxicity (not shown).

Salmonella-induced suppression. Spleen cells from mice receiving SL3235 were tested for capacity to respond to lipopolysaccharide (LPS) of Salmonella and *Escherichia coli*, as well as to other B- and T-cell mitogens, to see if immune C3H/HeJ animals were converted to responsiveness to phenol-water-extracted LPS. It was found that the responses of all three mouse strains to all mitogens tested were profoundly suppressed, that the suppression was maximal at 7 days post-SL3235 (Fig. 3), and that in C3H/HeJ mice, removal of macrophages could restore mitogenic responsiveness to *E. coli* LPS, and partially restore responsiveness to Salmonella LPS (Fig. 4). Removal of T- or B-cells by anti-Thy 1.2 or $F(ab')_2$ anti-IgG did not restore responsiveness (13). Thus, suppression appeared to be mediated by macrophages.

Table 2. Protection of Mice of the C3H Lineage by live or acetone-killed *S. typhimurium* SL3235

	60-day Survival (survivors/total)										
	C3H/HeJ mice				C3HeB/FeJ mice			C3H/HeNCrlBR mice			
	Challenge doses (cells)[c]										
Treatment	6	90	900	9000	120	1200	12,000	2.3×10^4	1×10^5	1×10^6	1×10^7
Live SL3235[a]	-	11/12	11/12	8/11	12/12	11/12	12/12	-	6/6	6/6	0/6
Saline	0/14	0/12	-	-	0/12	0/10	-	1/9	0/6	-	-
Acetone-killed SL3235[b]	5/14	-	-	-	-	3/10	-	10/10	-	-	-

[a]C3H/HeJ mice were immunized ip with 5×10^4 live, avirulent *S. typhimurium* SL3235 21 days before challenge. C3HeB/FeJ and C3H/HeNCrlBR mice received 7×10^4 organisms.

[b]Mice received two doses of 60 µg of acetone-killed cells ip (6×10^7 organisms) given 14 days apart, and were challenged 21 days later.

[c]Mice were challenged ip with virulent *S. typhimurium*, strain W118-2.

(Data on C3H/HeJ and C3HeB/FeJ mice using live SL3235 reprinted with permission of the *Journal of Immunology*. See ref. 12.)

Table 3. Long-Term Protection of C3H/HeJ Mice by SL3235 Against S. typhimurium and L. monocytogenes Challenges

Immunization[a]	Time of challenge[b]	S. typhimurium challenge[c]		L. monocytogenes challenge[d]	
		$LD_{50}s$	Survivors/ total	$LD_{50}s$	Survivors/ total
SL3235	4 weeks	870	5/6	98.0	3/6[e]
		87	6/6	9.8	3/6[e]
Saline		87	0/6	9.8	0/6
SL3235	12 weeks	1,000	6/6	100	0/6
		100	5/6	10	0/6
Saline		100	0/6	10	0/6
SL3235	28 weeks	2,000	4/6	ND[f]	ND
		200	6/6	ND	ND
Saline		200	0/6	ND	ND

[a]Mice were immunized ip with 7.5×10^4 live S. typhimurium strain SL3235 cells suspended in 0.5 ml saline or with saline alone as a control.
[b]Time after immunization.
[c]Mice were challenged ip with S. typhimurium strain W118-2 cells suspended in 0.5 ml of saline (1 LD_{50} is 1 cell). Survival was scored for 60 days.
[d]Mice were challenged ip with L. monocytogenes cells suspended in 0.5 ml of saline (1 LD_{50} is 6×10^3 cells). Survival was scored for 60 days.
[e]Not significant.
[f]ND, not done.

FIG. 1. Colonization of C3H/HeJ (●) and C3H/HeNCrlBR (o) spleens after infection with 5×10^5 S. typhimurium strain SL3235 cells. X, Infecting dose.

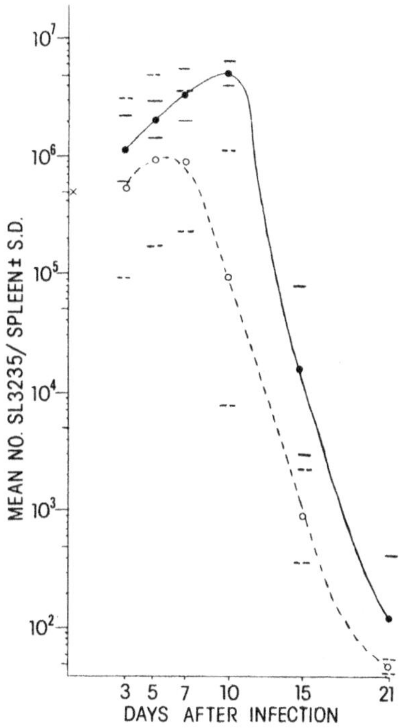

(Table 3 and Fig. 1 reprinted with permission from The American Society for Microbiology. See ref. 16.)

Table 4. Transfer of Protection to C3H/HeJ Mice Against *Salmonella* Challenge by Cells From Nylon Wool Fractions

Fraction[a]	Mitogenicity (Δcpm ± SD) Phytohemagglutinin	Trichloroacetic acid-lipopolysaccharide	Survivors/total[b]
Nonfractionated	45,377 ± 6,089	16,469 ± 5,257	7/8[c]
Plastic nonadherent	ND[d]	ND	4/8
Nylon wool nonadherent	130,670 ± 29,624	8,241 ± 426	0/8
Nylon wool adherent	7,578 ± 2,056	24,992 ± 1,333	0/8
Control	ND	ND	2/8

[a]A sample (2×10^7 cells) of each cell fraction in 1 ml of RPMI-1640 was injected i.p. Controls received 1×10^6 SL3235 cells in 1 ml of RPMI-1640.
[b]At 24 h after injection, mice were challenged with 22 LD_{50}s of virulent *S. typhimurium* strain W118-2.
[c]Significantly different from the control group ($P < 0.05$).
[d]ND, not done.

(By permission of The American Society for Microbiology. See ref. 16.)

Table 5. Transfer of Protection to C3H/HeJ Mice With Spleen Cell Populations Enriched for Macrophages

Fraction[a,b]	Total no. of cells transferred[c]	% Macrophages[d]	No. of macrophages transferred	Survivors/total[e]
Nonfractionated	2×10^7	30	6.0×10^6	6/6[f]
	1×10^7		3.0×10^6	4/6[f]
	5×10^6		1.5×10^6	2/6
Nonadherent	2×10^7	14	2.8×10^6	1/6
	1×10^7		1.4×10^6	1/6
	5×10^6		7.0×10^5	1/6
Adherent	2×10^7	68	1.4×10^7	6/6[f]
	1×10^7		7.0×10^6	3/6
	5×10^6		3.5×10^6	3/6
Control	None			0/7

[a]Donors were immunized i.p. with 1.8×10^6 SL3235 cells 1 week before challenge.
[b]Cells were fractionated by incubating on gelatin- and plasma-coated plates.
[c]Cells were suspended in 1 ml of RPMI-1640 and injected i.p. Controls were injected with RPMI-1640 only.
[d]Percentage of cells that ingested greater than 10 latex particles.
[e]Recipients were challenged i.p. 24 h after cell transfer with virulent *S. typhimurium* strain W118-2. Mice were challenged with 25 LD_{50}s.
[f]Statistically significant from controls ($P < 0.05$).

(By permission of The American Society for Microbiology. See ref. 16.)

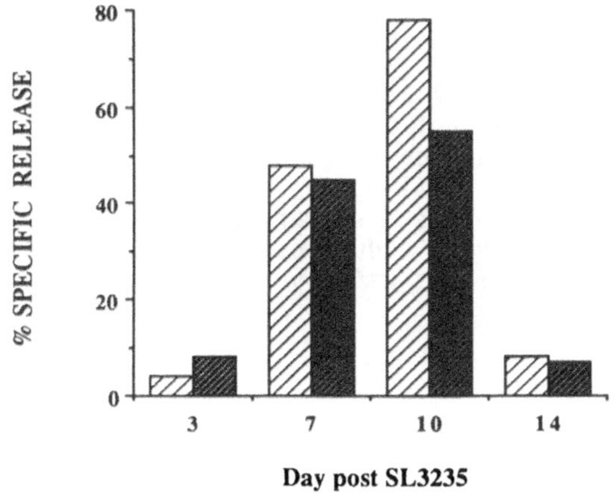

FIG. 2. Kinetics of tumor cytotoxicity of macrophages from SL3235-immunized mice. Peritoneal cells from C3HeB/FeJ (▨) or C3H/HeJ (▩) mice immunized with 5 x 10^5 SL3235 were harvested at 3, 7, 10, or 14 days post-injection, and the adherent peritoneal cells were incubated with ^{51}Cr-prelabeled P815 mastocytoma cells. Cytotoxicity was estimated by measuring ^{51}Cr release at 16 h and expressed as percent specific release.

(Reprinted with permission of Journal of Immunology. Schafer et al. 140:1638, 1988.)

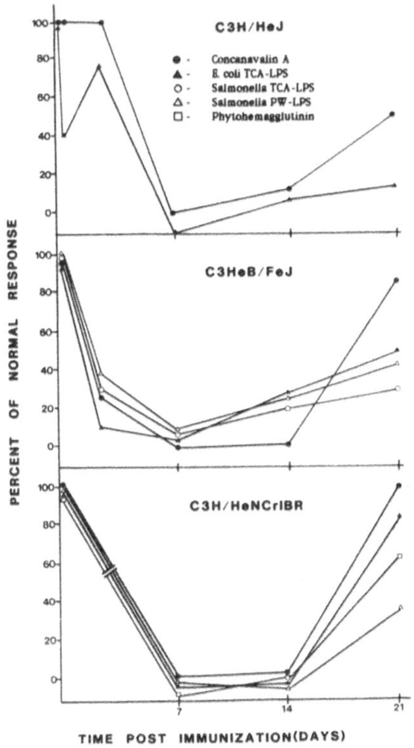

FIG. 3. Mitogenic suppression in spleen cells of C3H/HeJ, C3HeB/FeJ, and C3H/HeNCrlBR mice at various times after infection with SL3235.

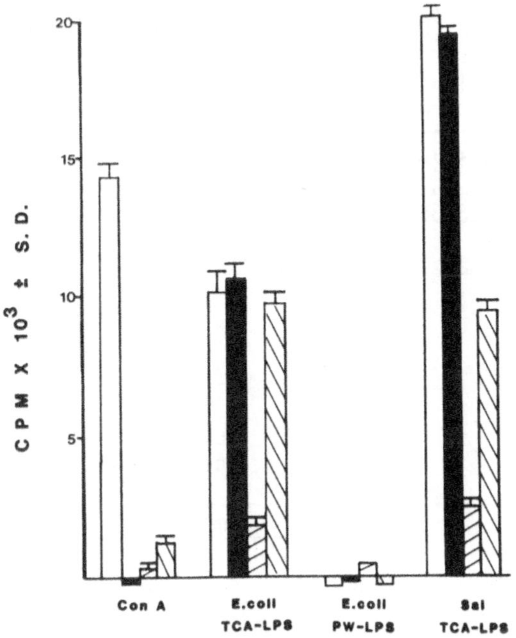

FIG. 4. Mitogenic response of unseparated and macrophage-depleted spleen cells from normal and SL3235-immune C3H/HeJ mice at 2 weeks post-infection. Spleen cells from normal mice (□); macrophage-depleted spleen cells from normal mice (■); spleen cells from SL3235-infected mice (///); macrophage-depleted spleen cells from SL3235-immune mice (\\\).

(Figs. 3 and 4 reprinted by permission of Cellular Immunology. See ref. 13.)

Suppression of the plaque-forming cell response to sheep red blood cells. C3HeB/FeJ mice given SL3235 showed a marked suppression of their in vivo PFC responses to SRBC given 7 days post-SL3235, the time of maximal mitogenic suppression (Table 6). The hemagglutinating titer in serum was similarly reduced in suppressed mice (data not shown). When in vitro immunization was carried out using Mishell-Dutton cultures, the response of cells taken from SL3235-infected mice was also markedly suppressed. Depletion of macrophages from immune cells resulted in partial restoration of the PFC responses in co-culture experiments using various ratios of normal and immune spleen cells (Table 7).

DISCUSSION

It is evident that live, attenuated Salmonella, strain SL3235, is able to confer superior protection on Salmonella-hypersusceptible mice, as compared with acetone-killed cells. Based on the cross-protection studies with Listeria, and analysis of the bacterial numbers in spleen with time after immunization, the mechanisms of immunity fit the classical picture of cellular immunity, first described by Mackaness, in which a primary infection with one intracellular pathogen engenders transient cross-protection to another such pathogen due to a state of temporary macrophage activation induced by the primary infection (22). However, the model would predict that immunized mice would develop sensitized T-cells to Salmonella which could be demonstrated by adoptive transfer studies, as has been done for Mycobacteria and Listeria (23,24). In the model using the C3H/HeJ mice, we were unable to demonstrate a population of splenic lymphocytes which would transfer protection. Transfer was, however, demonstrated with a fibronectin-adherent cell fraction, obtained 1 week after SL3235 administration, and enriched for splenic macrophages. Peritoneal macrophages taken one week to 10 days after SL3235 injection were also shown to be tumoricidal and Leishmaniacidal (latter data not shown). Thus, by a variety of indirect and direct assays, live SL3235 was found to be able to induce activated macrophages, even in the C3H/HeJ strain of mice which have a genetically determined defect in macrophage activation (25).

Table 6. Suppression of the In Vivo PFC Response of C3HeB/FeJ Mice by SL3235

Group	Treatment		PFC/spleen[c]	% Suppression
	SL3235[a] (day 0)	SRBC[b] (day 7)		
A	-	-	200	-
B	+	-	150	-
C	-	+	195,460	-
D	+	+	10,528	95

[a]Mice received $2x10^5$ SL3235 ip in 0.5 ml saline. Controls received saline alone.
[b]Mice received $5x10^8$ SRBC ip in 0.2 ml of saline on day +7 with respect to day of infection. Controls received saline alone.
[c]PFC determined 4 days post-antigen (SRBC or saline).

Table 7. Effect of Macrophage Depletion of SL3235-Infected Spleen Cells on the In Vitro Primary PFC Response to SRBC

Group		Treatment: SL3235[a] (in vivo)	Treatment: SRBC[b] (in vitro)	PFC/culture[c] (mean ± S.D.)	Suppression index[d]
Background		-	-	15 ± 7	
Saline		-	+	1,147 ± 472	
Infected control		+	-	26 ± 20	
Infected		+	+	126 ± 70	0.11
Cocultures					
%I[e]	%N[e]				
10	90	+	+	2,153 ± 273	1.88
25	75	+	+	1,070 ± 214	0.93
50	50	+	+	243 ± 6	0.21
Coculture control					
50	50	+	-	13 ± 13	
G-10 depletion of SL3235-infected spleen cells					
Infected, G-10-depleted (I*)[f]		+	+	383 ± 76	0.33
Cocultures					
%I*	%N				
10	90	+	+	2,780 ± 433	2.42
25	75	+	+	3,467 ± 1,419	3.02
50	50	+	+	3,389 ± 105	2.92
Coculture control					
50	50	+	-	27 ± 12	

[a]Mice received $2.2x10^5$ SL3235 ip in 0.5 ml of saline. Controls received saline alone.
[b]Spleen cells were cultured with 0.05 ml of a 0.1% SRBC suspension. Control cultures received 0.05 ml of tissue culture medium.
[c]PFC were determined on the fifth day of the Mishell-Dutton culture.
[d]Suppression index = PFC of culture/PFC of saline group.
[e]I = infected spleen cells (SL3235 injected); N = normal spleen cells (saline injected).
[f]I* = Sephadex G-10-depleted spleen cells from SL3235-immunized mice.

Spleen cells of mice taken 7 days post-SL3235 injection, were found to be highly suppressed in their responses to a panel of B- and T-cell mitogens, and in their plaque-forming cell responses to sheep red blood cells. Suppression of both responses was significantly alleviated by removal of G-10-adherent cells, presumed to be macrophages.

Taken together, these results present a paradox, in that SL3235-immunized mice demonstrate very high levels of protection against Salmonella infection, and substantial, although transient, protection against Listeria infection, while exhibiting parameters of profound immunosuppression, with both phenomena apparently being at least partially mediated by macrophages. Other investigators working with different intracellular pathogens have also observed macrophage-mediated immunosuppression, but in general, they have been using sublethal doses of virulent organisms, and have interpreted the immunosuppression as an adverse effect that the pathogen induces on the host (26-28). We have a unique system in that the live Salmonella are actually a vaccine strain, which allowed us to show that protection against virulent challenge, and suppression, can coexist in the immunized animal.

Major unanswered questions posed by these observations are: 1) Are the suppressive macrophages and the effector macrophages the same population of cells? 2) Teleologically, what is the meaning of the suppression? 3) Why could we not find a population of sensitized T-cells that would transfer protection, even though the long-term protection engendered by the vaccine against Salmonella infection suggests such a population must exist? and 4) Why are live cells so superior to killed cells in inducing protection in hypersusceptible mice?

In regard to the first question, no definitive answer is yet available. The cell transfer experiments were carried out with fibronectin-adherent spleen cells and the tumor cytotoxicity was measured on peritoneal cells. Evidence which suggests that they may represent two separate populations is obtained from the observation (data was not shown) that fibronectin-adherent spleen cells taken from immunized mice were not tumoricidal in the P815 mastocytoma assay. However, peritoneal macrophages, which are tumoricidal, have not been tested for their capacity to transfer protection. Dissection of the cell populations mediating the different biological phenomena may be complex, as shown in studies using the macrophage-activating agent, C. parvum, which also induces suppressor cells in the spleen (29,30).

If macrophage activation and protection coexist with suppression, it suggests that suppression may not be an adverse effect that the microbe induces in the host, but possibly a reflection of a strong immunomodulatory process which is characteristic of the host response to intracellular pathogens that parasitize macrophages. The suppression may be a marker for macrophage-mediated orchestration of the immune system, to channel host defenses against the invader. The mechanism of the suppression has not been determined, but the mitogenic suppression is not indomethacin inhibitable (13).

The failure to find T-cells in SL3235-immunized mice that would confer adoptive immunity is in accord with a paucity of reports in the literature in this regard for Salmonella, in spite of an extensive literature documenting successful transfers for other intracellular pathogens. Hochadel and Keller transferred B- and T-cell fractions from immune mice and found that the B-cell fraction from lymph nodes, but not the T-cell fraction from the thymus, was protective (31). A recent report claims that T-cells transfer immunity when given in high numbers, but none of the mice survived, and mean time to death was only marginally prolonged (32). There is one laboratory that has reported successful transfer of anti-Salmonella immunity with spleen cell "transfer factor" (33) and T-cell lines derived from peritoneal cells (34). In our studies, we did obtain some evidence for T-cells in peritoneal exudate cells of mice 1 to 3 months after SL3235 immunization, in that nylon-wool nonadherent cells responded with tritiated thymidine incorporation to acetone-killed cells and to a preparation of endotoxin-protein, but not to LPS (16). Why such T-cells were not detected in spleen cells in transfer experiments is speculative. Perhaps the T-rich population in the first few weeks of the infection contained a mixture of suppressor and effector cells, so that the suppressor cells neutralized the effector functions. Spleen cells taken after 21 days may have had low numbers of Salmonella-sensitized T-cells as the organisms were being cleared from the circulation at that time. Alternatively, sensitized T-cells may not be sufficient for host defense. The mechanism of immunity to Salmonella in the hypersusceptible mice is not mediated by humoral antibody, because hyperimmune serum raised to acetone-killed cells was unable to protect C3H/HeJ mice, and was only marginally protective for C3HeB/FeJ mice, although it was protective in the resistant C3H/HeNCrlBR mice (21). Further, serum taken from C3H/HeJ mice which had received live SL3235, and which themselves were so highly resistant to virulent challenge, was unable to transfer protection to naive C3H/HeJ mice (16).

Finally, the question must be addressed as to the differences in mechanisms between live and acetone-killed Salmonella in inducing immunity to virulent challenge. From studies of the growth kinetics of challenge organisms in mice vaccinated with live versus nonviable preparations, it has been appreciated for over 20 years that there are fundamental differences in the type of host response induced by the viable as compared with dead organisms (35,36). In the studies presented here, we have shown that acetone-killed cells differ from live cells in their capacity to activate macrophages of C3H/HeJ and C3HeB/FeJ mice, with live cells bringing macrophages of both strains to full tumoricidal capacity, but acetone-killed cells only able to prime the HeJ macrophages. If the ultimate effector cell against Salmonella is the macrophage, one would have expected that macrophage activation would be sufficient to induce resistance. However, the hypersusceptible mice were not protected by the killed preparation against challenge doses of 100 virulent cells, while the live organisms protected against 10,000 LD_{50} doses. The results suggest either that macrophage activation alone is not sufficient, or that the state of macrophage activation induced by the live and killed Salmonella, which appears to be identical as assessed by tumoricidal activity, is not really the same, i.e., the live cells may actually induce an even higher state of activation but the tumoricidal assay sees only the lower threshold. It would be interesting to see if macrophages activated by acetone-killed cells can transfer anti-Salmonella immunity. Following the first line of reasoning, it may be that the activated macrophages are sufficient to prolong the mean time to death, but that ultimately T-cells are needed, and the acetone-killed cells, for reasons unknown, are unable to induce a T-cell immunity, but the live cells have this capacity. It is interesting, however, that we were unable to detect a delayed-type hypersensivity (DTH) reaction in live SL3235-immunized C3H/HeJ or C3HeB/FeJ mice to a Salmonella supernatant elicitin, even though they were so highly protected (37,38). The elicitin was shown to be active in giving foot-pad responses in SL3235-immunized inherently Salmonella-resistant mouse strains (37). Thus, we seem to be engendering protection in the hypersusceptible strains without the obvious markers of cellular immunity: a positive DTH reaction to Salmonella antigens and a population of T-cells from immunized animals which can transfer immunity. Whether the sensitized T-cells are there and are difficult to find, or whether they are not necessary for host defense against this infection is yet to be determined.

CONCLUSIONS

These studies show that an attenuated strain of Salmonella confers superior levels of protection against challenge with virulent Salmonella. The vaccine strain also induces a profound immunosuppression of mitogenic responses of spleen cells and of in vivo and in vitro plaque-forming cell responses to sheep red blood cells. Macrophages seem to be significant mediators of the suppression. The vaccine also induces activated macrophages as shown by the tumoricidal activity of peritoneal macrophages taken from mice receiving the attenuated Salmonella, and by the capacity of a spleen cell population enriched for macrophages to transfer protection to virulent Salmonella challenge. The relationship between suppressor and effector macrophages in immunity to Salmonella infection remains to be investigated.

ACKNOWLEDGMENTS

This work was supported by Public Health Service grant AI15613 from the National Institutes of Health.

REFERENCES

1. Edelman, R., and M. M. Levine, Summary of an international workshop on typhoid fever, Rev. Inf. Dis. 8:329 (1986).
2. Eisenstein, T. K., and B. M. Sultzer, Immunity to Salmonella infection, in: "Host Defenses to Intracellular Pathogens," T. K. Eisenstein, P. Actor, and H. Friedman, eds., Plenum, New York (1983).
3. Ashcroft, M. T, A seven year field trial of two typhoid vaccines in Guyana, Lancet 2:1056 (1967).
4. Wahdan, M. H., C. Sérié, Y. Cerisier, S. Sallam and R. Germanier, A controlled field trial of live Salmonella typhi strain Ty 21a oral vaccine against typhoid: three-year results, J. Inf. Dis. 145:292 (1982).
5. Levine, M. M., R. E. Black, C. Ferreccio, M. L. Clements, C. Lanata, J. Rooney, and Chilean Typhoid Committee, The efficacy of attenuated Salmonella typhi oral vaccine strain Ty21a evaluated in controlled field trials, in: "Proceedings of the Nobel Conference on Recent Advances in Vaccines and Drugs against Diarrhoeal Diseases, Stockholm, 3-6 June 1985," J. Holmgren, A. Lindberg and R. Mollby, eds., Student Literatur, Gothenburg, Sweden (1986).
6. Silva, B. A., C. Gonzalez, G. C. Mora and F. Cabello, Genetic characteristics of the Salmonella typhi strain Ty21a vaccine, J. Inf. Dis. 155:1077 (1987).
7. Hoiseth, S. K., and B. A. D. Stocker, Aromatic-dependent Salmonella typhimurium are non-virulent and effective as live vaccines, Nature 291:238 (1981).
8. Smith, B. P., M. Reina-Guerra, B. A. D. Stocker, S. K. Hoiseth and E. Johnson, Aromatic-dependent Salmonella dublin as a parenteral modified live vaccine for calves, Am. J. Vet. Res. 45:2231 (1984).
9. Levine, M. M., D. Herrington, J. R. Murphy, J. G. Morris, G. Losonsky, B. Tall, A. A. Lindberg, S. Svenson, S. Baqar, M. F. Edwards and B. Stocker, Safety, infectivity immunogenicity, and in vivo stability of two attenuated auxotrophic mutant strains of Salmonella typhi, J. Clin. Invest. 79:888 (1987).
10. Clements, J. D., F. L. Lyon, K. L. Lowe, A. L. Farrand and S. El-Morshidy, Oral immunization of mice with attenuated Salmonella enteritidis containing a recombinant plasmid which codes for production of the B subunit of heat-labile Escherichia coli enterotoxin, Infect. Immun. 53:685 (1986).
11. Maskell, D., F. Y. Liew, K. Sweeney, G. Dougan and C. E. Hormaeche, Attenuated Salmonella typhimurium as live oral vaccines and carriers for delivering antigens to the secretory immune system, in: "Vaccines 86," R. A. Lerner, R. Channock and F. Brown, eds., Cold Spring Harbor Laboratory, Cold Spring Harbor, N.Y. (1986).
12. Eisenstein, T. K., L. M. Killar, B. A. D. Stocker and B. M. Sultzer, Cellular immunity induced by avirulent Salmonella in LPS-defective C3H/HeJ mice, J. Immunol. 133:958 (1984).
13. Lee, J-C., C. W. Gibson and T. K. Eisenstein, Macrophage-mediated mitogenic suppression induced in mice of the C3H lineage by a vaccine strain of Salmonella typhimurium, Cell. Immunol. 91:75 (1985).
14. Angerman, C. R., and T. K. Eisenstein, Comparative efficacy and toxicity of a ribosomal vaccine, acetone-killed cells, lipopolysaccharide, and a live cell vaccine prepared from Salmonella typhimurium, Infect. Immun. 19:575 (1978).
15. Eisenstein, T. K., L. W. Deakins, L. Killar, P. H. Saluk and B. M. Sultzer, Dissociation of innate susceptibility to Salmonella infection and endotoxin responsiveness in C3HeB/FeJ mice and other strains in the C3H lineage, Infect. Immun. 36:696 (1982).

16. Killar, L. M., and T. K. Eisenstein, Immunity to Salmonella typhimurium infection in C3H/HeJ and C3H/HeNCrlBR mice: studies with an aromatic-dependent live S. typhimurium strain as a vaccine, Infect. Immun. 47:605 (1985).
17. Freundlich, B., and N. Avdalovic, Use of gelatin/plasma coated flasks for isolating human peripheral blood monocytes, J. Immunol. Methods 62:31 (1983).
18. Ly, I. A., and R. I. Mishell, Separation of mouse spleen cells by passage through columns of Sephadex G-10, J. Immunol. Methods 5:239 (1974).
19. Cunningham, A. J., and A. Szenberg, Further improvements in the plaque technique for detecting single antibody-forming cells, Immunology 14:599 (1968).
20. Mishell, R. I., and R. W. Dutton, Immunization of dissociated spleen cell cultures from normal mice, J. Exp. Med. 126:423 (1967).
21. Eisenstein, T. K., L. M. Killar and B. M. Sultzer, Immunity to infection with Salmonella typhimurium: mouse-strain differences in vaccine- and serum-mediated protection, J. Inf. Dis. 150:425 (1984).
22. Mackaness, G. B., The immunological basis of acquired cellular resistance, J. Exp. Med. 120:105 (1964).
23. Orme, I. M., and F. M. Collins, Adoptive protection of the Mycobacterium tuberculosis-infected lung. Dissociation between cells that passively transfer protective immunity and those that transfer delayed-type hypersensitivity to tuberculin, Cell. Immunol. 84:113 (1984).
24. Mackaness, G. B., and W. C. Hill, The effect of anti-lymphocyte globulin on cell-mediated resistance to infection, J. Exp. Med. 129:993 (1969).
25. Ruco, L. P., and M. S. Meltzer, Defective tumoricidal capacity of macrophages from C3H/HeJ mice. J. Immunol. 120:329 (1978).
26. Wellhausen, S. R., and J. M. Mansfield, Characteristics of splenic suppressor cell-target-cell interaction in experimental Africal Trypanosomiasis, Cell. Immunol. 54:414 (1980).
27. Suzuki, Y., N. Watanaba and A. Kobayashi, Nonspecific suppression of primary antibody responses and the presence of plastic adherent suppressor cells in Toxoplasma gondii-infected mice, Infect. Immun. 34:30 (1981).
28. Tarleton, R. L., R. Schafer and R. E. Kuhn, Effects of extracts of Trypanosoma cruzi on immune responses: induction of a nonspecific suppressor factors, Infect. Immun. 41:978 (1983).
29. Shibata, Y., and A. Volkman, The effect of bone marrow depletion on prostaglandin E-producing suppressor macrophages in mouse spleen, J. Immunol. 135:3897 (1985).
30. Shibata, Y., and A. Volkman, The effect of hemopoietic microenvironment on splenic suppressor macrophages in congenitally anemic mice of genotype Sl/Sl^d, J. Immunol. 135:3905 (1985).
31. Hochadel, J. F., and K. F. Keller, Protective effects of passively transferred immune T- or B-lymphocytes in mice infected with Salmonella typhimurium, J. Inf. Dis. 135:813 (1977).
32. Chander, R., K. B. Sainis and N. F. Lewis, Role of thymus-derived lymphocytes in acquired immunity to salmonellosis in mice, Microbiol. Immunol. 30:1299 (1986).
33. Smith, R. A., A. Esa and M. Stiff, Transfer of Salmonella resistance and delayed hypersensitivity with murine-derived transfer factor, Infect. Immun. 36:271 (1982).
34. Paul, C., K. Shalala, R. Warren and R. Smith, Adoptive transfer of murine host protection to salmonellosis with T-cell growth factor-dependent, Salmonella-specific T-cell lines, Infect. Immun. 48:40 (1985).
35. Ushiba, D., Two types of immunity in experimental typhoid; "cellular immunity" and "humoral immunity," Keio J. Med. 14:45 (1965).

36. Blanden, R. V., G. B. Mackaness and F. M. Collins, Mechanisms of acquired resistance in mouse typhoid, J. Exp. Med. 124:585 (1966).

37. Killar, L. M., and T. K. Eisenstein, Differences in delayed-type hypersensitivity responses in various mouse strains in the C3H lineage infected with Salmonella typhimurium, strain SL3235, J. Immunol. 133:1190 (1984).

38. Killar, L. M., and T. K. Eisenstein, Delayed-type hypersensitivity and immunity to Salmonella typhimurium, Infect. Immun. 52:504 (1986).

INDUCTION OF IMMUNOSUPPRESSIVE B-LYMPHOCYTES WITH COMPONENTS OF CANDIDA ALBICANS

Christopher F. Cuff, Beryl Packer, Victor Rivas, Christina M. Rogers, Antonio Cassone, Raymond Donnelly, and Thomas J. Rogers

Department of Microbiology and Immunology, Temple University School of Medicine, Philadelphia, PA 19140 and Laboratory of Bacteriology and Medical Mycology Instituto Superiore di Sanita, Rome, Italy

INTRODUCTION

Infections with Candida albicans are associated with a depressed immune response. The immunological profile present during candidiasis is extremely complex. Certain individuals with a congenital defect in the development of a normal cellular immune system are frequently the subject of clinical Candida disease involving mucocutaneous tissues (reviewed in 1). On the other hand, disseminated candidiasis is frequently encountered in individuals suffering with polymorphonuclear leukocyte function such as chronic granulomatous disease, myeloperoxidase deficiency, or Chediak-Higashi Syndrome (2,3,4). Individuals who manifest both mucocutaneous and disseminated forms of candidiasis are rare. The mode of resistance against these two forms of candidiasis presents a paradox since immune mechanisms effective in the first case apparently do not operate in the other.

The immune status of individuals with chronic mucocutaneous candidiasis (CMC) is itself quite heterogeneous. These individuals exhibit a range of immunodeficiencies which may be either antigen (Candida)-specific, or non-specific (5). The immunological profile may include a failure to manifest normal delayed-type hypersensitivity (DTH) responses to antigens from Candida, as well as certain dermatophytes, mumps virus, or Streptococci. There may also be a failure to exhibit a positive contact sensitivity response to agents such as dinitrochlorobenzene sulfonic acid. In vitro cellular responses in these individuals may also be depressed. This may include a failure to mount a normal lymphocyte transformation response to Candida antigen specifically, or to various T-cell mitogens. In addition, the generation of the lymphokine macrophage migration inhibitory factor may also be depressed. Finally, some individuals with CMC may not exhibit any apparent immunological impairment whatsoever.

These suppressed cellular responses are occasionally in contrast to antibody levels in CMC patients. These patients frequently manifest elevated immunoglobulin levels in general, as well as increased levels of antibody specific for Candida. Moreover, the Candidiasis Endocrinopathy syndrome is occasionally associated with autoimmune antibody, suggesting the presence of inadequate (or at least altered) immunoregulatory function. On the other hand, depressed specific antibody levels in CMC have been documented as well.

The association of CMC with certain congenital defects in the cellular immune response is an obvious example of disease resulting from infection by an opportunistic microbe in a compromised host. It should be pointed out, however, that both clinical and experimental evidence suggests that infection with *Candida* may be responsible for (or at least contribute to) the immunosuppressed status of the host (6-8). This evidence includes data which show that immunological responses may return to normal following anti-fungal antibiotic therapy and clinical clearance of the infectious agent (6).

EXPERIMENTAL ANIMAL STUDIES

Experimental Infection

A variety of reports have suggested that infection with *Candida* results in a diminished immune response. Reports from a number of investigators have suggested that experimental animals infected with *C. albicans* manifest a reduced capacity to resist infection by a variety of bacteria (9-11, and reviewed in 1). Additional results have also shown that DTH responses (12), as well as antibody responses to T-dependent (but not T-independent) antigens (13), are suppressed following infection with *C. albicans*.

This laboratory has been involved for some time in studies of the immunosuppressive activity of *C. albicans*. We have shown that lymphocytes from mice intravenously infected with *Candida* exhibit a transient decline in the ability to respond to T-cell-, but not B-cell-, specific mitogens. The ability of these mice to develop a response to PPD, after vaccination with *Mycobacterium bovis* strain BCG, is also impaired. Finally, mice infected with *C. albicans* also manifest a transient decline in the ability to respond *in vitro* to *Candida* antigens (14).

Induction of Suppressor Cells

The suppression induced by *C. albicans* is due, at least in part, to the induction of suppressor cells by a component(s) of the organism. Lymphocytes from animals injected with non-viable *Candida* fail to manifest a normal response to Phytohemagglutinin (PHA) or Concanavalin A (Con A), while the response to LPS remains normal (15)(Figure 1). The presence of suppressor cells in the *Candida*-primed population was revealed by performing co-culture experiments. Results show that co-cultures consisting of *Candida*-primed cells together with normal cells fail to respond to either PHA or Con A (15). Again, co-cultures containing *Candida*-primed cells manifest a normal response to LPS (Packer, B.;C.F. Cuff, and T.J. Rogers, manuscript in preparation).

We have recently extended these studies and we have found that suppressor cells may be induced by simply culturing lymphoid cells with non-viable *Candida in vitro* (16). Co-cultures containing cells primed with *Candida in vitro* also inhibit both the proliferative response of normal cells to PHA, as well as the antibody response to the T-dependent antigen TNP-sheep erythrocytes (TNP-SRBC). The results show that co-cultures

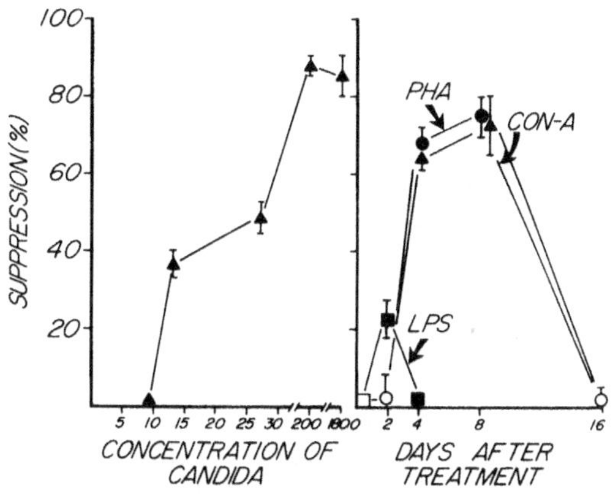

Figure 1A. Dose-response curve for formalin-killed Candida treated mice. Mice were injected i.v. with various doses of Candida and sacrificed 4 days later. The splenocytes were cultured with PHA (2ug/ml). The average PHA response of normal cells was 76,434 CPM. Figure 1B. Mice were sacrificed at various time intervals after treatment with Candida (12ug). Cells were incubated with optimal doses of PHA, LPS and Con A(Reprinted with permission from the Journal of Immunology.)

containg 10% Candida-primed cells exhibit a significantly reduced response to the TNP-SRBC (as assessed by measuring both the accumulation of specific antibody, as well as the number of antibody-producing B-cells).

Characterization of the Suppressor Cell Population

Experiments to characterize the nature of suppressor cell induced by Candida have shown that the inhibitory activity is due primarily to the generation of a lymphocyte population which is apparently a member of the B-cell lineage. The activity of the suppressor cell population is not sensitive to treatment with monoclonal anti-Thy 1 antibody, yet the suppressor cell population is inactivated by treatment with monoclonal anti-Lyb 2 antibody (Figure 2). The suppressor cell population adheres specifically to plastic dishes coated with anti-Ig, but does not adhere to dishes coated with monoclonal anti-Mac 1 (a macrophage-granulocyte marker) antibody (15,16). Furthermore, the suppressor cell is not depleted by passage through Sephadex G-10 (16). These characteristics are possessed by cells primed either in vitro or in vivo.

Our characterization of these suppressor cells has recently been extended to an analysis of the susceptibility of these cells to the monoclonal antibody J11D (17). This antibody recognizes a marker on erythrocytes, neutrophils, 80-90% of B-cells, and >90% of immature T-cells. This marker is apparently absent on mature T-cells. Contrary to what might be expected, experiments with this monoclonal antibody have shown that the Candida-primed suppressor cell is J11D-negative (Table 1). It has been suggested that the J11D marker may be associated with resting B-cells (17,18). The failure to express the marker is transient (17), and

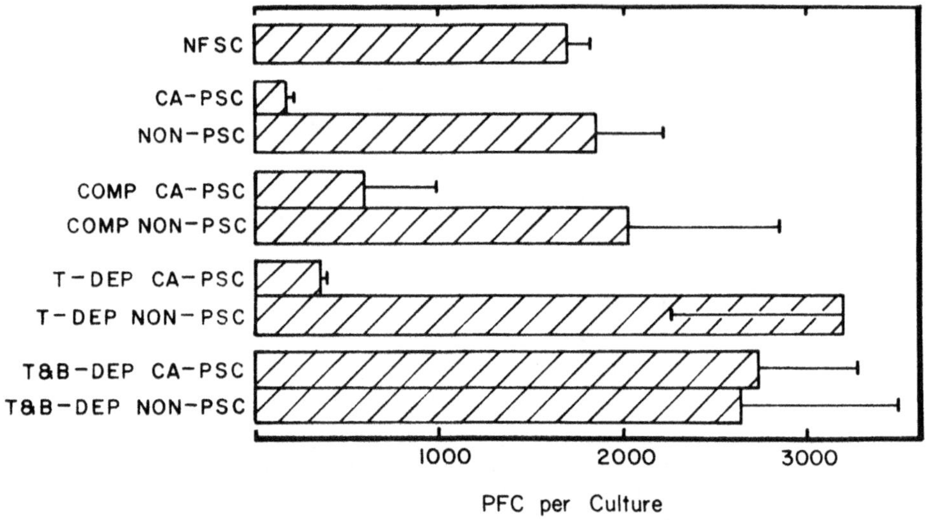

Figure 2. Depletion of suppressor cell activity with anti-Lyb 2. Suppressor cells were generated *in vitro*. Both CA-PSC and NON-PSC were treated with either anti-Thy 1 (T-DEP) or a combination of anti-Thy 1 and anti-Lyb 2 (TB-DEP). Co-cultures consisted of 10% CA-PSC or NON-PSC. (Reprinted with permission from *Cellular Immunology*)

Table 1. *Candida*-Primed Suppressor B-Cells Do Not Exhibit the J11D Cell Surface Marker.

Group	Mean PFC/Culture	%Suppression
100% Normal	9700	--
10% CA-PSC	3080	68
10% NON-PSC	9380	3
10% J11D-dep CA-PSC	4333	55
10% J11D-dep NON-PSC	9266	4

Cells were primed *in vitro* with *Candida* and co-cultured with normal cells in a Mishell-Dutton assay. The antibody response was measured on day 5. Cells were depleted with monoclonal antibody J11D.

these results suggest that the suppressor cell population is member of a sub-population of activated B-lymphocytes.

We have carried out a series of experiments in collaboration with Dr. James Kenny (National Cancer Institute) with C.CBA/N mice which carry the X-linked immunodeficiency gene (*xid*). These mice appear to lack or exhibit a defect in the Lyb 5 B-cell lineage (19). Our results show that splenocytes from the *xid* mice manifest suppressive activity following priming with *Candida*. These results suggest that Lyb 5-negative cells are capable of developing suppressive activity following priming. It is not clear at this time whether Lyb 5-positive cells in normal mice are also capable of manifesting suppressive activity. The answers to this question must await the availability of highly specific anti-Lyb 5 antibody.

Until recently, we have been unable to demonstrate the presence of any suppressor T-cell activity in the Candida-primed population. This is somewhat surprising given the results obtained by others with various Candida-derived products (20-22). We have recently obtained some evidence that suppressor T-cell activity may exist within our Candida-primed cultures. When the primed cells are added on day 0 of a 5-day Mishell-Dutton culture assay, little or no detectable suppressive activity is observed in the T-cell component (16). At the same time, the primed B-cell populations manifest significant suppressive activity. On the other hand, if primed cells are added late in an ongoing Mishell-Dutton culture (i.e. day 3 of a 5 day assay), the primed T-cell component exhibits suppressive activity, while the primed B-cell component does not. These data suggest that early events in the antibody response are susceptible to the action of the primed B-cells, while late events are susceptible to the action of the suppressor T-cell.

Cellular Requirements for the Development of Suppressor B-Cells

We have analyzed the requirements for both T-cells and macrophages in the development of suppressor B-cell activity. First, we have found that cultures depleted of T-cells with monoclonal anti-Thy 1 prior to priming with Candida are unable to develop suppressive activity. These results suggest that T-cells are required for the induction of suppressor B-cells. The Candida component(s) responsible for induction of suppressor cell activitation is therefore a T-dependent antigen.

We have also found that splenocyte cultures depleted of macrophages by passage over Sephadex G-10 are also unable to develop suppressive activity. As would be expected, the generation of suppressor B-cell activity is dependent on accessory cell function.

We have attempted to replace the requirement for T-cells in the priming cultures with supplementary exogenous interleukin 2 (IL-2). Splenocyte cultures were depleted of T-cells with anti-Thy 1, and exogenous IL-2 was added prior to priming with Candida. The results show that the IL-2-supplemented T-cell-depleted cultures fail to develop suppressive activity following priming. The source of IL-2 was a de-lectinated supernatant from rat splenocytes stimulated with Con A. The concentration of IL-2 in the supplemented cultures (about 1 unit) may not have been sufficient to compensate for the absence of T-cells in the priming cultures. In addition, the Con A supernatant may very well be lacking in a necessary "helper" factor which would permit the activation of the suppressor B-cell activity.

In an additional set of experiments we have carried out studies to assess the nature of the role of macrophages in the priming period. The results described above demonstrated a requirement for macrophages in the induction of suppressor B-cell activity. We attempted to determine whether the macrophage could be replaced by interleukin 1 (IL-1) in the priming cell cultures. Using supernatants from LPS-induced RAW 264 cells as a source of IL-1, we have found that this monokine alone is apparently not sufficient for the replacement of macrophages in the priming cultures. These results must be evaluated in light of the limitations discussed above for supplementary IL-2. However, the results suggest that the role of the macrophages in the priming cell cultures extends beyond the simple production of IL-1.

Target of the Suppressor B-Cell Activity

Our results up to this point have shown that the Candida-primed B-cells are capable of inhibiting both the antibody response to a T-cell-dependent antigen (SRBC), as well as the proliferative response to the

T-cell-dependent mitogens PHA and Con A. Given the apparent activity of the suppressor B-cells on T-cell function, we attempted to determine whether other T-cell functions were susceptible to the effects of the suppressor B-cells.

Our studies were first directed toward an analysis of the effect of the suppressor B-cells on the development of cytotoxic T-cell activity. The Candida-primed cells were co-cultured at the initiation of a mixed-lymphocyte culture consisting of normal splenocytes and irradiated allogeneic stimulator cells. The results showed that the development of cytotoxic T-cell activity was not inhibited by the Candida-primed cells. These results indicate that this population of T-cells was apparently insensitive to the effects of the suppressor B-cells.

We assessed the effect of the suppressor B-cells on the production of IL-2. Candida-primed cells were added at culture initiation to normal cells together with Con A and the production of IL-2 was assessed 48 hours later. The results show that the suppressor B-cells have no effect on the production of IL-2. We have also found that the production of IL-2 in mixed-lymphocyte cultures is not inhibited by the suppressor B-cells. Here again, the suppressor B-cells do not appear to act by inhibiting T-helper cell function. It should be pointed out, of course, that the production of other helper factors may be inhibited by the suppressor B-cells. Alternatively, it is possible that the existence of both susceptible and non-susceptible populations of T-helper cells would also be consistent with these results.

The results obtained with T-helper cells (at least as assessed by IL-2 production) are somewhat surprising in light of experiments conducted recently. Analysis of the suppressor B-cell activity shows that the antibody response to the T-independent antigens TNP-LPS and TNP-ficoll, unlike the response to T-dependent antigens, is not inhibited. It is now fairly well established that the antibody response to T-independent antigens is not entirely "T-independent." Differences in the T-cell function involved in the response to the T-dependent versus T-independent do exist, however (23). Nevertheless, our results suggest that the target cell in the suppression of antibody production is within the T-cell population.

In an attempt to take our results up to this time into account, we have proposed the following model to explain the suppression of the antibody response. Candida is capable of activating a population of B-cells which have suppressive activity. We propose, on the basis of purely preliminary data, that these B-cells suppress by producing antibody. This antibody acts on specific sub-populations of T-cells and inhibits the activity of these cells. A portion of the T-cell arm of the immune response escapes the activity of this antibody (e.g. T-cytotoxic cell activity and IL-2 producing T-helper cells). The function of these target T-cells is inhibited and this results in the reduced response to T-dependent antigens.

The generation of antibody specific for T-helper cells has been reported for a high percentage of chronic Candida vaginitis patients (24). This is consistent with the experimental studies just reviewed.

Nature of the Component which Induces Suppressor B-cells

The identification of components of the yeast which are responsible for altering immune responses has been the focus of a great deal of the work in our laboratory as well as the work of a variety of other investigators. There is clinical evidence to suggest that the immunosuppression which is observed in patients with chronic mucocutaneous candidiasis (CMC) is due at least in part to the presence of inhibitory factors in the serum of CMC patients (5,6). These factors can suppress the *in vitro* proliferative responses of human lymphocytes to *Candida* antigens. The factors appear to consist in part of mannan-containing polysaccharide *Candida* antigens, but in experimental systems, both mannan and non-mannan components of *Candida* have been shown to have immunosuppressive properties. Fischer and co-workers have characterized a suppressive component which was found in the serum of patients with CMC (25). This factor inhibited the proliferative response of normal lymphocytes to *Candida* antigens. The activity was characterized as non-dialysable, thermostable, and absorbable with Con A-coupled agarose columns. The factor was found in patients with normal responses to PPD or streptokinase, but negative skin test reactions to *Candida* antigens. Although most of these patients had measurable titers of anti-*Candida* antibody in their serum, lymphocytes from these patients uniformly failed to proliferate in response to *Candida* antigens *in vitro*. In addition, these investigators produced mannan-rich extracts of *C. albicans* which inhibited the proliferative responses of normal lymphocytes to *Candida* antigens. This group later reported that the specific cellular non-responsiveness to *Candida* antigens in patients with CMC was due to an intrinsic defect in the ability of patients' monocytes to process mannan-containing *Candida* antigens (26).

In studies by Piccolella and co-workers (20-22,27), polysaccharide fractions prepared from heat-killed *Candida* by ethanol precipitation were found to have a number of immunoregulatory effects on human lymphocytes. The preparation, labeled Mangion purified polysaccharide (MPPS) consisted mainly of glucan and mannan. In addition to being mitogenic for human lymphocytes, MPPS was also found to induce suppressor T-cells which could directly inhibit the proliferative response of fresh human lymphocytes to MPPS *in vitro*. The diversity of activities attributed to MPPS may be due to the heterogeneity of these preparations and the cell populations affected by MPPS.

Although mannans have been implicated as immunosuppressive components of *C. albicans*, other investigators have demonstrated the suppressive activity of non-mannan containing *Candida* components. A report by Carrow and Domer (28) indicates that the treatment of mice with mannan had no effect on the delayed-type hypersensitivity (DTH) responses to glycoprotein extracts or membrane derived antigens in mice previously immunized with viable *C. albicans*. In contrast, water soluble glycoprotein extracts of *Candida* cell walls did have immunomodulatory properties. This material (termed GP) was shown to inhibit the DTH response to GP in mice immmunized with viable *Candida* (28). The immunosuppressive component of this material appeared to be sensitive to papain and heat treatment, suggesting that it is a protein.

As part of our studies on *Candida*-induced immunoregulation, we have attempted to extract and identify components of *Candida* which exhibit the capacity to suppress the immune response. We have consistently observed that cell wall preparations possess the ability to induce suppressor B-cell activity. On the other hand, cell cytosol preparations exhibit highly variable activity in this regard.

Our attempts to determine the specific component of the cell wall responsible for the suppressor-inducer activity was directed toward mannan preparations. In our studies, mice treated with purified mannans failed to manifest normal antibody responses to the T-dependent antigen sheep erythrocytes (SRBC), yet the response to the T-independent antigen TNP-ficoll remained normal (Table 2). In these studies, the mannan treatment failed to induce active suppressor cells in that lymphocytes from mannan treated mice failed to suppress the antibody responses of normal

Table 2. *In vitro* Antibody Response of Splenocytes From *Candida*-Treated Mice

Group	Antibody response (PFC/culture)	
	anti-SRBC	anti-DNP-ficoll
Normal	1885	1321
Mannan-treated	445	1200
50% mannan-treated	1895	1545
25% mannan-treated	1825	2325

Mice were treated with 400 ug of mannan-enriched material. Splenocytes were obtained after sacrifice 8 days later. Some groups of treated splenocytes were co-cultured with normal splenocytes.

Table 3. Failure to Induce Suppressor Cells With Mannan.

Group	Response to PHA(2ug/ml)
Normal cells	105,668
Mannan-treated cells	87,770
25% Normal B-cells	52,808
25% Mannan-treated B-cells	55,265

Mice were primed with 400 ug of mannan.

Table 4. Suppressor cell induction with GMP.

Group	anti-SRBC antibody (PFC/culture)
Normal	1220
10% NON-PSC	1153
10% GMP-PSC	673
10% T-dep GMP-PSC	446
10% ALK-M-PSC	1006
10% T-dep ALK-M-PSC	1073

Cells were primed *in vitro* with either GMP or a hot-alkaline extract mannan preparation (ALK-M). Some groups were depleted with monoclonal anti-Thy 1.

cells in *in vitro* co-cultures. In contrast, cells taken from mice treated with formalin-killed *Candida* actively suppressed the anti-SRBC response of normal immune mice as well as the *in vitro* proliferative responses to the T-cell mitogens PHA and Con A (15). Cells from mice primed with mannan also failed to inhibit the proliferative response to PHA (Table 3).

We have found that a soluble glucan-mannan-containing glycoprotein extract of *Candida* cell walls termed GMP (29) did induce suppressor cell activity *in vitro* (Table 4). Hot alkali-extracted mannan failed to exhibit any activity in this regard. Normal spleen cells cultured with this extract could inhibit the anti-SRBC response of normal immmune mouse lymphocytes *in vitro* in Mishell-Dutton cultures.

More recently, we have successfully produced extracts of *Candida* cell walls which can induce suppressor cells *in vitro*. An ethylene diamine glycoprotein extract fom *Candida* cell walls has been found to be immunosuppressive. This material consists of approximately 3% protein and 97% carbohydrate by dry weight. The carbohydrate component has been analyzed by gas chromatography and has been found to consist of 73% glucose, 24% mannose, and 3% N-acetylglucosamine. In addition, western blot analysis shows that this material reacts with serum from a patient with CMC. The soluble glycoprotein extract can induce suppressor cells in a dose dependent manner, and appears to be non-toxic at effective doses. Although it is not yet known if the glycoprotein is inducing the same B-suppressor cell population found in cell populations which are primed with formalin-killed whole cell preparations, the suppressor cells induced by the extract are plastic non-adherent, and resistant to treatment with anti-Thy-1 antibody plus complement. The immunosuppressive component of the glycoprotein extract fails to bind to Con A-linked Sepharose columns indicating that the immunosuppresive component of this extract is not mannan. Because of the high carbohydrate content of this extract, further characterization of the protein component has been difficult.

A second procedure has also been used to extract cell wall components of *C. albicans*. Using procedures described by Jones and co-workers (30), we have extracted glycoproteins from *Candida* cell walls using the reducing agent dithiothreitol(DTT). This DTT also induces suppressor cells which inhibit the anti-SRBC response of normal immune spleen cells *in vitro*. The DTT extract consists of approximately 25% protein and 75% carbohydrate by dry weight. Interestingly, gas chromatographic analysis of this material indicates that it contains little or no detectable mannose. The DTT extract reacts with serum from a patient with CMC by western blot analysis. Serum from this patient recognizes distinct bands which constitute major protein components found in the DTT extract. Future experiments on the DTT extract will focus on ascribing the immunosuppressive activity to the protein or carbohydrate component of the material and further biochemical and serological characterization of this material. In addition, the phenotype of the suppressor cells induced by the DTT extract will be determined.

CONCLUSIONS

A number of fundamental questions must be answered before these findings can be applied to the treatment of candidiasis. The immunosuppression by *Candida* in humans *in vivo* could be due to at least 3 distinct mechanisms. First, it appears that some products of the *Candida* cell inhibit the activity of responder cells directly. In addition, *Candida* components may induce specific and/or non-specific suppressor cells which inhibit effector cell responses. Finally, the immune response to some *Candida* components may result in the production of cross-reactive antibodies to "self" determinants found in the host's own immune system. Indeed, the appearance of anti-T-cell antibodies in the serum of women with chronic vaginal candidiasis has been documented(24). Thus, it is conceivable that part of the immune response to *Candida* results in an autoimmune response resulting in generalized or specific non-responsiveness. In this case, therapy may be designed to inhibit the production of a cross-reactive autoimmune response. The manner in which the immune system of a host responds to various *Candida* components may be an important factor in determining whether or not chronic infections are established in such a host. An understanding of the immunomodulatory properties of *Candida* and, of equal importance, an understanding of the mechanism of this suppression may result in the development of techniques to identify individuals who are at risk of developing chronic infection as well as designing effective therapy to combat infection.

ACKNOWLEDGEMENTS

The authors acknowledge the generous gift of C.CBA/N mice from Dr. James Kenney. This work was supported by Public Health Service grants AI-19045 and RR-05417.

REFERENCES

1. Rogers, T. J., and E. Balish. 1980. Immunity to Candida albicans. Microbiol. Rev. 44:660-682.

2. Lehrer, R. I. 1970. Measurement of candidacidal activity of specific leukocyte types in mixed cell populations. I. Normal myeloperoxidase deficient, and chronic granulomatous disease neutrophils. Infect. Immun. 2:42-47.

3. Lehrer, R. I. 1971. Measurement of candidacidal activity of specific leukocyte types in mixed cell poulations. II. Normal and chronic granulomatous disease eosinophils. Infect. Immun. 3:800-802.

4. Anderson, W. D. 1971. Pathology. C. V. Mosby Co., St. Louis.

5. Valdimarsson, H., J. Higgs, R. Wells, M. Yamamura, J. Hobbs, and P. Holt. 1973. Immune abnormalities associated with chronic mucocutaneous candidiasis. Cell. Immunol. 11:348-361.

6. Paterson, P., R. Semo, B. Blumenschein, and J. Swetlstad. 1971. Mucocutaneous anergy and a plasma inhibitor of cellular immunity: reversal after amphotericin B therapy. Clin. Exp. Immunol. 9:595-602.

7. Kirkpatrick, C., R. Rich, and J. Bennett. 1971. Chronic mucocutaneous candidiasis: model-building in cellular immmunity. Ann. Intern. Med. 74:955-978.

8. Budtz-Jorgensen, E. 1973. Cellular immunity in acquired candidiasis of the palate. Scand. J. Dent. Res. 81:372-382.

9. Fischer, G., and L. Horbach. 1958. Untersuchungen uber Promunitat und Infektionsimmunitat bei der experimentallen Soorinfektion. Arch. Hyg. Bakteriol. 142:14-25.

10. Mankiewicz, E., E. Stackiewicz, and M. Liivak. 1959. A polysaccharide isolated fom Candida albicans as a growth promoting factor for tuberculosis. Can. J. Microbiol. 5:261-267.

11. Mankiewicz, E., and M. Liivak. 1960. Effect of Candida albicans on the evolution of experimental tuberculosis. Nature (London) 187:250-251.

12. Ferrante, A., and T. H. Thong. 1980. The effect of amphotericin B treatment on Candida albicans-induced imunosuppression in mice. Immunol. Lett. 1:321-323.

13. Vardinon, N., and E. Segal. 1979. Suppressive action of Candida albicans on the immune system in mice. Exp. Cell. Biol. 47:275-280.

14. Rogers, T., and E. Balish. 1978. Suppression of lymphocyte blastogenesis by Candida albicans. Clin. Immunol. Immunopathol. 10:298-305.

15. Rivas, V. and T. Rogers. 1983. Studies on the nature of *Candida albicans*-induced suppression. J. Immunol. 130:376-379.

16. Cuff, C., C. Rogers, B. Lamb, and T. Rogers. 1986. Induction of suppressor cells *in vitro* by *Candida albicans*. Cell. Immunol. 100:47-56.

17. Bruce, J. F. Symington, T. McKearn, and J. Sprent. 1981. A monoclonal antibody discriminating between subsets of T and B cells. J. Immunol. 127:2496-2501.

18. Raychaudhuri, S., and M. Cancro. 1985. Cellular basis for neonatally induced T-suppressor activity. J. Exp. Med. 161:816-829.

19. Smith, H., L. Jaffe, D. Kastner, and A. Steinberg. 1986. Evidence that Lyb-5 is a differentiation antigen in normal and *xid* mice. J. Immunol. 136:1194-1200.

20. Piccolella, E., G. Lombardi, and R. Morelli. 1981. Generation of suppressor cells in the response of human lymphocytes to a polysaccharide from *Candida albicans*. J. Immunol. 126:2151-2155.

21. Picolella, E., G. Lombardi, and R. Morelli. 1981. Mitogenic response of human peripheral blood lymphocytes to a purified *C. albicans* polysaccharide fraction: lack of helper activities is responsible for the *in vitro* unresponsiveness to a second antigenic challenge. J. Immunol. 126:2156-2160.

22. Lombardi, G., D. Vismara, E. Picolella, V. Colizzi, and G. Asherson. 1985. Non-specific inhibitor produced by *Candida albicans* activated T-cells impairs cell proliferation by inhibiting interleukin-1 production. Clin. Exp. Immunol. 60:303-310.

23. Mond, J., J. Farrar, W. Paul, J. Fuller-Farrar, M. Schaefer, and M. Howard. 1983. T-cell dependence and factor reconstitution of *in vitro* antibody responses to TNP-*B. abortus* and TNP-Ficoll: restoration of depleted responses with chromatographed fractions of a T-cell-derived factor. J. Immunol. 131:633-637.

24. Mathur, S., J. Melchers III, E. Ades, H. Williamson, and H. Fudenberg. 1980. Anti-ovarian and anti-lymphocyte antibodies in patients with chronic vaginal candidiasis. J. Reprod. Immunol. 2:247-262.

25. Fischer, A., J. Ballet, and C. Griscelli. 1978. Specific inhibition of *in vitro Candida*-induced lymphocyte proliferation by polysaccharide antigens present in the serum of patients with chronic mucocutaneous candidiasis. J. Clin. Invest. 62:1005-1013.

26. Fischer, A., L. Pichat, M. Audinot, and C. Griscelli. 1982. Defective handling of mannan by monocytes in patients with chronic mucocutaneous candidiasis resulting in a specific cellular unresponsiveness. Clin. Exp. Immunol. 47:653-660.

27. Piccolella, E., G. Lombardi, and R. Morelli. 1980. Human lymphocyte activating properties of a purified polysaccharide from *Candida albicans*: B and T cell cooperation in the mitogenic response. J. Immunol. 125:2082-2088.

28. Carrow, E., and J. Domer. 1985. Immunoregulation in experimental murine candidiasis:specific suppression induced by *Candida*

albicans cell wall glycoprotein. Infect. Immun. 49:172-181.

29. Cassone, A., P. Marconi, F. Bistoni, E. Mattia, G. Sbaraglia, E. Garaci, and E. Bonmassar. 1981. Immunoadjuvant effects of *Candida albicans* and its cell wall fractions in a mouse lymphoma model. Clin. Immunol. Immunother. 10:181-190.

30. Smail, E. and J. Jones. 1984. Demonstration and solubilization of antigens expressed primarily on the surfaces of *Candida albicans* germ tubes. Infect. Immun. 45:74-81.

IMMUNOMODULATION OF MURINE LEISHMANIASIS WITH CYCLOSPORIN A

Nancy C. Behforouz and Charlotte D. Wenger

Biology Department, Ball State University, Muncie
Indiana 47306

The fungal metabolite, cyclosporin A (CsA), is an undecapeptide with novel immunosuppressive effects as well as anti-parasitic and anti-inflammatory properties (1,2). CsA is particularly effective in preventing activation of T helper and T cytotoxic cells at the induction phase of T cell responses both *in vitro* and *in vivo* (3). Although the mode of action of CsA is not yet entirely clear, it has been shown to inhibit the production of IL-2 and may have effects on other lymphoid communication signals and responsiveness (2-4). Cyclosporin A has been shown to have unexpected beneficial effects on certain parasitic infections in animal models of human disease. In murine malaria, cyclosporin A exhibited potent activity against *P. yoelii* and *P. berghei* when administered to mice either prophylactically or therapeutically (5,6). Furthermore, CsA also markedly inhibited the growth of *Plasmodium falciparum* in cultured human erythrocytes (6). In this work, both the therapeutic and prophylactic effects of the drug were thought to be due to the direct effect of the CsA on the *Plasmodium* parasites. Surprisingly, CsA also had protective effects in mice infected with the helminth *Schistosoma mansoni*. Animals were protected both from primary infections and secondary challenges (7,8). In these studies, however, no direct effect of the drug on the parasite was observed, and it was concluded that the drug evoked a stimulation of host mechanisms directed against the parasite (8). In contrast to these studies, CsA treatment of *Trypanosoma cruzi* infected mice was found to exacerbate the disease (9).

Previous work in our own laboratory has shown that CsA given prophylactically, but not therapeutically, dramatically enhanced resistance to *Leishmania major* in the genetically susceptible Balb/c mice and induced immunity to challenge (Fig. 1) (10). Extracellular *Leishmania* promastigotes were not found to be sensitive to physiologically achievable levels of CsA. The mechanism of the CsA induced protection in this model is not clear and may involve several different modes of action working in concert to produce immunity rather than severe disease.

Firstly, it is possible that this CsA-mediated protection is due to an immunomodulatory effect on the T helper subset which appears to normally undergo excessive activation in the early stages of *L. major* infection in Balb/c mice (11). In fact, a variety of other prophylactic immune manipulations including thymectomy, irradiation, and bone marrow reconstitution; B cell depletion; *in vivo* anti-L3T4 treatment; or sublethal irradiation will all cause these highly susceptible mice to exhibit enhanced resistance to

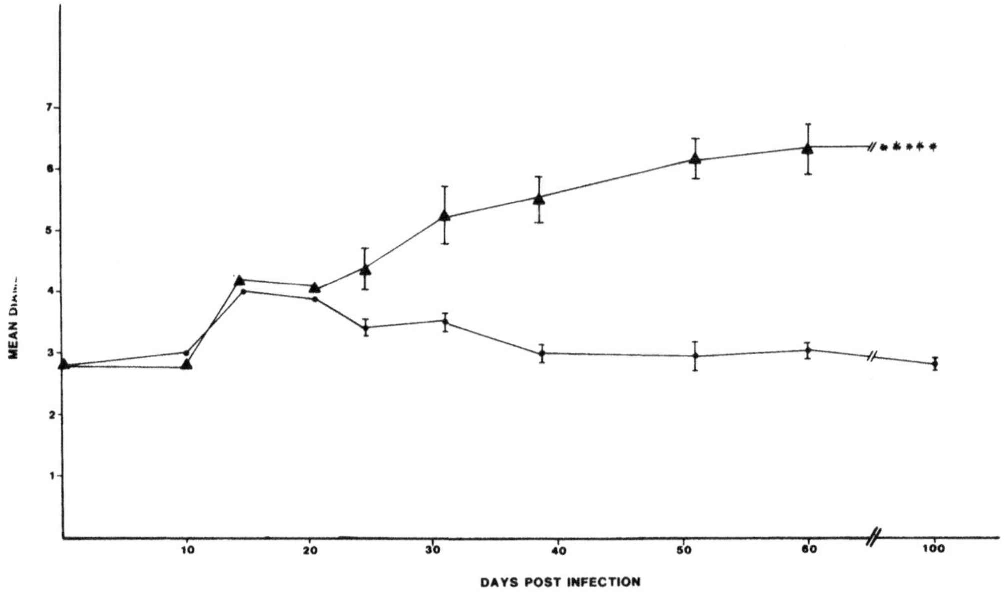

Figure 1. Prophylactic effect of CsA on L. major infections. Mice were infected with 1x10^6 promastigotes in the left hind footpad. On day -1 through 5, these mice received daily injections of either diluent alone (▲) or CsA (●) at a dosage of 100 mg/kg. The footpad diameters of both groups of mice were measured at regular time intervals after infection.

infection with L. major (11-14). All of these treatments were shown to affect, either directly or indirectly, early T cell activation which apparently allows for the development of a curative immune response in these otherwise susceptible animals. Secondly, it is also possible that cyclosporin A, acting as an anti-inflammatory agent, allows for protective immunity to develop against L. major. Hoover and Nacy have suggested that inflammation may be detrimental to host defense against L. major (15). They found that the ability of inflammatory macrophages to kill the intracellular amastigotes was markedly lower than that of resident peritoneal macrophages when exposed to activating lymphokines. Indeed, indomethacin administered to these mice in drinking water dramatically slowed metastasis of the parasites to the spleen (16). Thirdly, it may be that cyclosporin A has a direct toxic effect on the intracellular growth or survival of amastigotes in the phagolysosomes of the macrophages or stimulates the phagocytes in their ability to kill the intracellular parasites.

In order to address this third, macrophage-linked possibility, we examined the in vitro effect of cyclosporin A on intracellular survival of Leishmania major. Resident peritoneal macrophages were allowed to adhere overnight on culture slides and were infected in vitro with Leishmania promastigotes. Duplicate cultures of these adherent cells were treated with various concentrations of cyclosporin A or diluent beginning 24 hours before infection and continuing throughout the culture period. The percentage of infected macrophages was determined microscopically in the different Giemsa stained treatment groups, and the microbicidal activity of the CsA treated macrophages was determined by the formula described in the legend of Fig. 2.

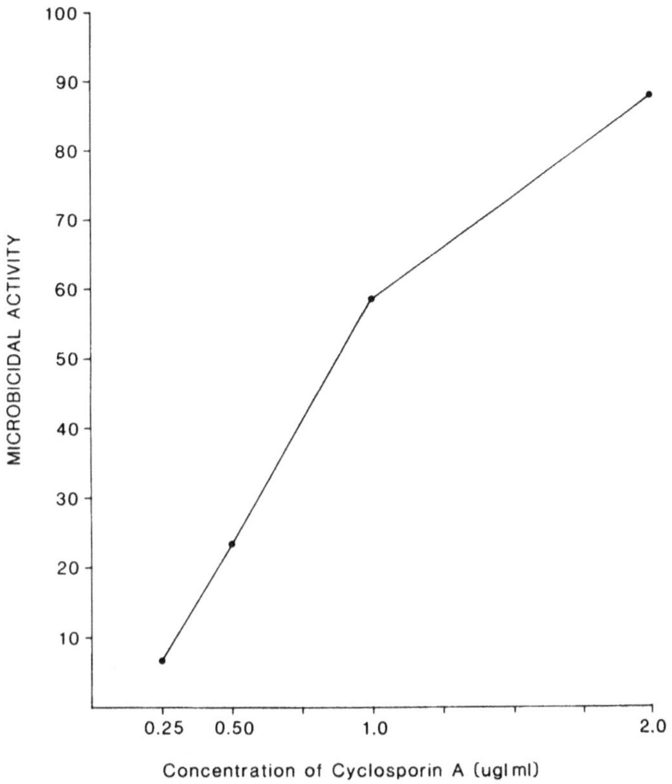

Figure 2. Effect of cyclosporin A on microbicidal activity of macrophages toward Leishmania major. Resident peritoneal macrophages were harvested from Balb/c mice, allowed to adhered, washed and cultured for a total of 7 days at 37°C in 5% CO_2. The macrophages were treated continuously with diluent or CsA beginning 24 hours before infection with 2-3 L. major promastigotes per macrophage and throughout the 7 day culture period. Cultures treated with diluent alone contained 21.5+1.2% infected macrophages after incubation. Microbicidal activity was calculated by the formula:

$$\frac{\text{\% infected control macrophages} - \text{\% infected treated macrophages}}{\text{\% infected controls}} \times 100$$

Table 1. Treatment of cultured Balb/c macrophages with CsA and its analogue B-5-49 following infection.[a]

Treatment	Percent Infected Macrophages	Microbicidal Activity
Diluent	29 ± 0.1	0
B-5-49		
1 ug/ml	31 ± 6.5	0
2 ug/ml	26 ± 4.0	10
CsA		
1 ug/ml	7.5 ± 2.0	73.6[b]
2 ug/ml	1.0 ± 0.2	96.5[b]

[a]Resident peritoneal macrophages were harvested and cultured for 24 hours and were infected with *L. major* for 2 hours. Following infection and extensive washing, either diluent, cyclosporin A or the cyclosporin analog, B-5-49, was added to duplicate culture wells. The infected treated macrophages were then re-cultured for 6 additional days.

[b]Denotes microbicidal activities that exceeded 95% confidence limits for triplicate diluent control cultures.

Macrophages cultured in increasing concentrations of cyclosporin showed a dose-dependent increase in microbicidal activity towards *Leishmania*. Cultures exposed to 1 or 2 ug/ml CsA showed increasing microbicidal activity of 59 and 88%, respectively, as compared to diluent treated macrophages. Thus, it appears that cyclosporin A has a profound effect on the survival of *Leishmania* in macrophage cultures.

In order to determine whether cyclosporin was simply preventing infection, cultured resident peritoneal macrophages were harvested, allowed to adhere and infected with *L. major*. Cyclosporin A, diluent, or the non-immunosuppressive CsA analog B-5-49 was added to washed duplicate culture wells following the two-hour infection period. Six days later, the cultures were examined microscopically for percent infected macrophages (Table 1).

Although the cyclosporin A analog B-5-49 induced no significant anti-leishmanial activity in infected macrophage cultures over that seen in diluent treated cultures, macrophages treated with CsA itself exhibited considerable microbicidal activity. After 6 days in culture, only 1% of the post-infection treated cells were infected whereas 29% of the diluent treated controls carried *Leishmania*.

It appears, therefore, that cyclosporin A can affect the survival of amastigotes intracellularly following infection, and the anti-leishmanial activity observed *in vitro* is not simply due to lowering the infectivity of the parasite for cultured macrophages.

Table 2. Pulse treatment of macrophages with CsA following infection.[a]

CsA Treatment	Percent Infected Macrophages	Microbicidal Activity
None	24 ± 4.0	0
7 day-continuous	1.3 ± 0.3	95[b]
96 hr.-pulse	8.3 ± 1.0	67[b]
48 hr.-pulse	7.2 ± 3.0	70[b]

[a]Resident peritoneal macrophages were harvested, cultured, infected and washed as described previously. Following infection, cyclosporin A, (1 ug/ml) or an equivalent amount of diluent was added to all macrophage cultures. The infected macrophages were cultured for a total of 7 days. At either 48 or 96 hours following infection, some of the duplicate wells were washed, fresh medium added and the cultures were reincubated for the remainder of the culture period.

[b]Denotes microbicidal activities that exceeded 95% confidence limits for quadruplicate diluent control wells.

In order to further analyze the effect which CsA has on microbicidal activity, macrophages were pulse treated for 48 or 96 hours immediately following infection with CsA as shown in Table 2. Although continuous exposure to cyclosporin for the 7 day culture period induced the highest level of microbicidal activity, the pulse treatments also caused significant microbicidal activity over that in control diluent treated cultures.

In conclusion, it appears that CsA, but not the B-5-49 analog, has a profound, dose dependent effect on the survival of intracellular *Leishmania major* in macrophages *in vitro*. This decreased survival is apparently not related to a decrease in infectivity. CsA can induce a dramatic microbicidal activity in macrophages when added to 7 day cultures for as little as 48 hours in a post-infection pulse. It is possible that CsA activates macrophages to kill *Leishmania* with increased efficiency just as lymphokines, particularly interferon, have been shown to do (17). It is also possible that the drug has a direct toxic effect on the intracellular amastigote form which lessens its ability to survive in its host macrophage. These two possibilities are now under investigation in our laboratory. The *in vitro* phenomenon of CsA induced microbicidal activity which we have documented here may play a role in the increased resistance to *Leishmania major* expressed by Balb/c mice prophylactically treated with cyclosporin A.

ACKNOWLEDGEMENT

This work was supported in part by grants from the University Research Committee of Ball State University and grant 1-R15 AI-23141-01 from the National Institutes of Health.

REFERENCES

1. Borel, J.F., C. Magnee and H. Stahelin. 1976. Effects of the new anti-lymphocytic peptide cyclosporin A in animals. Immunology 32:1017-1025.
2. Thomson, A.W. 1983. Immunobiology of cyclosporin A-a review. Aust. J. Exp. Bio. Med. Sci. 61:147-172.
3. Shevach, E.M. 1985. The effects of cyclosporin A on the immune system. Ann. Rev. Immunol. 3:397-423.
4. Palacios, R. and G. Moler. 1981. Cyclosporin A blocks receptors for HLA-DR antigens on T cells. Nature 290:792-794.
5. Thommen-Scott, K. 1981. Antimalarial activity of cyclosporin A. Agents Actions 11:770-773.
6. Nickell, S., L. Scheibel and G. Cole. 1982. Inhibition by cyclosporin A of rodent malaria *in vivo* and human malaria *in vitro*. Infect. Immun. 37:1093-1100.
7. Bueding, E., J. Hawkins and Y.-N Cha. 1981. Antischistosomal effects of cyclosporin A. Agents Actions 11:380-383.
8. Bout, D., D. Deslee and A. Capron. 1983. Protection against schistosomiasis produced by cyclosporin A. Am. J. Trop. Med. Hyg. 33:185-186.
9. Kierszenbaum, F., C. Gottlieb and D. Budzko. 1983. Exacerbation of *Trypanosoma cruzi* infection in mice treated with the immunoregulatory agent cyclosporin A. Tropenmed. Parasit. 34:4-6.
10. Behforous, N., C. Wenger and B. Mathison. 1986. Prophylactic treatment of Balb/c mice with cyclosporin A and its analog B-5-49 enhances resistance to *Leishmania major*. J. Immunol. 136:3067-3075.
11. Titus, R., R. Ceredig, J. Cerottini and J. Louis. 1985. Therapeutic effect of anti-L3T4 monoclonal antibody Gk 1.5 on cutaneous leishmaniasis in genetically susceptible Balb/c mice. J. Immunol. 135:2108-2114.
12. Howard, J., C. Hale and F. Liew. 1980. Immunological regulation of cutaneous leishmaniasis. III. Nature and significance of specific suppression of cell-mediated immunity in mice highly susceptible to *Leishmania tropica*. J. Exp. Med. 152:594-607.
13. Sacks, D., P. Scott, R. Asofsky, and F. Sher. 1984. Cutaneous leishmaniasis in anti-IgM-treated mice. Enhanced resistance due to functional depletion of a B cell dependent T cell involved in the suppressor pathway. J. Immunol. 132:2072-2077.
14. Howard, J., C. Hale and F. Liew. 1981. Immunological regulation of experimental cutaneous leishmaniasis. IV. Prophylactic effect of sublethal irradiation as a result of abrogation of suppressor T cell generation in mice genetically susceptible to *Leishmania tropica*. J. Exp. Med. 153:557-568.
15. Hoover, D. and C. Nacy. 1984. Macrophage activation to kill *Leishmania tropica*: defective intracellular killing of amastigotes by macrophages elicited with sterile inflammatory agents. J. Immunol. 132:1487-1491.
16. Mock, B., M. Potter, R. Nordan and C. Nacy. 1986. The effects of anti-inflammatory agents on *Leishmania* infections. 6th International Congress of Immunology. Abstract 5.22.41, p. 627.
17. Nacy, C., A. Fortier, M. Meltzer, N. Buchmeier and R. Schreiber. 1985. Macrophage activation to kill *Leishmania major*: activation of macrophages for intracellular destruction of amastigotes can be induced by both recombinant interferon- and non-interferon lymphokines. J. Immunol. 135:3505-3511.

AUTHOR INDEX

SUBJECT INDEX

GPSR Compliance

The European Union's (EU) General Product Safety Regulation (GPSR) is a set of rules that requires consumer products to be safe and our obligations to ensure this.

If you have any concerns about our products, you can contact us on ProductSafety@springernature.com

In case Publisher is established outside the EU, the EU authorized representative is:

Springer Nature Customer Service Center GmbH
Europaplatz 3
69115 Heidelberg, Germany

Batch number: 10838521

Printed by Printforce, the Netherlands